50 Studies Every Orthopaedic Surgeon Should Know

50 STUDIES EVERY DOCTOR SHOULD KNOW

50 Studies Every Doctor Should Know: The Key Studies that Form the Foundation of Evidence Based Medicine, Revised Edition
Michael E. Hochman

50 Studies Every Internist Should Know
Kristopher Swiger, Joshua R. Thomas, Michael E. Hochman, and Steven Hochman

50 Studies Every Neurologist Should Know
David Y. Hwang and David M. Greer

50 Studies Every Pediatrician Should Know
Ashaunta T. Anderson, Nina L. Shapiro, Stephen C. Aronoff, Jeremiah Davis, and Michael Levy

50 Imaging Studies Every Doctor Should Know
Christoph I. Lee

50 Studies Every Surgeon Should Know
SreyRam Kuy, Rachel J. Kwon, and Miguel A. Burch

50 Studies Every Intensivist Should Know
Edward A. Bittner

50 Studies Every Palliative Care Doctor Should Know
David Hui, Akhila Reddy, and Eduardo Bruera

50 Studies Every Psychiatrist Should Know
Ish P. Bhalla, Rajesh R. Tampi, and Vinod H. Srihari

50 Studies Every Anesthesiologist Should Know
Anita Gupta, Michael E. Hochman, and Elena N. Gutman

50 Studies Every Ophthalmologist Should Know
Alan D. Penman, Kimberly W. Crowder, and William M. Watkins, Jr.

50 Studies Every Urologist Should Know
Philipp Dahm

50 Studies Every Obstetrician and Gynecologist Should Know
Constance Liu, Noah Rindos, and Scott Shainker

50 Studies Every Doctor Should Know: The Key Studies that Form the Foundation of Evidence-Based Medicine, 2nd Edition
Michael E. Hochman and Steven D. Hochman

50 Studies Every Occupational Therapist Should Know
Elizabeth A. Pyatak and Elissa S. Lee

50 Studies Every Orthopaedic Surgeon Should Know
Kapil Sugand and Hani B. Abdul-Jabar; Illustrated by Konstantinos Doudoulakis

50 Studies Every Orthopaedic Surgeon Should Know

EDITED BY

Kapil Sugand, PhD CSci M-CCT/FST/SET F-EBOT/ICR/IET/RCS (T&O)/RSA/RSPH SICOT
Peripheral Nerve & Musculoskeletal Surgery Fellow, Royal National Orthopaedic Hospital, UK
Honorary Clinical Research Fellow & Senior Clinical Teacher—Imperial College London, UK

Hani B. Abdul-Jabar, BSc FRCS
Consultant Trauma & Orthopaedic Surgeon—London North West University Healthcare NHS Trust, UK
Senior Clinical Lecturer—Imperial College London, UK

SERIES EDITOR

Micheal E. Hochman

EXPERT ILLUSTRATOR

Konstantinos Doudoulakis, MSc FEBOT
Senior Trauma & Orthopaedic Fellow—Imperial College Healthcare NHS Trust, UK

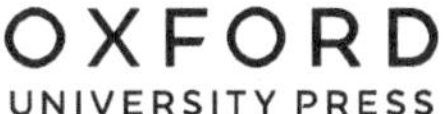

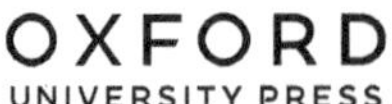

Oxford University Press is a department of the University of Oxford. It furthers the University's objective of excellence in research, scholarship, and education by publishing worldwide. Oxford is a registered trade mark of Oxford University Press in the UK and certain other countries.

Published in the United States of America by Oxford University Press
198 Madison Avenue, New York, NY 10016, United States of America.

Library of Congress Cataloging-in-Publication Data
Names: Sugand, Kapil, editor. | Abdul-Jabar, Hani B. (Hani Basil), editor.
Title: 50 studies every orthopaedic surgeon should know /
edited by Kapil Sugand, Hani B. Abdul-Jabar.
Other titles: Fifty studies every orthopaedic surgeon should know |
50 studies every doctor should know (Series)
Description: New York, NY : Oxford University Press, [2024] |
Series: Fifty studies every doctor should know series |
Includes bibliographical references and index.
Identifiers: LCCN 2023049386 (print) | LCCN 2023049387 (ebook) |
ISBN 9780190096656 (paperback) | ISBN 9780190096670 (epub) |
ISBN 9780190096687 (online)
Subjects: MESH: Orthopedic Procedures | Fractures, Bone—surgery |
Musculoskeletal Diseases—surgery | Case Reports
Classification: LCC RD755 (print) | LCC RD755 (ebook) | NLM WE 168 |
DDC 617.9—dc23/eng/20231215
LC record available at https://lccn.loc.gov/2023049386
LC ebook record available at https://lccn.loc.gov/2023049387

DOI: 10.1093/med/9780190096656.001.0001

Printed by Marquis Book Printing, Canada

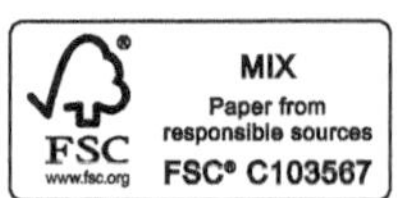

KS: *To my family, Poonam and Rahul, friends and colleagues for their undying support and encouragement.*

HAB: *To my wife and family for their continued support and limitless belief in me.*

We are also grateful to the following parties:

- *Our expert content contributors consisting of both Fellows and Attendings*
- *Our loyal team at Oxford University Press, especially Dr. Michael Hochman (series editor) and Ms. Marta Moldvai (editor). Thank you for supporting our vision and having faith in our abilities.*
- *We wholeheartedly thank our dedicated expert surgeons for reviewing the selection of studies featured in this book: Mr. Hani Abdul-Jabar, Mr. Simon Newman, Mr. Ahsan Sheeraz, and Mr. Paddy Subramaniam.*
- *We are eternally grateful to our expert illustrator, Mr. Konstantinos Doudoulakis, for his valuable contribution to make the content more user-friendly.*

CONTENTS

PREFACE

Trauma and orthopaedic surgery is an essential hospital specialty and encompasses surgery on the musculoskeletal system, from the cervical spine down to the toenail. In the past two decades, literature in the field has grown by leaps and bounds, through high-quality studies that have ultimately led to standardized clinical guidelines from professional and international orthopaedic bodies.

Yet to ensure that these research advances lead to real-world gains for patients, it is necessary to disseminate findings to the front-line clinicians. A common challenge faced by many orthopaedic trainees—and even practicing clinicians—is finding the time to review the research. Hence, there was a need to consolidate the most important studies and summarize the key results within a digestible, manageable, and reader-friendly template.

We are pleased to publish the first edition of *50 Studies Every Orthopaedic Surgeon Should Know*. This is a compilation of landmark studies in all subspecialities within emergency and elective orthopaedic practice that have influenced clinical decision-making. Though many of the studies are technical in nature, we strove to write the book to also be accessible to a broad array of practicing experts, healthcare students, allied healthcare professionals, and even the inquisitive general public. Each chapter has been reduced to the critical points, while listing all definitions and avoiding unnecessary jargon. Unlike similar books, we have focused on crucial information that is often overlooked, including study funding sources and conflicts of interest, criticisms and limitations, and results from associated studies, along with tables and figures showcasing the study design. Each chapter concludes with a case study, offering the reader the opportunity to contextualize the findings.

The formidable task of choosing the 50 studies for the book was done thoroughly and conscientiously. Like other books in the *50 Studies* series, we used objective selection criteria, including citations/year, impact factor of the journals, high level of evidence, clinical studies and trials, and a 3-stage Delphi review by international experts in the field.

Finally, this has been a work of passion for us. We are excited to receive feedback, advice, and comments. As clinical practice continues to evolve, there will undoubtedly be updates and revisions, making this book a perpetual work in progress but still topical and timely. Nevertheless, we hope you enjoy reading this first volume, and that it helps you gain a foundation for evidence-based practice in the field of orthopaedics.

ABBREVIATIONS

[]	Concentration
X°	Angle/degree
AAOS	American Association of Orthopaedic Surgeons
ACFAS	American College of Foot and Ankle Surgeons
ACI	Autologous Chondrocyte Implantation
ACL	Anterior Cruciate Ligament
ACR	American College of Rheumatology
ACS	American College of Surgeons
ADL	Activities of Daily Living
AIMS2	Arthritis Impact Measurement Scales (score)
AKS	Australian Knee Society
AMTS	Abbreviated Mental Test
AO	Arbeitsgemeinschaft für Osteosynthesefragen
AOFAS	American Orthopaedic Foot and Ankle Society
AP	Anteroposterior
APTA	American Physical Therapy Association
ASA	American Society of Anesthesiologists
ASES	American Shoulder and Elbow Surgeons
ASIA	American Spinal Injury Association
AUC	Area Under the Curve
AVN	Avascular Necrosis
BASK	British Association for Surgery of the Knee
BASS	British Association of Spine Surgeons
BCIS	Bone Cement Implantation Syndrome
BMD	Bone Mineral Density
BMI	Body Mass Index
BOA	British Orthopaedic Association
BOAST	British Orthopaedic Association Standards for Trauma

BPT	Best Practice Tariff
BSAP	Bone-Specific Alkaline Phosphatase
BSSH	British Society for Surgery on the Hand
BTHA	Big femoral head diameter Total Hip Arthroplasty
CAT	Computed Axial Tomography
CCC	Close Contact Casting
CES	Cauda Equina Syndrome
Cl	Confidence Interval
CM	Constant-Murley (score)
COPD	Chronic Obstructive Pulmonary Disease
CR	Cruciate Retaining (TKR)
CRIF	Closed Reduction and Internal Fixation
CRP	Complement Reactive Protein
CS	Cancellous Screws
CSAW	Can Shoulder Arthroscopy Work (trial)
CTHA	Constrained liner Total Hip Arthroplasty
CTX	C-terminal Telopeptide of type 1 collagen
DASH	Disabilities of the Arm, Shoulder, and Hand (score)
DCP	Dynamic Compression Plating
DHS	Dynamic Hip Screw
DMTHA	Dual Mobility Total Hip Arthroplasty
DNAR	Do Not Attempt Resuscitation
DRAFFT	Distal Radius Acute Fracture Fixation Trial
DRC-ICPMS	Dynamic Reaction Cell Inductively Coupled Plasma Mass Spectrometry
DVT	Deep Vein Thrombosis
EDTA	Ethylenediaminetetraacetic Acid
EQ-5D	EuroQol 5D (score)
ESR	Erythrocyte Sedimentation Rate
ESSKA	European Society of Sports Traumatology, Knee Surgery, and Arthroscopy
EULAR	European Alliance of Associations for Rheumatology
FAITH	Fixation using Alternative Implants for the Treatment of Hip fractures
FCR	Flexor Carpi Radialis
FIT	Fracture Intervention Trial
FLEX	Fracture intervention trial Long-term Extension (trial)
FRAX	Fracture Risk Assessment tool
F/U	Follow-Up
FWB	Full Weight Bearing
GA	General Anesthesia

GIRFT	Getting It Right First Time
HA	Hemiarthroplasty
Hb	Hemoglobin
HEALTH	Hip Fracture Evaluation with Alternatives of Total Hip Arthroplasty versus Hemi-Arthroplasty (trial)
HES	Hospital Episode Statistics
HHS	Harris Hip Score
HORIZON	Health Outcomes and Reduced Incidence with Zoledronic acid ONce yearly (trial)
HVA	Hallux Valgus Angle
ICER	Incremental Cost-Effectiveness Ratio
ICRS	International Cartilage Repair Society
IKDC	International Knee Documentation Committee
IMA	Intermetatarsal Angle
IMN	Intramedullary Nail
IV	Intravenous
K-wire	Kirschner wire
KOOS	Knee injury and Osteoarthritis Outcome Score
KSPS	Knee Specific Pain Scale (score)
KSS	Knee Society Score
LCP	Locking Compression Plate
LOS	Length of Stay
LS	Lysholm Score
MCL	Medial Collateral Ligament
MEPS	Mayo Elbow Performance Score
MF	Microfracture
MHRA	Medicines and Healthcare products Regulatory Agency
MI	Myocardial Infarction
MIPO	Minimally Invasive Plate Osteosynthesis
MIS	Minimally Invasive Surgery
Mm	Millimeters
MOM	Metal-on-Metal
MPFL	Medial Patellofemoral Ligament
MRI	Magnetic Resonance Imaging
MSCC	Metastatic Spinal Cord Compression
MSK	Musculoskeletal
MUA	Manipulation under Anesthesia
NHS	National Health Service
NICE	National Institute for Health and Care Excellence
NJR	National Joint Registry
NNT	Numbers Needed to Treat

NOF	Neck of Femur
NS	Not Significant
NSAID	Nonsteroidal Anti-Inflammatories
NTX	N-terminal Telopeptide of type 1 collagen
NWB	Non–Weight Bearing
OA	Osteoarthritis
OARSI	Osteoarthritis Research International
ODI	Oswestry Disability Index
OHS	Oxford Hip Score
OKS	Oxford Knee Score
OMAS	Olerud-Molander Ankle Score
ONS	Office for National Statistics
Op	Operative(ly)
OPD	Outpatient Department
OR	Odds Ratio
ORIF	Open Reduction and Internal Fixation
OSS	Oxford Shoulder Score
OTA	Orthopaedic Trauma Association
p=	Probability value
P1NP	Procollagen type 1 N-Propeptide
PCL	Posterior Cruciate Ligament
PE	Pulmonary Embolism
PEMS	Patient Evaluation Measure Score
PFT	Pivotal Fracture Trial
PKA/R	Partial Knee Arthroplasty/Replacement
PLC	Posterolateral Corner
PMMA	Polymethylmethacrylate
POP	Plaster of Paris
POSSUM	Physiological and Operative Severity Score for the enUmeration of Mortality and Morbidity (score)
ppb	Parts per Billion
PROFHER	Proximal Fracture of the Humerus Evaluation by Randomization
PROM	Patient-Reported Outcome Measure
PRWE	Patient-Rated Wrist Evaluation (score)
PS	Posterior-Stabilized (TKR)
QALY	Quality-Adjusted Life Year
QOL	Quality of Life
RCT	Randomized Controlled Trial
RHD	Right-Hand Dominant
ROC	Receiver Operating Characteristic

ROM	Range of Movement/Motion
RR	Relative Risk
RTSA/R	Reverse Total Shoulder Arthroplasty/Replacement
SD	Standard Deviation
SE	Standard Error
SF	Short Form
SHR	Subhazard Ratio
SHS	Sliding Hip Screw
SLAP	Superior Labral tear from Anterior to Posterior
SPORT	Spine Patient Outcomes Research Trial
STAR	Scandinavian Total Ankle Replacement
STHA	Standard Total Hip Arthroplasty
SUCRA	Surface under Cumulative Ranking Curve
TAA	Total Ankle Arthroplasty
TAD	Tip-Apex Distance
TAS	Tegner Activity Scale (score)
TEA	Total Elbow Arthroplasty
THA/R	Total Hip Arthroplasty/Replacement
TKA/R	Total Knee Arthroplasty/Replacement
TOPKAT	Total or Partial Knee Arthroplasty Trial
UHMWPE	Ultra-High-Molecular-Weight Polyethylene
UKA/R	Unicondylar Knee Arthroplasty/Replacement
UK HeFT	UK Heel Fracture Trial
US	Ultrasound
VAS	Visual Analog Scale
VMO	Vastus Medialis Oblique
VS.	Versus
VTE	Venous Thromboembolic Event
WOMAC	Western Ontario and McMaster Universities Osteoarthritis Index (score)
WOMET	Western Ontario Meniscal Evaluation Tool (score)
WOOS	Western Ontario Osteoarthritis of the Shoulder (score)
WOSI	Western Ontario Shoulder Instability Index (score)
XLPE	Highly Cross-Linked Polyethylene

CONTRIBUTORS

Hani B. Abdul-Jabar, London North West University Healthcare NHS Trust

Amin Abukar, Whipps Cross University Hospital

Arash Aframian, Imperial College Healthcare NHS Trust

David Ahearne, Hillingdon Hospitals

Raju Ahluwalia, Kings College Hospital

Mudassar Ahmad, Whittington Hospital

Khalid Al-Dadah, Kingston Hospital

Garth Allardice, London North West University Healthcare NHS Trust

Bilal Al-Obaidi, Hillingdon Hospital

Abtin Alvand, University of Oxford

Angelos Assiotis, Lister Hospital

Matthew Barry, University Hospital Southampton

Peter Bates, Royal London Hospital, Barts Health NHS Trust

Rebecca Emily Beamish, University Hospital Southampton

Ghias Bhattee, London North West University Healthcare NHS Trust

Nicola Blucher, London North West University Healthcare NHS Trust

Henry Edmund Bourke, Frimley Health NHS Foundation Trust

Sara Boutong, Whittington Hospital

Chris Brown, Royal Berkshire NHS Trust

Sophia Burns, North East Thames UCLH Rotation

Duncan Coffey, Royal London Hospital

James Dalrymple, North Middlesex University Hospital NHS Trust

Donald Davidson, Royal National Orthopaedic Hospital

Andrew Davies, Imperial College Healthcare NHS Trust

Rishi Dhir, Princess Alexandra Hospital

Peter Domos, Royal Free NHS Trust

Thomas C. Edwards, MSk Lab, Imperial College

Sherif El-Tawil, London North West University Healthcare NHS Trust

Mike Elvey, University College London NHS Foundation Trust

Rafik Nabil Fanous, Nottingham University Hospitals NHS Trust

David A. George, Princess Alexandra Hospital

Asim Ghafur, London North West University Healthcare NHS Trust

Subhajit Ghosh, West Hertfordshire Hospitals NHS Trust

Ian Gill, Kingston Hospital NHS Trust

Ben Gooding, Nottingham University Hospitals NHS Trust

Borna Guevel, West Middlesex University Hospital

Zakir Haider, Whipps Cross Hospital

Thomas W. Hamilton, University of Oxford

John Hardman, Imperial College Healthcare NHS Trust

Hamid Hassany, Imperial College Healthcare NHS Trust

Ian Holloway, London North West University Healthcare NHS Trust

Shireen Ibish, Hillingdon Hospital

Edward Ibrahim, Chelsea and Westminster NHS Foundation Trust

Edmund Ieong, West Hertfordshire NHS Trust

Arjuna Imbuldeniya, West Middlesex University Hospital

Luke D. Jones, Chelsea and Westminster Hospital, London

Monil Karia, Royal Berkshire NHS Trust

Akib Majed Khan, Frimley Health NHS Foundation Trust

Yasmeen Khan, Oxford University Hospitals

Ashish Khurana, Aneurin Bevan University Health Board

Iris H. Y. Kwok, Royal London Hospital, Barts Health NHS Trust

Shirley Anne Lyle, Royal National Orthopaedic Hospital NHS Trust

Ahmed Mabrouk, Huddersfield Royal Infirmary

Henry Magill, Chelsea and Westminster Hospital

Alexander Magnussen, London North West University Healthcare NHS Trust

Piyush Mahapatra, West Hertfordshire Hospitals NHS Trust

Tim Maheswaran, Imperial College Healthcare NHS Trust

Daoud Makki, West Middlesex University Hospital

Alexander Martin, Trauma and Orthopaedic Rotation, Oxford Deanery

Simon Mellor, Royal Free NHS Trust

Kashif Memon, Frimley Health NHS Foundation Trust

Irfan Merchant, London North West University Healthcare NHS Trust

Lydia Milnes, Kingston Hospital NHS Foundation Trust

Chris Mitchell, University College London Hospital NHS Trust

Reza Mobasheri, Imperial College Healthcare NHS Trust

Abdul Nazeer Moideen, Cardiff and Vale University Health Board

Mohammed Monem, Imperial College Healthcare NHS Trust

Catrin Morgan, London North West University Healthcare NHS Trust

John Paul Murphy, London North West University Healthcare NHS Trust

Ali Z. Naqvi, Imperial College Healthcare NHS Trust

Dinesh Nathwani, Imperial College Healthcare NHS Trust

Cenk Oguz, London North West University Healthcare NHS Trust

Andrew Osborne, London North West University Healthcare NHS Trust

Piers Page, Frimley Park Hospital

Anna Panagiotidou, Royal National Orthopaedic Hospital NHS Trust

Chang Park, London North West University Healthcare NHS Trust

Shelain Patel, Royal National Orthopaedic Hospital NHS Trust

Michael Pearse, Imperial College Healthcare NHS Trust

Ravi Popat, West Hertfordshire Hospitals NHS Trust

Michael Rafferty, London North West University Healthcare NHS Trust

Palanisamy Ramesh, Kingston Hospital NHS Foundation Trust

Naeem Raza, Frimley Health NHS Foundation Trust

Peter Reilly, Imperial College Healthcare NHS Trust

Barry Rose, Eastbourne District General Hospital

Branavan Rudran, Chelsea and Westminster Hospital NHS Foundation Trust

Sanjeeve Sabharwal, Imperial College Healthcare NHS Trust

Khaled M. Sarraf, Imperial College Healthcare NHS Trust

Shalin Shaunak, Ashford and St Peter's Hospitals NHS Foundation Trust

Sameh A. Sidhom, Huddersfield Royal Infirmary

Ashok Singh, Imperial College Healthcare NHS Trust

Kewal Singh, Hillingdon Hospital

Sanjay Sinha, North Middlesex University Hospital NHS Trust

Tim Sinnett, Chelsea and Westminster Hospital

Dominic Spicer, Imperial College Healthcare NHS Trust

Kesavan Sri-Ram, Whipps Cross Hospital

Robin K. Strachan, Imperial College Healthcare NHS Trust

Kapil Sugand, Royal National Orthopaedic Hospital

Quen O. Tang, West Middlesex University Hospital

Dushan Thavarajah, Taunton and Somerset NHS Foundation Trust

Anthony Janahan Thayaparan, Imperial College Healthcare NHS Trust

Haider Twaij, West Middlesex University Hospital

Harpal Singh Uppal, Lister Hospital

Bernard H. van Duren, Huddersfield Royal Infirmary

Rupert Wharton, Kingston Hospital NHS Foundation Trust

Paul Whittingham-Jones, Watford General Hospital

Warran Wignadasan, University College London Hospitals NHS Foundation Trust

1

The Value of the Tip-Apex Distance in Predicting Failure of Fixation of Peritrochanteric Fractures of the Hip

DAVID A. GEORGE AND PAUL WHITTINGHAM-JONES

> None of the screws with a tip-apex distance (TAD) of ≤25 mm cut out, but there was a very strong statistical relationship between an increasing TAD and cut-out regardless of other variables ($p<0.0001$). An increasing age of the patient, unstable fracture, poor reduction, and use of a high-angle side-plate were also associated with a significantly increased risk of failure.
>
> —BAUMGAERTNER ET AL.[1]

Citation: Baumgaertner MR, Curtin SL, Lindskog DM, Keggi JM. The value of the tip-apex distance in predicting failure of fixation of peritrochanteric fractures of the hip. J Bone Joint Surg Am. 1995;77(7):1058–64.

Research Question: What are the main predictive factors that led to failure of fixation of peritrochanteric hip fractures?

Funding: Support from Smith and Nephew

Year Study Began: Unknown

Year Study Published: 1995

Study Location: Yale University, USA

Who Was Studied: Patients were identified from a database of all consecutively treated neck of femur fractures at their institute ($N = 336$). Inclusion criteria included:

- Treated with a fixed-angle sliding hip screw for a peritrochanteric hip fracture
- Complete radiographic and clinical data available
- Minimum follow-up (F/U) of 3 months or early failure of fixation

Who Was Excluded: 138 patients with fractures who had inadequate documentation (80 had complete perioperative data but F/U information was lacking). There was no significant difference between this group and the study group with respect to the stability of the fracture ($p = 0.25$) or the quality of reduction ($p = 0.35$), with an average TAD of 25.3 mm ($p = 0.76$).

How Many Patients: 193 patients (198 fractures)

Study Overview: See Figure 1.1.

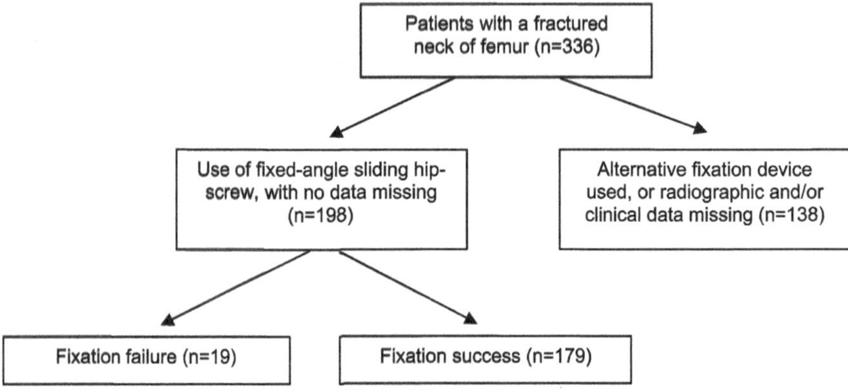

Figure 1.1. Summary of study design.

Study Intervention: The study was a retrospective review of hip fracture fixation, with the cases defined as those which failed fixation (i.e., screw cutout) and controls defined as those that had not, at a minimum of 3-month F/U. To observe for the risk factors of fixation, a thorough review of pre- and intraoperative details was conducted and analyzed using multivariate logistic regression. This required the intraoperative radiographs to be scrutinized for the position of the screw within the femoral head, quality of fracture reduction, and TAD. This is based upon intraoperative anteroposterior (AP) and lateral radiographs (Figure 1.2) and describes the sum of the distance from the tip of the lag screw to the apex of the femoral head. The cutoff for TAD of 25 mm or less (Figure 1.3) was further reviewed between both groups. Patients were followed up in the clinic with plain radiographs until either the fixation had failed or the fracture had united.

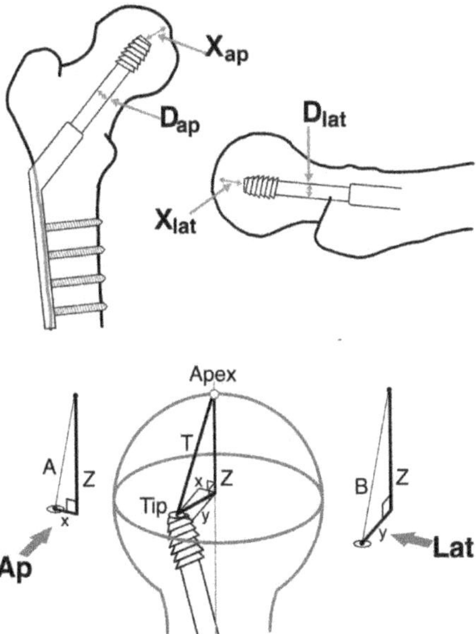

Figure 1.2. Calculating TAD in AP and lateral projections as well as zones of femoral head.

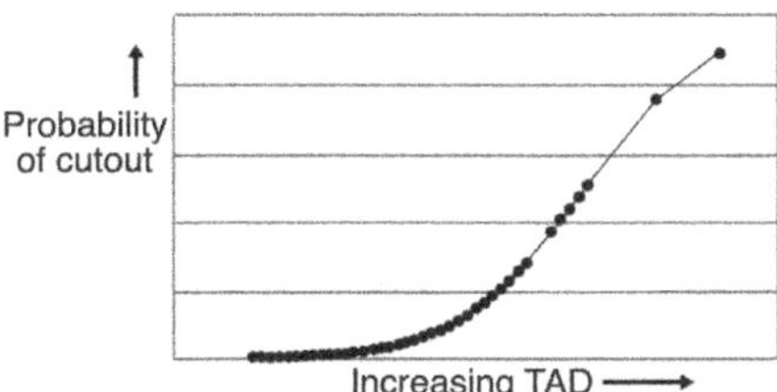

Figure 1.3. Baumgartner's curve for cutout depending on TAD.

Follow-Up: Mean of 13 months (range 3–48)

Endpoints:

Primary outcome: Failure of fixation (screw cutting out of femoral head, non-union, other reasons for failure).

Secondary outcomes:

- Factors that may be correlated with this failure (e.g., patient factors, fracture configuration, intraoperative fracture reduction, location of the screw within the femoral head zones described by Cleveland et al.[2])
- Effect of both interobserver and intraobserver variability on the TAD to assess the reproducibility of the measurement

RESULTS (TABLE 1.1)

- *Mode of failure:* 19 fixations failed (9.6%), 16 due to cutout (84.2%; defined as "cases"), nonunion with a broken side plate (*n* = 1, 5.3%), deep infection (*n* = 1, 5.3%), or complete collapse of the hip screw with resultant need for hemiarthroplasty (*n* = 1, 5.3%).
- *TAD:* There was an increased risk of screw cutout with increasing TAD: no cutout at TAD ≤ 25 mm (*n* = 120), 2% of screws with a TAD < 30 mm cut out (3 of 150 screws), 27% of screws with a TAD > 30 mm cut out (13 of 48 screws), and 60% of screws with a TAD > 45 mm cut out (6 of 10 screws).
- *Gender and comorbidities:* There was no associated risk of cutout based upon gender or patients' medical status or comorbidities.
- *Age:* Mean age of those with cutout was 85 (range 67–95) years old vs. 76 (range 19–100) years among those with intact fixation that progressed to union.
- *Unstable and malreduced fractures:* Significantly more cutouts were associated with unstable vs. stable fractures and those with a poor reduction.
- *Plates:* 10 side-plate devices cut out; 5 had a barrel angle of 150 degrees (used in a total of 24 fractures; 20.8% cutout rate), compared to 5 in the remaining 118 side plates with a lower varus angle (only 4.2%).
- *Screw positioning:* Based upon the 9 zones within the femoral head, screw positioning within the posterior-inferior (2 of 6) and anterior-superior (2 of 7) zones had a significant increased risk of cutout compared to the central zone. Yet, multivariate analysis of the zone of placement had no predictive value for or against cutout, especially for center-center or posterior-inferior placement.
- *Reproducibility:* There was high reproducibility of the TAD measurement when comparing between each author (SD 1.7 mm; range 0.3–5.1) and when reviewing the individual author's measurements following a

2–4-month period and remeasuring the same radiographs (SD 1.2 mm; range 0–5.7).

- *Cutout subanalysis:* With use of bivariate and multivariate model, TAD remained a strong independent predictor. In the multivariate model that included all variables, TAD, patient age, instability of the fracture, and a 150-degree side plate were significant *independent* predictors for cutout, whereas the quality of the fracture reduction and the location of the screw according to femoral head zone were insignificant.

Table 1.1 SUMMARY OF STUDY RESULTS AND KEY POINTS

Outcome		*n*
Failed fixation	Yes	19
	No	179
Time from surgery until cut-out (< 12 weeks)	Yes	14
	No	2
Tip-apex distance (mm)	Mean	25
	Minimum	9
	Maximum	63

Analysis of cases and controls

	Cases (*n* = 16)	**Controls (*n* = 182)**	***p* Value**
	Tip-apex distance (mm)		
Mean	38	24	0.0001
Minimum	28	9	
Maximum	48	63	
	Age (y)		
Mean	85	76	0.02
Minimum	67	19	
Maximum	95	100	

Criticisms and Limitations: A range of fixed-angle devices (i.e., plate vs. nail) possess differing biomechanical properties, including the moment arm and ability of the lag screw to slide within the nail or plate if the screw was locked in situ (as seen in Stryker Gamma intramedullary nails), which may influence the rate of failure. The assessment of the reproducibility of the TAD should have been undertaken by a range of surgeons of different experience and not solely based on the authors, due to obvious confounding factors and potential for bias. This is also a retrospective study.

Other Relevant Studies and Information:

- Andruszkow et al.[3] further reviewed the 25-mm cutoff and demonstrated a 24 times higher cutout rate if the TAD was above 25 mm (odds ratio [OR] 24.1; 95% CI: 1.01–1.41; $p < 0.003$) with either a dynamic hip screw (DHS) or Gamma intramedullary nail fixation. Furthermore, they showed that a valgus neck shaft angle of 5–10 degrees reduced screw cutout but without statistical significance ($p = 0.09$) and anterior screw placement significantly increased cutout ($p = 0.047$).
- Focused solely on intramedullary devices for intertrochanteric and subtrochanteric hip fractures, Geller et al.[4] reiterated the role of TAD and a cutoff of 25 mm ($p < 0.001$), whereas Caruso et al.[5] set their limit at 30.7 mm (OR 4.51).
- A biomechanical study[6] showed that positioning the lag screw in a low-center compared to a center-center position did not alter the rate of cutout despite the increased TAD, and was advantageous to reduce fracture translation ($p = 0.004$) and gap distraction ($p < 0.001$).
- A level IV study[7] confirmed that posterior and inferior locations of the sliding screw may help to support the posteromedial cortex and calcar in unstable fractures and reduce the risk of cutout failure.

Summary and Implications: This is the first study to highlight the correlation between TAD and the risk of screw cutout from the femoral head. The findings support achieving a TAD ≤ 25 mm, provided adequate fracture reduction as well as use of an appropriately angled device. This concept has become the gold standard for any fixed-angle device, and these recommendations continue to be justified and strengthened by supporting studies.

CLINICAL CASE: SURGICAL FIXATION IN INTERTROCHANTERIC NECK OF FEMUR FRACTURES

Case History

An 88-year-old male patient sustained an isolated pertrochanteric neck of femur fracture (Figure 1.4) following a mechanical fall in his nursing home. He has a history of hypertension and dementia and normally mobilizes with a Zimmer frame with assistance but has had a series of recurrent falls recently. His blood results are within normal range. Based upon the results of Baumgaertner's study,[1] what surgical considerations should be taken into account?

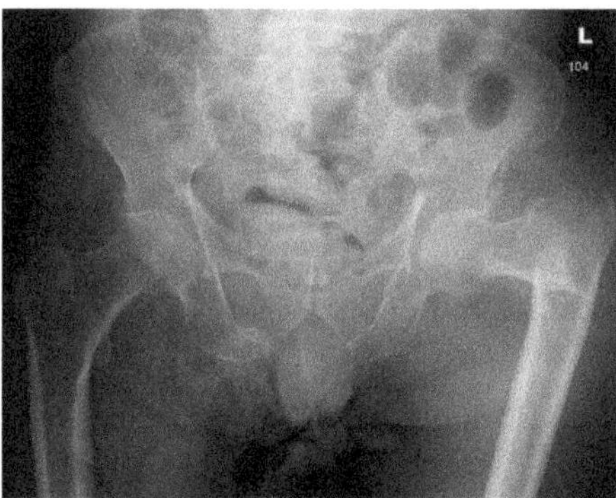

Figure 1.4. Plain radiograph of AP pelvis.

Suggested Answer

The image is an AP radiograph of the pelvis, with a shortened and displaced left per/intertrochanteric neck of femur fracture. His initial management in the Emergency Department should include an assessment of his neurovascular status, he should be given analgesia (including a fascia iliacus block), and traction or a box splint should be applied. Management options should be discussed with the patient (taking into account his capacity due to dementia) and his relatives, but an operation is advisable. Based upon this study, ensure that the fracture is reduced anatomically on the fracture/traction table, confirmed on both AP and lateral radiographs, and ensure that the TAD is within 25 mm. I would also ideally avoid using a 150-degree plate with a preference of a standard 130-degree DHS and place the lag screw in a center-center position of the head (avoiding the anterior-superior more than the posterior-inferior zones).

References

1. Baumgaertner et al. The value of the tip-apex distance in predicting failure of fixation of pertrochanteric fractures of the hip. J Bone Joint Surg Am. 1995;77(7): 1058–64.
2. Cleveland et al. A ten-year analysis of intertrochanteric fractures of the femur. Bone and Joint Surg. 1959;41-A:1399–408.
3. Andruszkow et al. Tip apex distance, hip screw placement, and neck shaft angle as potential risk factors for cut-out failure of hip screws after surgical treatment of intertrochanteric fractures. Int Orthop. 2012;36:2347–54.
4. Geller et al. Tip-apex distance of intramedullary devices as a predictor of cut-out failure in the treatment of pertrochanteric elderly hip fractures. Int Orthop. 2010;34: 719–22.

5. Caruso et al. 6-year retrospective analysis of cut-out risk predictors in cephalomeduallary nailing for pertrochanteric fractures. Bone Joint Res. 2017;6(8):481–8.
6. Kane et al. Is tip apex distance as important as we think? A biomechanical study examining optimal lag screw placement. Clin Orthop Rel Res. 2014;472(8):2492–8.
7. Güven et al. Importance of screw position in intertrochanteric femoral fractures treated by dynamic hip screw. Orthop Traumatol Surg Res. 2010;96(1):21–7.

2

Arthroscopic Partial Meniscectomy versus Sham Surgery for a Degenerative Meniscal Tear

AKIB MAJED KHAN AND HENRY EDMUND BOURKE

> Arthroscopic partial medial meniscectomy provides no significant benefit over sham surgery in patients with a degenerative meniscal tear and no knee osteoarthritis.
>
> —FIDELITY (FINNISH DEGENERATIVE MENISCAL LESION STUDY) GROUP[1]

Citation: Sihvonen R, Paavola M, Malmivaara A, Itälä A, Joukainen A, Nurmi H, Kalske J, Järvinen TL; Finnish Degenerative Meniscal Lesion Study (FIDELITY) Group. Arthroscopic partial meniscectomy versus sham surgery for a degenerative meniscal tear. N Engl J Med. 2013;369(26):2515–24.

Research Question: What is the efficacy of arthroscopic partial meniscectomy compared to sham arthroscopy in patients with an arthroscopy-confirmed degenerative tear of the medial meniscus but without knee osteoarthritis (OA)?

Funding: Sigrid Juselius Foundation, Competitive Research Fund of Pirkanmaa Hospital District, Academy of Finland, Finnish Orthopaedic Research Foundation

Year Study Began: 2007

Year Study Published: 2013

Study Location: 5 centers in Finland

Who Was Studied: Patients aged between 35 and 65 years with pain located over the medial joint line for more than 3 months. On clinical examination, the patients were required to have pain on palpation/compression of the medial joint line and/or a positive McMurray's test. Patients had a magnetic resonance imaging (MRI) scan indicating medial meniscal tear, which was ultimately confirmed as a degenerative tear at the time of arthroscopy.

Who Was Excluded: Patients who had acute trauma (including fractures), locking of the knee, previous surgery to the knee joint, OA of the medial compartment determined on American College of Rheumatology clinical criteria,[2] Kellgren-Lawrence[3] score > 1, reduced range of movement in knee, instability, MRI-confirmed tumor, or other condition requiring surgery.

How Many Patients: 146

Study Overview: See Figure 2.1.

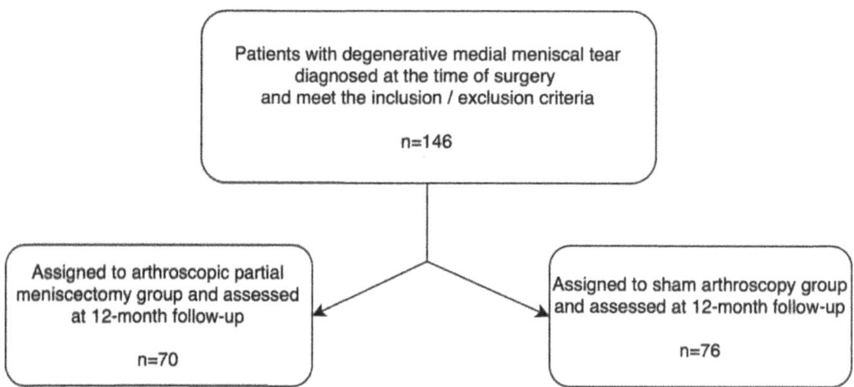

Figure 2.1. Study overview.

Study Intervention: Patients were randomized once they were confirmed to be eligible at the time of arthroscopy. A research nurse opened an envelope and showed the operating surgeon whether the patient would receive arthroscopic partial meniscectomy or sham surgery. During arthroscopic partial meniscectomy the meniscus was debrided using a punch and arthroscopic shaver until stable (confirmed on probing) meniscal tissue was reached. Loose and unstable fragments were also removed. No other procedure was performed. During sham surgery the patient's knee was manipulated as if a meniscectomy was being performed. The surgeon asked for all of the equipment required for a meniscectomy and inserted an arthroscopic shaver without a blade into the knee. The patient was kept in the operative room for the same duration as if an arthroscopic partial meniscectomy was being performed. Statistical analysis was performed on an intention-to-treat basis. No per-protocol analysis was performed because the frequency of crossover was low.

Follow-Up: 12 months

Endpoints: Patient questionnaires were performed at baseline and at 2, 6, and 12 months. The primary outcomes were the presence or absence of knee pain after exercise, Lysholm knee score,[4] and Western Ontario Meniscal Evaluation Tool (WOMET) score,[5] all assessed at 12-month follow-up. Secondary outcomes included the same 3 primary outcome measures at 2 and 6 months postoperatively, a quality of life measurement tool (15D),[6] and knee pain at rest at 12 months.

RESULTS (TABLE 2.1)

- *Selection:* 205 patients were eligible for the study but 59 (28.8%) were excluded, resulting in 146 (71.2%) patients randomized to arthroscopic partial meniscectomy (*n* = 70 [47.9%]) or sham arthroscopy (*n* = 76 [52.1%]).
- *1-year outcome:* There was marked improvement in the 3 primary outcome measures in both the arthroscopy and sham group at the 12-month stage from baseline, but no between-group differences.
- *< 1-year outcome:* At the 2- and 6-month follow-up there was a trend for the arthroscopic partial meniscectomy group to have a higher WOMET score and less pain after exercise, but these were used only to illustrate the trajectory of the treatment response (Figure 2.2).
- *Insignificance:* Additionally, there was no statistically significant difference between the groups for the following:
    - Lysholm knee score, WOMET score, or knee pain after exercise
    - Any of the other secondary outcome measures
    - The need for subsequent knee surgery or serious adverse events
    - Patients guessing which group they were assigned to

● Arthroscopic partial meniscectomy ■ Sham surgegy

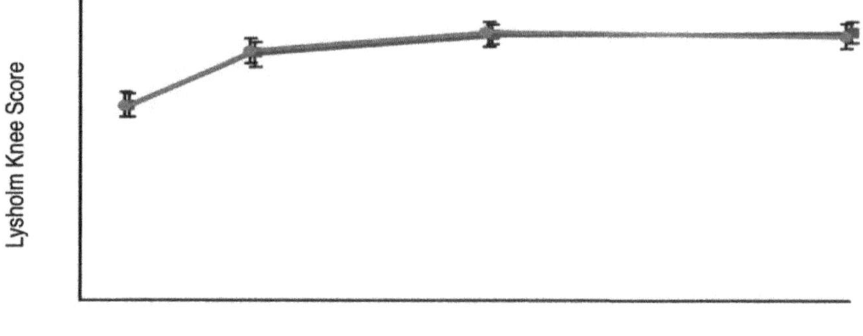

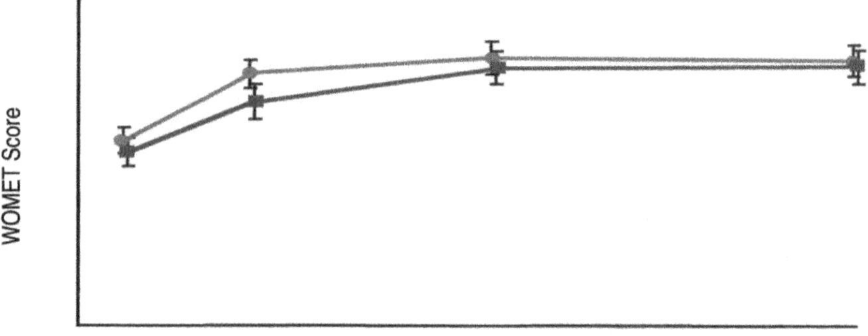

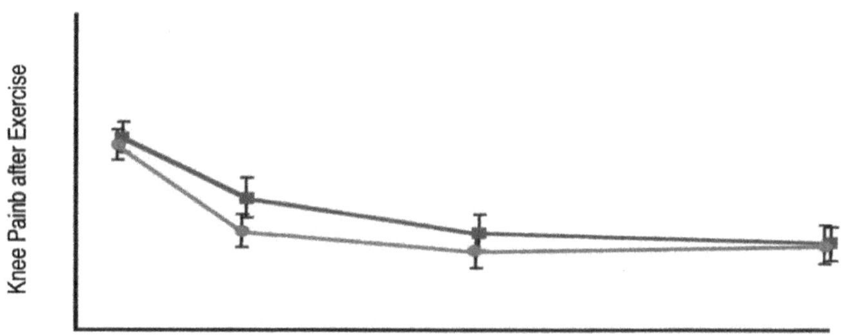

Figure 2.2. Primary outcomes in the partial meniscectomy group and the sham surgery group. x-axis = time (months) and y-axis = score.

Table 2.1 Summary of Arthroscopic Partial Meniscectomy versus Sham Surgery for Degenerative Meniscal Tear Findings at 12 Months[1]

Outcome	Partial Meniscectomy ($n = 70$)	Sham Surgery ($n = 76$)	Between-Group Difference in Improvement from Baseline (Partial Meniscectomy vs. Sham)
Primary Outcome (95% CI)			
Lysholm Knee Score	82.2 (78.4–85.9)	83.4 (80.3–86.5)	−1.6 (−7.2–7.0)
WOMET Score	81.0 (76.1–85.9)	79.9 (75.1–84.7)	−2.5 (−9.2–4.1)
Knee pain after exercise	2.7 (2.1–3.3)	2.9 (2.3–3.4)	−0.1 (−0.9–0.7)
Secondary Outcome (95% CI)			
15D Score	0.94 (0.92–0.95)	092 (0.90–0.93)	0.01 (−0.01–0.02)
Knee pain at rest	1.6 (1.0–2.1)	1.9 (1.4–2.5)	0.0 (−0.9–1.0)

Criticisms and Limitations:

- Patients with history of injury or mechanical symptoms were excluded from this study.
- The longevity of symptoms prior to meniscectomy/sham arthroscopy was not mentioned.
- The sham arm of this study still underwent a therapeutic procedure. It is unclear what exactly was performed inside the knee whilst the patient was kept in the operating room for the amount of time required to perform a partial meniscectomy (i.e., did arthroscopic lavage occur?). It is unclear whether instrumentation of the knee may also have had a therapeutic effect.
- In the meniscectomy group it is unclear about the proportion of the meniscus removed.
- The quality of life impact on patients prior to the 12-month mark was not studied. It is possible that 1 group may have experienced a high quality of life faster than the other.

Other Relevant Studies and Information:

- As an extension of the FIDELITY trial,[1] the study authors followed up with patients at the 2-year mark and found no difference between the arthroscopic partial meniscectomy and sham groups in the Lysholm knee score, WOMET score, and knee pain after exercise.

- A large UK registry study found that the risks of performing arthroscopic partial meniscectomy are low but include serious 90-day complications including pulmonary embolism (0.078%) and deep infections (0.135%).[7]
- A previous randomized controlled trial showed no difference between arthroscopic debridement, arthroscopic lavage, and sham surgery in patients with OA of the knee.[8]
- The European Society of Sports Traumatology, Knee Surgery, and Arthroscopy (ESSKA) developed a consensus algorithm in 2016 for patients with degenerative meniscal tears. This algorithm suggests arthroscopic partial meniscectomy should be performed in patients with no OA on plain radiographs or MRI if they have failed nonoperative treatment with or without injections for at least 3 months.[9]
- The British Association for Surgery of the Knee developed guidelines in 2018 that recommend arthroscopic meniscectomy in patients with locked knee, acute injury with meniscal target on MRI, and meniscal target on MRI with corresponding symptoms or signs if present for > 3 months. Otherwise, optimal nonoperative treatment and reassessment in patients with either a possible meniscal target on MRI or a clear meniscal target on MRI with corresponding symptoms or signs if present for < 3 months were recommended.[10]

Summary and Implications: This study found that those patients who undergo partial meniscectomy have the same function, knee pain, and quality of life outcomes at 12 months postoperatively compared to patients receiving an arthroscopic sham procedure.

CLINICAL CASE: DEGENERATIVE MENISCAL TEAR

Case History

A 40-year-old gentleman presents to the clinic complaining of medial joint line pain and swelling. He denies any mechanical symptoms. He first noticed the pain the day after playing football with some friends in the park 6 months ago but cannot recall a specific traumatic event. He is keen on getting back to football but is struggling to run. He has no previous knee pathology. He takes no medicines, smokes, and has a desk-based job. On clinical examination he has a full range of movement but tenderness to palpation of the medial joint line, a small effusion, and positive McMurray's test. Radiographs show no OA, and an MRI scan confirms a degenerative medial meniscal tear with no displaced flaps. How will you manage this patient?

Suggested Answer

This patient has a degenerative medial meniscal tear without mechanical symptoms. He should undergo at least 3 months of conservative management including analgesia and physiotherapy. If he continues to have significant symptoms following this period, the following should be discussed with the patient: (1) further physiotherapy, (2) joint injection, or (3) arthroscopy ± partial meniscectomy.

If the patient is managed with arthroscopy, intervention should occur if there are other surgically treatable abnormalities or a different type of meniscal tear is identified (i.e., displaced flaps). If only a degenerative meniscal tear is identified, the surgeon may make a choice to either debride or leave the meniscal tear as the functional and quality of life outcomes at 12 months are similar regardless. However, the ESSKA guidelines[9] suggest that performing a partial meniscectomy at this stage would be justifiable and appropriate surgical treatment.

References

1. Sihvonen et al. Arthroscopic partial meniscectomy versus sham surgery for a degenerative meniscal tear. N Eng J Med. 2013;369(26):2515–24.
2. Altman et al. Development of criteria for the classification and reporting of osteoarthritis: classification of osteoarthritis of the knee. Arthritis Rheum. 1986;29(8): 1039–49.
3. Lysholm et al. Evaluation of knee ligament surgery results with special emphasis on use of a scoring scale. Am J Sports Med. 1982;10(3):150–4.
4. Kellgren et al. Radiological assessment of osteo-arthrosis. Ann Rheum Dis. 1957;16(4): 494–502.
5. Kirkley et al. The development and validation of a quality of life-measurement tool for patients with meniscal pathology: the Western Ontario Meniscal Evaluation Tool (WOMET). Clin J Sport Med. 2007;17(5):349–56.
6. Sintonen. The 15D instrument of health-related quality of life: properties and applications. Ann Med. 2001;33(5):328–36.
7. Abram et al. Adverse outcomes after arthroscopic partial meniscectomy: a study of 700 000 procedures in the national Hospital Episode Statistics database for England. Lancet. 2018;392(10160):2194–202.
8. Moseley et al. A controlled trial of arthroscopic surgery for osteoarthritis of the knee. N Eng J Med. 2002;347(2):81–8.

9. European Society of Sports Traumatology, Knee Surgery, and Arthroscopy. ESSKA Meniscus Consensus Project: degenerative meniscus lesions. 2016. https://www.esska.org/news/555974/ESSKA-consensus-on-degenerative-and-traumatic-meniscus-lesions.htm
10. British Association for Surgery of the Knee. BASK meniscal guideline. 2018. www.baskonline.com/professional/wp-content/uploads/sites/5/2018/07/BASK-Meniscal-Surgery-Guideline-2018.pdf

3

How Long Does a Hip Replacement Last?

A Systematic Review and Meta-Analysis of Case Series and National Registry Reports with More Than 15 Years of Follow-Up

HAIDER TWAIJ, KASHIF MEMON, AND NAEEM RAZA

> Using available arthroplasty registry data, we estimate that about three quarters of hip replacements last 15–20 years and just over half of hip replacements last 25 years in patients with osteoarthritis.
>
> —EVANS ET AL.[1]

Citation: Evans JT, Evans JP, Walker RW, Blom AW, Whitehouse MR, Sayers A. How long does a hip replacement last? A systematic review and meta-analysis of case series and national registry reports with more than 15 years of follow-up. Lancet. 2019;393(10172):647–54.

Research Question: How long does a total hip arthroplasty (THA) last?

Funding: National Institute for Health Research, National Joint Registry (NJR; for England, Wales, Northern Ireland, and Isle of Man), and Royal College of Surgeons of England

Year Study Began: 2017

Year Study Published: 2019

Study Location: Musculoskeletal Research Unit, Translational Health Sciences, Bristol Medical School, Southmead Hospital, Bristol

Who Was Studied: This was a meta-analysis reviewing all articles considering patients who underwent THA for primary osteoarthritis (OA) alone. Only articles reviewing predominantly unselected patients were considered.

Who Was Excluded: Any non-English articles or conference abstracts reviewing complex primary THA, revision THA, resurfacing, or procedures performed for reasons other than OA. Implant construct survivorship from registry data, pooled data from the reviews (to avoid duplication), and articles without follow-up (F/U) or survivorship data were also excluded.

How Many Patients: 228 888

Study Overview: See Figure 3.1.

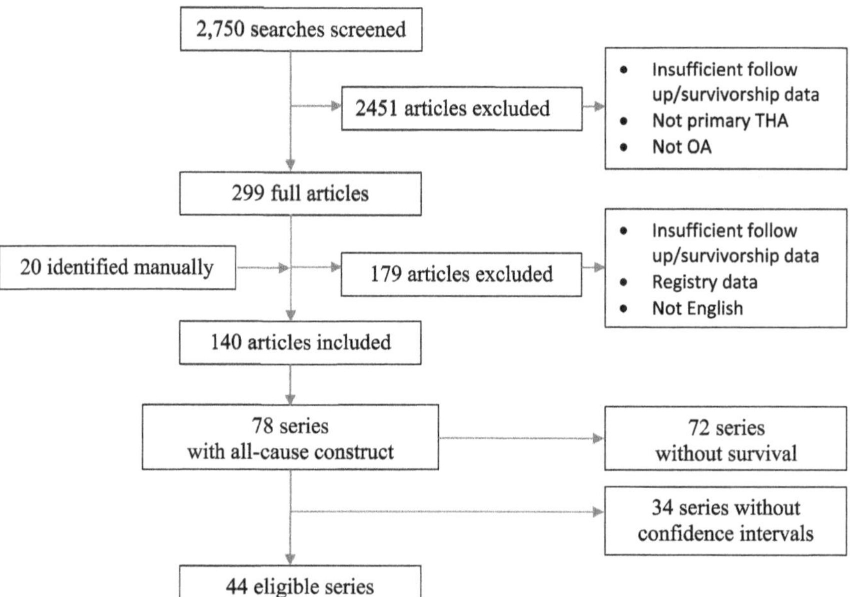

Figure 3.1. Summary of study intervention.

Table 3.1 Summary of Inclusion Criteria and Demographics

	Individual Case Series	**Australian Orthopaedic Association NJR (2017)**	**Finnish Arthroplasty Report (November 2017)**
Location	16 countries	Australia	Finland
No. of series (*n*)	44	36	56
Year of publication	1993–2017	2017	2017
THA (*n*)	13 212	121 384	94 292
Mean age (y)	57.9	67.7	65–74
% of implants for OA	61.8	88.5	Not reported

Study Intervention: This was a systematic review and meta-analysis of case series and cohort studies. All data considering unselected patients undergoing primary conventional THA using any prosthesis were assessed for implant survival with respect to specific implant, brand, or construct. There was no control group. A second meta-analysis was conducted of the national joint replacement registries (from Australia, Denmark, Finland, New Zealand, Norway, and Sweden) with > 15 years F/U, reported in English and available within the Medline and Embase databases.

Follow-Up: Variable depending on the study but > 15 years of F/U for registry data

Endpoints: The sole endpoint was the revision of any part of the THA construct for any reason as this marks the end of survivorship of the implant. No secondary outcomes were recorded. This was recorded either via the NJR or from the case-series searches.

RESULTS (TABLE 3.1)

- *Initial search*: The search yielded 4195 references, which were screened to 44 useable case series (see Figure 3.1). These were reviewed and articles were excluded for insufficient F/U, poor survival analysis, using registry data, using language other than English, using alternative outcomes, or procedures not for primary hip OA.
- *Final analysis:* The 44 case series represent all-cause construct survival in 13 212 THAs (range 73–2000) with F/U ranging from 15 to 40 years.
- *Pooled analysis*: Data from case series of THA reported at exactly 15, 20, and 25 years showed all-cause survivorship of 85.7% (95% CI: 85.0–86.5) at 15 years, 78.8% (95% CI: 77.8–79.9) at 20 years, and 77.6% (95% CI: 76.0–79.2) at 25 years (Table 3.2, Figure 3.2).

- *Survival analysis:*
  - Case series that did not have these time points were rounded down to the nearest time point to increase the data set. This gave a pooled survival of 87.9% (95% CI: 87.2–88.5) at 15 years, 78.0 (95% CI: 77.9–80.0) at 20 years, and 76.6% (95% CI: 75.1–78.2) at 25 years.
  - The NJR reports yielded 92 series, in which all individually reported survival analyses at 15 years (215 676 THAs [100%]), 43 series reported survival analyses at 20 years (73 057 THAs [34%]), and 29 series reported survival analyses at 25 years (51 359 THAs [24%]).
  - Women have slightly better construct survivorship at all ages than men.

Table 3.2 Summary of Key Findings from Pooled Survival Data

Survivorship Mean (95% CI)	**15 Years (95% CI)**		**20 Years (95% CI)**		**25 Years (95% CI)**	
Study	**Series** (%)	**Registry** (%)	**Series** (%)	**Registry** (%)	**Series** (%)	**Registry** (%)
THA	87.9% (87.2–88.5)	89.4% (89.2–89.6)	78.9% (77.9–80.0)	70.2% (69.7–70.7)	76.6% (75.1–78.2)	57.9% (57.1–58.7)

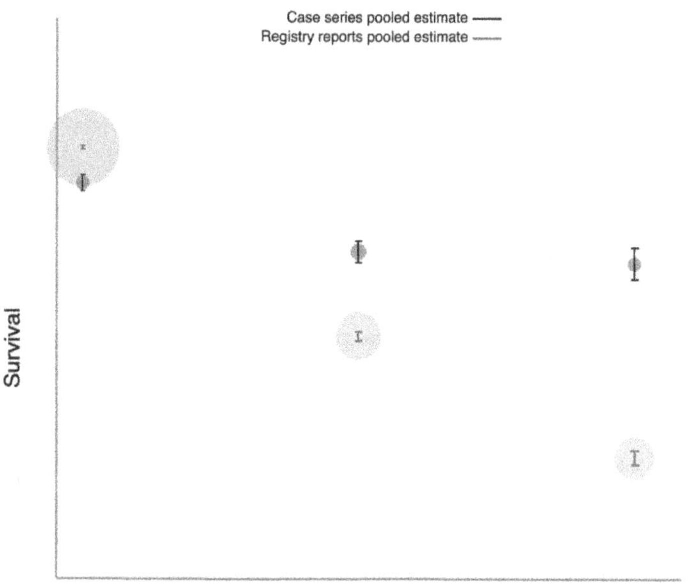

Figure 3.2. Comparison of pooled survival estimates from case series and registry reports at 15 years, 20 years, and 25 years respectively. The size of each circle is proportional to the total number of hip replacements at the start of all the series contributing to that pooled estimate.

Criticisms and Limitations: The quality of published case series was low, indicating that 24 (54.5%) of 44 series were consecutive, none were multicenter, 5 (11.4%) had < 20% F/U, and 7 (15.9%) used multivariable analyses. Pooled data from the authors' search was not adjusted or stratified by patient demographics that could have influenced survivorship. Pooled survival observed from case series showed a more optimistic estimate than pooled registry data, but the authors believed the registry data to be the more accurate. Furthermore, the registry results were drawn from Australia and Finland only. Survival analysis from registry data beyond 20 years was limited to Finnish data alone and may not be representative. Registry data is heavily dependent on linkage of the primary arthroplasty to a revision procedure, but threshold for revision surgery may differ between centers, registries, and countries. Excluding non-English articles removed 13 further series, which could have altered the pooled results. Data generated for long-term F/U is historic and as such may not represent the expected outcomes of implants being used in modern practice (i.e., metal-on-metal [MOM] bearings).

Other Relevant Studies and Information:

- The same research group repeated their analysis through a systematic review and meta-analysis for total knee arthroplasty (TKA) and unicondylar knee arthroplasty (UKA), which showed the following:[2]
  - *TKA:* Survivorship was studied at 15 years (47 case series, 299 291 TKAs), 20 years (20 case series, 88 532 TKAs), and 25 years (14 case series, 76 651 TKAs). The pooled survival from registry data showed an all-cause construct survivorship of 93.0% (95% CI: 92.8–93.1) at 15 years, 90.1% (95% CI: 89.7–90.4) at 20 years, and 82.3% (95% CI: 81.3–83.2) at 25 years.
  - *UKA:* Survivorship was studied at 15 years (5 case series, 7714 UKAs), 20 years (4 case series, 3395 UKAs), and 25 years (4 case series, 3935 UKAs). The pooled survival from registry data showed an all-cause construct survivorship of 76.5% (95% CI: 75.2–77.7) at 15 years, 71.6% (95% CI: 69.6–73.6) at 20 years, and 69.8% (95% CI: 67.6–72.1) at 25 years.

Summary and Implications: This systematic review and meta-analysis showed that the 25-year pooled survival of THA from 44 case series was 77.6% (95% CI: 76.0–79.2) and 57.9% (95% CI: 57.1–58.7) from national joint replacement registries (from Finland and Australia). Patients and surgeons can expect a conventional THA indicated for primary OA to last 15–20 years in about three-quarters and last 25 years in over half of patients.

CLINICAL CASE: COUNSELING A PATIENT AND THEIR RELATIVE ON THE LONGEVITY OF A THA

Case History

A 65-year-old man with severe end-stage right hip OA has attended the clinic with his daughter (Figure 3.3). Conservative measures including physiotherapy, analgesia, and a walking aid have failed to improve walking distance. A diagnostic hip injection gave him 2 weeks of pain relief. He has agreed to a THA after discussing the risks and benefits including the chance of revision surgery. His daughter has numerous questions and would like to know how long the hip replacement will last and which implant will be used. Based on the results of the study, how should the patient and his daughter be counseled?

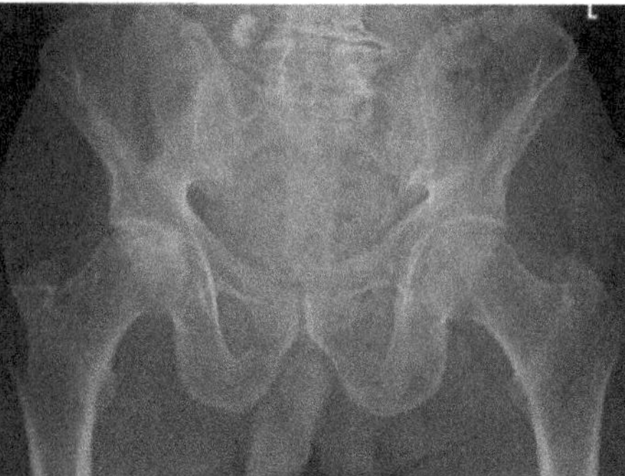

Figure 3.3. Plain radiograph of the pelvis and hips.

Suggested Answer

This is a typical question that patients or their families ask. They are likely to know someone who has had either a primary or revision arthroplasty surgery, or they may have looked up hip replacement surgery on the Internet and longevity may show up as a late complication. Quite commonly they may ask about the implant such as its brand and constituents. There are a number of reasons a hip replacement may need revision, ranging from infection to instability. Also note the severe lower lumbar degenerative spondylosis affecting spinal alignment. A high-level study has shown that three-quarters of all THAs—regardless of implant design or technique—will last 20 years, and just over half will last 25 years.

References

1. Evans et al. How long does a hip replacement last? A systematic review and meta-analysis of case series and national registry reports with more than 15 years of follow-up. Lancet. 2019;393:647–54.
2. Evans et al. How long does a knee replacement last? A systematic review and meta-analysis of case series and national registry reports with more than 15 years of follow-up. Lancet. 2019; 393:655–63.

4

Timing for Surgery for Hip Fractures

DUNCAN COFFEY AND RAJU AHLUWALIA

> Delaying surgery may not affect mortality, but it is likely to increase morbidity, particularly the incidence of pressure sores and will increase hospital stay. Therefore, patients admitted to hospital with a hip fracture, in whom there are no conditions that can be improved prior to surgery, should have their surgery as soon as possible after admission.
>
> —Khan et al.[1]

Citation: Khan SK, Kalra S, Khanna A, Thiruvengada MM, Parker MJ. Timing of surgery for hip fractures: a systematic review of 52 published studies involving 291,413 patients. Injury. 2009;40(7):692–7.

Research Question: Is there a difference in mortality and complication rates in regard to timing of surgery for hip fractures?

Funding: None reported

Year Study Began: Data collection 1960–2007

Year Study Published: 2009

Study Location: Peterborough and Stamford National Health Service Foundation Trust, UK

Who Was Studied: All studies from 1960 to 2007 were included if they reported on the timing of surgery to outcomes of mortality (within the follow-up period of that study), postoperative medical complications, hospital length of stay (LOS), or proportion of patients discharged home. An objectively scored assessment of the methodological quality was performed for all included studies.

Who Was Excluded: Studies that related to fracture healing complications, patients who had surgery delayed for medical reasons, and non-English published literature.

How Many Patients: 291 413

Study Overview: See Figure 4.1.

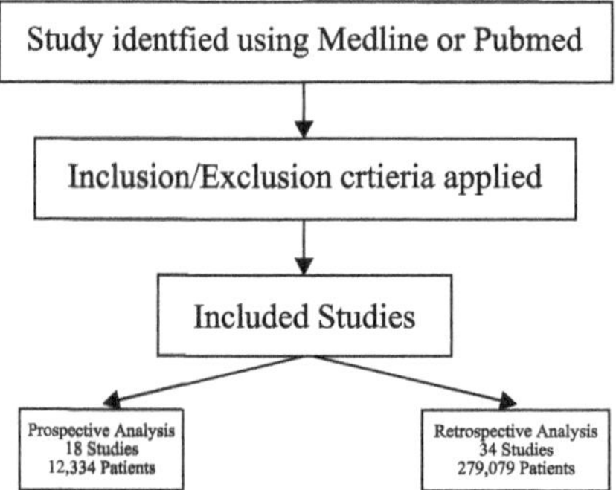

Figure 4.1. Study overview.

Study Intervention: Included studies were categorized into prospective or retrospective data collection (see Figure 4.1). If this was unclear, then the data was considered to be retrospective. Retrospective studies were then subdivided into review of case notes or evaluation of a central database. Confounding factors that could influence mortality or morbidity included age, mental status, residential status, American Society of Anesthesiologists grade, walking ability, and associated medical comorbidities.

Prospective studies were considered as the foremost methodology, which excluded operations delayed to improve fitness for surgery as well as statistical adjustment for confounding factors that were associated with mortality. The next favorable methodology consisted of prospective data and statistical adjustment but no exclusion of those initially considered unfit for surgery, followed by those studies that had retrospective data collection but with statistical adjustment. Other studies that used statistical adjustment were retrospective reviews of central databases or patient hospital episode registers. Those studies that used no statistical adjustment for confounding factors were separated into those that had prospective or retrospective collection of data and those that used hospital episode registers. Each study was scored using a validated assessment of methodological quality. The study defined surgery within 24 hours of admission as day 1, surgery between 24 and 48 hours of admission as day 2, and surgery between 48 and 72 hours of admission as day 3.

Follow-Up: Up to 10 years within included studies

Endpoints: Reported outcomes were mortality, medical complications, LOS, and failure to return home.

RESULTS (TABLE 4.1)

- *Final analysis:* 52 published studies were identified for inclusion in the final analysis.
- *Mortality:* 22 studies reported reduced mortality with early surgery (defined differently in each study), 25 studies reported no effect with early surgery, and 2 studies reported increased mortality with early surgery.
- *Medical complications:* 9 studies reported reduced medical complications with early surgery, and 9 studies reported no effect with early surgery.
- *LOS:* 13 studies reported a reduced hospital stay with early surgery, and 6 studies reported no effect with early surgery.
- *Failure to return home:* 2 studies reported a reduction in failure to return home with early surgery, and 2 studies reported no effect from early surgery.

Table 4.1 Summary of Results of the Effect of Early Surgery on Outcomes

	Reduced (% Studies)	**No Effect (% Studies)**	**Increased (% Studies)**	**Not Reported (% Studies)**
Mortality	42.3	40.1	3.8	5.8
Medical complications	17.3	17.3	0	65.4
LOS	25	11.5	0	63.5
Failure to return home	3.8	3.8	0	92.4

Criticisms and Limitations: Level 1 studies randomizing patients into early or late surgery had not been performed at the time of this study but would have been ideal in addressing the research question. Pain was not addressed, which may affect speed of rehabilitation. Issues related to the timing of surgery for intracapsular neck of femur (NOF) fractures were also not addressed. The authors never defined the quality of methodological scores but only found 3 studies to have optimum methodology. Studies that failed to adjust for confounding variables were more likely to find adverse effects from delay to surgery, particularly for mortality.

Other Relevant Studies and Information:

- 3 prospective cohort studies[2–4] have reported that early surgery can reduce the risk of (1) mortality, (2) LOS, and (3) postoperative medical complications.
- A prospective observational study[5] looking at the effect of early surgery in patients > 90 years of age who present with NOF fractures reported that both mortality and morbidity were reduced with early surgery. Moreover, elevated orthopaedic Physiological and Operative Severity Score for the Enumeration of Mortality and Morbidity scores[6] correlated with a higher mortality in late surgery.
- In a study of circa 40 000 hip fractures,[7] the overall mortality at 30 days was 7% with supporting information from the British Orthopaedic Association Standards for Trauma[8] guidelines that indicates a 10% mortality at 30 days and up to 30% mortality at 1 year. Propensity-score-matched patients of circa 13 000 who received surgery < 24 hours vs. > 24 hours had a significantly higher 30-day mortality risk (% absolute risk difference = 0.79 [95% CI: 0.23–1.35]) and composite outcome (i.e., composite of mortality or any medical complication such as myocardial infarction, venous thromboembolic event, and pneumonia; % absolute risk difference = 2.16 [95% CI: 1.43–2.89]). Nevertheless, there are studies that do not show any compelling evidence to support this statement.
- The HIP ATTACK trial[9] is currently ongoing; it is a multicenter, international, parallel-group randomized controlled trial (RCT) comparing early surgery vs. standard care. The primary outcomes reported will be mortality and morbidity.
- Analysis of just under 130 000 hip fractures from Hospital Episode Statistics by Bottle et al.[10] indicated a delay in surgery was associated with an increased risk of death but not readmission, despite adjustment for comorbidity, and with a wide variation between hospitals.
- A 5-year retrospective review[11] of delay in fracture fixation in 82 elderly (> 65 years) patients, who were physiologically stable on admission,

demonstrated a significant increase in morbidity (i.e., infections and LOS) and mortality and adversely affected resource utilization (i.e., total hospital cost). Time to surgery was stratified as early (< 24 hours), intermediate (24–72 hours), or late (> 72 hours).

- National Institute for Health and Care Excellence guidelines for the management of hip fractures in adults include the aforementioned 3 prospective cohort studies[2–4] as evidence for timing for surgery.[12] The Best Practice Tariff in the United Kingdom recommends operating on hip fractures within a 36-hour window.

Summary and Implications: This systematic review of observational studies provides modest support that early surgery in patients with NOF fractures can reduce postoperative medical complications, distress, and LOS. However, the results indicate that delayed surgery may not *adversely* affect mortality. The HIP ATTACK trial[9] is an ongoing RCT that will evaluate the benefits of early surgery vs. standard treatment.

CASE STUDY: WHEN SHOULD I HAVE MY HIP FRACTURE FIXED, DOCTOR?

Case History

A 76-year-old male presents with a fractured neck of the femur (Figure 4.2). He is otherwise medically stable. He has no significant past medical history or any allergies. He is scared since his wife passed away after hip surgery 2 years ago in the same hospital. He pleads to have a few days to think about the surgery and when to have it. The patient is keen on obtaining a second opinion from his next of kin, his son, who is returning from abroad a few days later. What are the risks and benefits of early vs. delayed surgery according to this study?

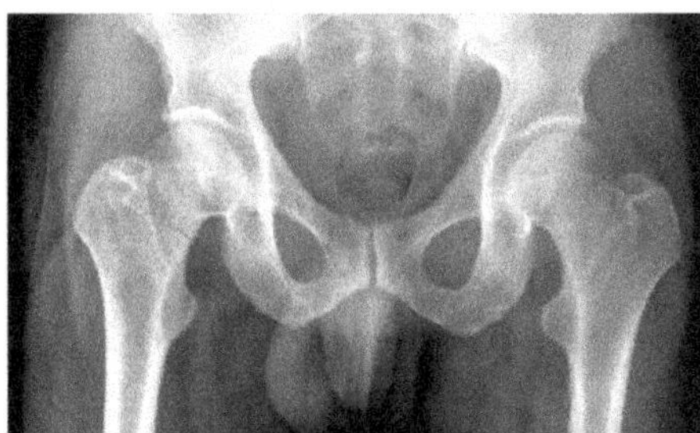

Figure 4.2. AP radiograph of pelvis and hips demonstrating a minimally displaced transcervical NOF.

Suggested Answer

It is important that a patient has surgery when they have had time to understand and weigh their options to offer their informed consent in writing. In the case of surgery for a fractured NOF there is evidence that suggests that early surgery can reduce the risk of death postoperatively as well as reducing medical complications and LOS and increasing the chance to get the patient back home. It would be important to explain this to the patient so that he can make a reasoned judgement on when he would like to proceed with the operation. There is enough statistical and clinical evidence to support early timing to surgery to reduce risk of mortality and postoperative complications.

References

1. Khan et al. Timing for surgery for hip fractures: a systematic review of 52 published studies involving 291,413 patients. Injury. 2009;40:692–7.
2. Orosz et al. Association of timing of surgery for hip fracture and patient outcome. JAMA. 2004;291:1738–43.
3. Moran et al. Early mortality after hip fracture: is delay before surgery important. J Bone Joint Surg Am. 2005;87(3):483–9.
4. Siegmeth et al. Delay to surgery prolongs hospital stay in patients with fractures of the proximal femur. J Bone Joint Surg Br. 2005;87(8):1123–26.
5. Hapuarachchi et al. Neck of femur fractures in the over 90s: a select group of patients who require prompt surgical intervention for optimal results. J Orthopaed Traumatol. 2014;15(1):13–19.
6. Copeland et al. POSSUM: a scoring system for surgical audit. Br J Surg. 1991;78(3):355–60.
7. Pincus et al. Association between wait time and 30-day mortality in adults undergoing hip fracture surgery. JAMA. 2017;318(20):1994–2003.
8. British Orthopaedic Association. British Orthopaedic Standards for Trauma (BOAST) 1 guideline. Patients sustaining a fragility hip fracture. January 2012. https://www.boa.ac.uk/asset/067568A1%2D9138%2D490E%2DBD346A2D8AFCC79D/
9. Borges et al. Rationale and design of the HIP fracture Accelerated surgical TreaTment And Care tracK (HIP ATTACK) trial: a protocol for an international randomised controlled trial evaluating early surgery for hip fracture patients. BMJ Open. 2019;9:e028537.
10. Bottle et al. Mortality associated with delay in operation after hip fracture: observational study. BMJ. 2006;332:947–51.
11. Rogers et al. Early fixation reduces morbidity and mortality in elderly patients with hip fractures from low-impact falls. J Trauma. 1995;39:261–5.
12. National Institute for Health and Care Excellence. Hip fracture: management. Clinical guideline (CG124). 2017. www.nice.org.uk/guidance/cg124

5

Treatment for Acute Anterior Cruciate Ligament Tears

NICOLA BLUCHER AND GHIAS BHATTEE

> In young, active adults with an acute ACL tear, a strategy of structured rehabilitation plus early ACL reconstruction did not result in better patient-reported outcomes at 2 years than a strategy of rehabilitation plus optional delayed ACL reconstruction in those with symptomatic instability.
>
> —FROBELL ET AL.[1]

Citation: Frobell R, Roos E, Roos H, Ranstam J, Lohmander L. A randomized trial of treatment for acute anterior cruciate ligament tears. N Engl J Med. 2010;363:331–42.

Research Question: Is a strategy of structured rehabilitation + early anterior cruciate ligament (ACL) reconstructive surgery superior to a strategy of structured rehabilitation with delayed ACL reconstruction for young, active, adult patients who continue to have symptomatic knee instability following acute ACL tears?

Funding: Swedish Research Council and the Medical Faculty of Lund University and others

Year Study Began: 2002

Year Study Published: 2010

Study Location: Lund, Sweden: Helsingborg Hospital and Lund University Hospital

Who Was Studied: Adults, aged 18–35 years, who presented with recent rotational knee trauma within the preceding 4 weeks. ACL insufficiency as determined by clinical examination. Tegner Activity Scale[2] (TAS) score 5–9 (indicating participation in recreational sports, including competitive sports at a nonprofessional level).

Who Was Excluded: Previous knee injury or surgery; associated posterior cruciate ligament, medial collateral ligament grade III, or lateral/posterolateral corner injury; pregnancy; and history of deep vein thrombosis. Postrandomization; patients with an intact ACL, total collateral ligament rupture, or a full-thickness cartilage lesion on magnetic resonance imaging (MRI). Intact ACL found intraoperatively or extensive fixation of large meniscal tears requiring a change in postoperative rehabilitation.

How Many Patients: 141

Study Overview: See Figure 5.1.

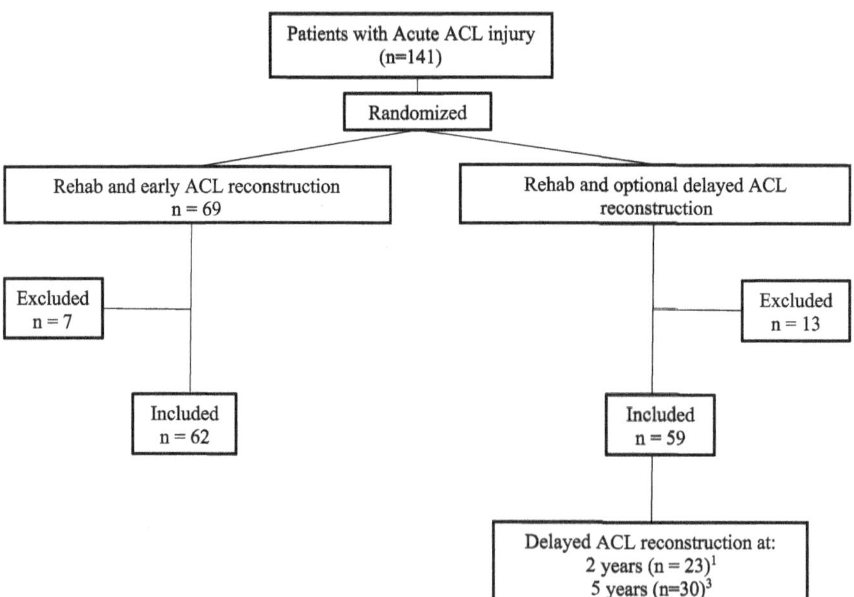

Figure 5.1. Summary of study design.

Study Intervention: All patients followed a rehabilitation protocol; this was commenced before or at the time of randomization and supervised by experienced physical therapists. The protocol was goal focused and progressive. Patients in the rehabilitation and early ACL reconstruction group underwent surgery within 10 weeks of injury by 1 of 4 surgeons. The choice of procedure was based on surgeon's preference (patella tendon n = 25, hamstring tendon n = 36). Patients in the rehabilitation + optional delayed ACL reconstruction group followed the rehabilitation protocol. If prespecified criteria were met (self-reported symptomatic instability and positive pivot shift test), patients were referred for delayed ACL reconstruction. This was performed by the same surgeons as the early reconstruction group.

Follow-Up: 2 years

Endpoints: Primary outcome consisted of change from baseline to 2 years in the average score for 4 of the 5 Knee injury and Osteoarthritis Outcome Score ($KOOS_4$) (0–100) subscales.[3] Secondary outcomes consisted of results on the following:

- 5 KOOS subscales (self-administered survey evaluating both short-term and long-term consequences of knee injury that holds 42 items in 5 separately scored subscales: pain, other symptoms, function in daily living, function in sport and recreation, and knee-related quality of life)
- SF-36 physical and mental components[4] (a survey evaluating health-related quality of life by measuring 8 scales: physical functioning, role physical, bodily pain, general health, vitality, social functioning, role emotional, and mental health. There are 2 distinct concepts measured by the SF-36: Physical Component Summary and Mental Component Summary)
- TAS[2] scores (1-item score that graded activity based on work and sports activities on a scale of 0–10; 0 represents disability because of knee problems and 10 represents national or international level sport participation)

Knee stability as determined with the Lachman test, pivot shift, and KT1000 knee arthrometry was also recorded.

RESULTS (TABLE 5.1)

- *Comparison:* Both treatment groups had improvement over the 2-year period. There were no significant differences in the change in $KOOS_4$ score from baseline to 2 years between the cohorts (mean scores 39.2 and 39.4 respectively; $p = 0.96$; Figure 5.2).
- *Early group:* Patients in the *early* group had a higher frequency of meniscal surgery than the *delayed* group (50 vs. 40 respectively; $p = 0.20$).
- *Delayed group:* Of the 59 patients, 23 (38.9%) underwent ACL reconstruction at an average of 11.6 months after randomization.
- *At 2 years:*
  - There were no significant between-group differences for any patient-reported secondary outcomes (KOOS, SF-36, or TAS).
  - Patients in the rehabilitation + *early* ACL reconstruction group had greater knee stability (KT1000 $p = 0.001$, Lachman $p < 0.001$, pivot shift $p = 0.003$).
- *Complications:* Surgery produced adverse events in both groups ($p = 0.06$):
  - *Early group:* 3 ACL graft ruptures and 1 arthrofibrosis
  - *Delayed group:* 1 ACL graft rupture

Table 5.1 Summary of Key Findings

Variable	**Rehabilitation + *Early* ACL Reconstruction ($n = 62$)**	**Rehabilitation + *Optional Delayed* ACL Reconstruction ($n = 59$)**	***p* Value**
		KOOS[a]	
Mean change in $KOOS_4$ score	39.2	39.4	0.96
		Mean SF-36 score[b]	
Physical component	82.1	78.0	0.11
Mental component	88.3	83.8	0.17
		TAS[c]	
Return to preinjury activity level or higher	27	21	0.37

[a] $KOOS_4$ includes four subscales: pain, symptoms, function in sports and recreation, and knee-related quality of life; scores range from 0 to 200, with higher scores indicating better results.

[b] Scores on the SF-36 range from 0 to 100, with higher scores indicating better results.

[c] TAS assesses activity level with specific emphasis on the knee. Scores range from 1 (least strenuous activity) to 10 (high knee-demanding activity on a professional level).

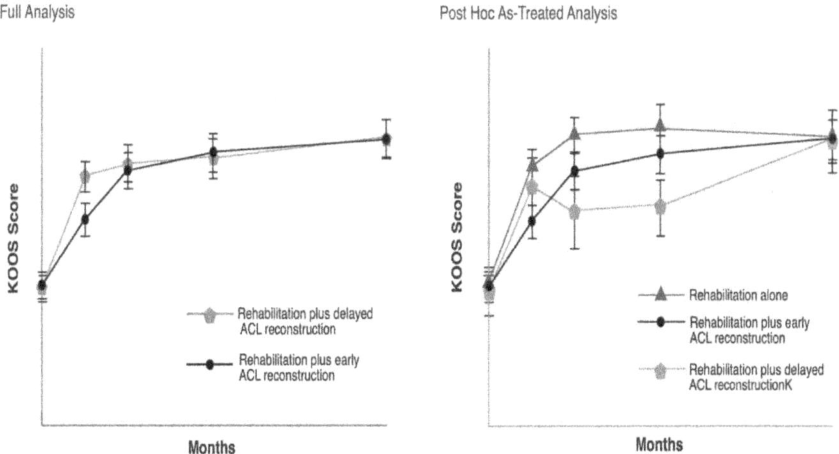

Figure 5.2. Mean $KOOS_4$ scores during the 2-year study period, according to treatment group.

Criticisms and Limitations: Both surgeons and patients were not blinded to their treatments, potentially introducing bias. Although the patient population was young adults with high preinjury activity levels, it did not include professional athletes. Follow-up was short at 2 years; continued follow-up is required to assess longer-term outcomes including the risk of osteoarthritis (OA).

Other Relevant Studies and Information:

- Systematic review[5] assessed the effects of surgical vs. conservative interventions for treating ACL injuries. After all titles and abstracts were screened for eligible studies, Frobell et al.[1] was the only study identified to be included. Using Grading of Recommendations, Assessment, Development, and Evaluations (GRADE) methodology,[6] they concluded that the overall quality of evidence was low across the different outcomes assessed.
- Frobell et al.[7] extended follow-up to 5 years; a further 7 patients had a *delayed* ACL reconstruction (n = 30). There remained no statistically significant difference between the groups in outcome scores. Hence, one treatment was not more harmful than the other over 2–5 years.
- Long-term implications of ACL deficiency include high risk of developing early-onset OA.[8]

- There are 2 ongoing randomized controlled trials; NTR2746[9] is examining clinical and cost effectiveness of *early* surgery vs. conservative management, and ACL SNNAP[10] is examining clinical and cost effectiveness of surgery vs. conservative management in patients with nonacute (> 4 months) ACL deficiency. Both will offer the option of *delayed* surgery. ACL SNNAP demonstrated that surgical reconstruction in nonacute ACL injury with persistent symptoms of instability was clinically superior and more cost effective in comparison with rehabilitation management.

Summary and Implications: This study indicates that in young, active adults with an *acute* ACL tear, patient-reported outcomes at 2 years are not statistically different between patients who undergo structured rehabilitation + *early* ACL reconstruction and those with symptomatic knee instability who undergo rehabilitation + *optional delayed* ACL reconstruction. Adopting a more conservative approach emphasizing initial structured rehabilitation, with surgical repair reserved only for those with persistent symptomatic joint instability, might reduce both the number of surgical procedures and associated complications. These findings do not necessarily apply to professional athletes, and the study does not show long-term follow-up results or implications.

CLINICAL CASE: ACUTE ACL INJURY

Case History

A 23-year-old female sustained an injury to her knee when playing netball a fortnight ago; she landed after a jump on an extended knee. She heard an audible "popping" sound and experienced immediate pain, swelling, and difficulty mobilizing. She works as an accountant and plays netball for a local team, attends the gym 3–4 times a week, and enjoys entering triathlons. She attends the clinic after being referred from the Emergency Department and wants to know about her treatment options. Her MRI (Figure 5.3) was performed elsewhere to prove a complete midsubstance ACL tear. She has done some research online, has spoken to friends who have had similar injuries, and wonders if she should undergo a course of rehabilitation first or have early surgical reconstruction. According to the results of this study, how should the patient be counselled?

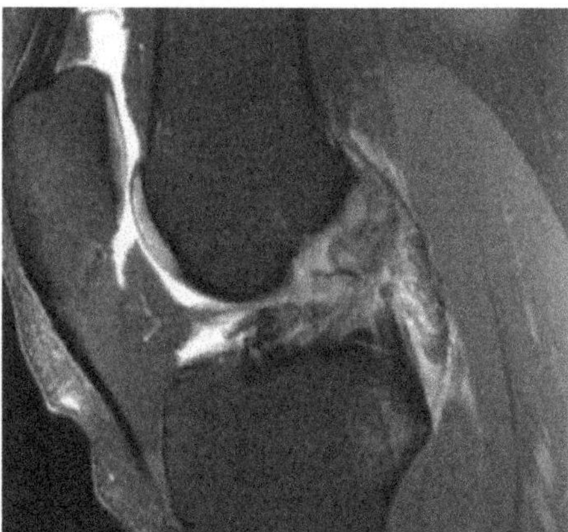

Figure 5.3. Sagittal T2-weighted MRI demonstrating ACL injury with loss of contour, increased signal intensity, and posterior translation of tibia relative to femur. There is also evidence of a retropatellar effusion as well as increased marrow signal changes in the anterior femur and posterior tibia indicating a likely pivot-shift mechanism of injury.

Suggested Answer

This study has shown that patients report similar outcomes of knee function at 2 years following either *acute* ACL reconstruction or structured rehabilitation with *delayed* ACL reconstruction if symptomatic. Approximately 40% of patients who were initially treated conservatively underwent delayed ACL reconstruction by 2 years. We are not fully aware of the long-term implications, but there is some evidence to indicate an increased risk of developing early-onset OA in ACL-deficient knees. With regards to surgical intervention, the procedure, complications, and risks should be explained to the patient so that she can make an informed decision prior to consenting.

References

1. Frobell et al. A randomized trial of treatment for acute anterior cruciate ligament tears. N Engl J Med. 2010;363:331–42.
2. Tegner et al. Rating systems in the evaluation of knee ligament injuries. Clin Orthop Relat Res. 1985;198:43–9.
3. Roos et al. Knee Injury and Osteoarthritis Outcome Score (KOOS)—development of a self-administered outcome measure. J Orthop Sports Phys Ther. 1998;28:88–96.
4. Ware et al. The MOS 36-item Short-Form health survey (SF-36). Conceptual framework and item selection. Med Care. 1992;30:473–83.

5. Monk et al. Surgical versus conservative interventions for treating anterior cruciate ligament injuries. Cochrane Database Syst Rev. 2016;4:CD011166.
6. Guyatt et al. GRADE: an emerging consensus on rating quality of evidence and strength of recommendations. BMJ (Clin Res Ed). 2008;336(7650):924–6.
7. Frobell et al. Treatment for acute anterior ligament tear: five year outcome of randomized trial. Br J Sports Med. 2015;49:700.
8. Lohmander et al. The long-term consequences of anterior cruciate ligament and meniscus injuries osteoarthritis. Am J Sports Med. 2007;35(10):1756–69.
9. Eggerding et al. ACL reconstruction for all is not cost-effective after acute ACL rupture. Br J Sports Med. 2022;56(1):24–8.
10. Beard et al. ACL SNNAP Study Group. Rehabilitation versus surgical reconstruction for non-acute anterior cruciate ligament injury (ACL SNNAP): a pragmatic randomised controlled trial. Lancet. 2022;400(10352):605–15.

6

UK DRAFFT

A Randomized Controlled Trial of Percutaneous Fixation with Kirschner Wires versus Volar Locking Plate Fixation in the Treatment of Adult Patients with a Dorsally Displaced Fracture of the Distal Radius

CHRIS MITCHELL, MONIL KARIA, AND PETER DOMOS

Study's Nickname: UK DRAFFT

> Contrary to the existing literature, and against the increasing use of locking-plate fixation, this trial shows that there is no difference between Kirschner wires and volar locking plates for patients with dorsally displaced extra-articular fractures of the distal radius. A Kirschner wire fixation is less expensive and quicker to perform.
>
> —Costa et al.[1]

Citation: Costa ML, Achten J, Plant C, Parsons NR, Rangan A, Tubeuf S, Yu G, Lamb SE. UK DRAFFT: a randomised controlled trial of percutaneous fixation with Kirschner wires versus volar locking-plate fixation in the treatment of adult patients with a dorsally displaced fracture of the distal radius. Health Technol Assess. 2015;19(17):1–124, v–vi.

Research Question: How do the functional outcomes and cost effectiveness compare between Kirschner-wire (K-wire) fixation and locking plate fixation in patients with acute dorsally displaced extra-articular fractures of the distal radius?

Funding: The National Institute for Health Research Health Technology Assessment Program

Year Study Began: January 2011–July 2012

Year Study Published: February 2015

Study Location: 18 centers in the UK

Who Was Studied: Patients ≥ 18 years old with a dorsally displaced extra-articular fracture of the distal radius that was < 2 weeks old and within 3 cm of the radiocarpal joint that the surgeon believed would benefit from surgical fixation.

Who Was Excluded: Patients < 18 years of age, unable to give consent, with contraindication to anesthetic, or unable to adhere to trial procedures; open fractures, > 2-week-old fractures, fractures extending > 3 cm from radiocarpal joint, and fractures not requiring fixation or an open approach to reduce.

How Many Patients: 461

Study Overview: See Figure 6.1.

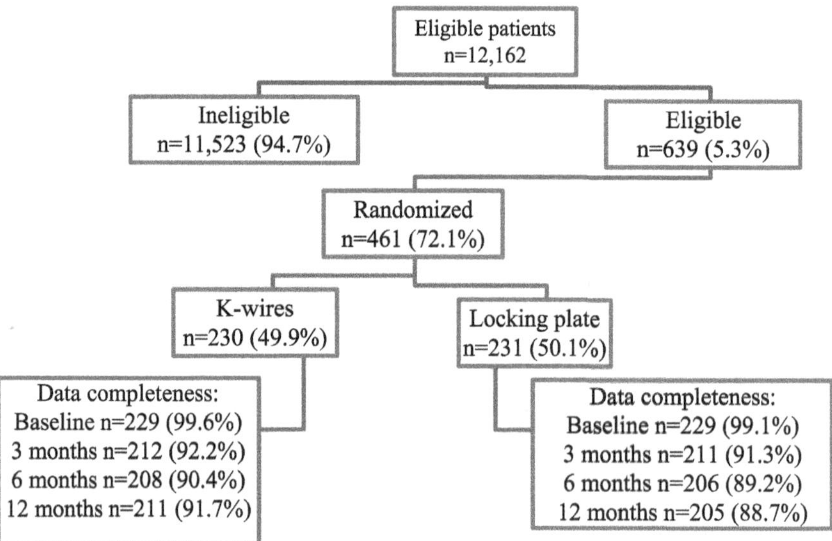

Figure 6.1. Summary of study design.

Study Intervention: Patients were randomized to either K-wire fixation or volar locking plate fixation. Differences between treatment groups were assessed on an intention-to-treat basis. The method of K-wire fixation was left to the preference of the operating surgeon and was then supplemented with plaster casting for 6 weeks when the cast and wires were removed. Volar locking plates were applied using a volar approach. The plate, screw configuration, and specifics of approach and postoperative immobilization were left to the operating surgeon's preference. Radiographic follow-up (F/U) was standardized at 6 weeks postoperatively and 12 months postoperatively. All patients received standardized written physiotherapy advice and were permitted to mobilize as soon as out of plaster. Any other rehabilitation was left to the surgeon's discretion.

Follow-Up: 12 months

Endpoints: The primary outcome measure was the Patient Rated Wrist Evaluation (PRWE)[2] score, which provides a brief, reliable, and valid measure of patient-rated pain and disability. Secondary outcome measures included:

- Disabilities of the Arm, Shoulder, and Hand[3] (DASH; 30-item, self-report questionnaire designed to assess degree of difficulty in performing different physical activities, severity of symptoms, and impact of the problem of social functioning because of arm, shoulder, and hand problems)
- EQ-5D[4] (self-assessed, health-related, quality of life questionnaire using a 5-component scale including mobility, self-care, usual activities, pain/discomfort, and anxiety/depression)
- Record of complications/rehabilitation or other interventions and economics questionnaire

The above questionnaires were collected at 3, 6, and 12 months. Complications were also recorded at 6 weeks. Radiographic evaluation of degree of palmar tilt, ulnar variance, and metaphyseal comminution were recorded at presentation, 6 weeks postinjury, and 12 months postinjury.

RESULTS (TABLE 6.1)

Questionnaire scores

- Postoperative wrist scores in both groups were similar, although function in both groups failed to return to baseline, with PRWE scores 15% worse than baseline in both groups.

- There was no statistically significant difference in PRWE questionnaires or EQ-5D or complications between the groups at any time point.
- There was a marginally insignificant ($p = 0.051$) but small treatment effect in favor of locking plate for DASH questionnaire at 12 months only.

Radiological parameters

- Dorsal angulation was significantly better in the locking plate group at 6 weeks by 3 degrees. There was also 0.75 mm less shortening. This persisted at 12 months, although it was deemed unlikely to be clinically significant (Figure 6.2).

Cost effectiveness and economic evaluation

- Mean cost of surgical fixation was higher in the locking plate (£818) group compared to the K-wire (£54) group. Societal costs were marginally higher by £70 in the K-wire group. The use of other health resource groups was comparable between groups (£1525 vs. £1590 respectively).
- There was no difference in health-related quality of life at 12-month F/U. There was a 0.008 quality-adjusted life year (QALY) gain to favor locking plate fixation.
- Locking plate fixation was not deemed to be cost effective. The incremental cost-effectiveness ratio of locking plates vs. K-wires was £89 322/QALY.

Table 6.1 A Comparison of Mean Radiographic, Functional, and Cost Outcomes at 12 Months between K-Wire Group and Locking Plate Group (Standard Deviations Are Shown in Brackets)

Outcome at 12 Months	**K-Wire Group**	**Locking Plate Group**	***p* Value**
Mean dorsal angle change (°)	−0.49 (12.45)	−5.20 (8.24)	< 0.001[a]
Ulnar variance (mm)	2.43 (2.31)	1.32 (2.02)	< 0.001[a]
PRWE score	15.3 (15.8)	13.9 (17.1)	NS
DASH score	16.2 (17.9)	13.0 (15.6)	0.051
EQ-5D score	0.83 (0.19)	0.85 (0.19)	NS
Total QALYs	0.734 (0.17)	0.742 (0.16)	NS
Total cost (£)	3440 (2539)	4145 (2203)	< 0.001

NS, not significant.

[a] Indicates statistical significance ($p < 0.05$).

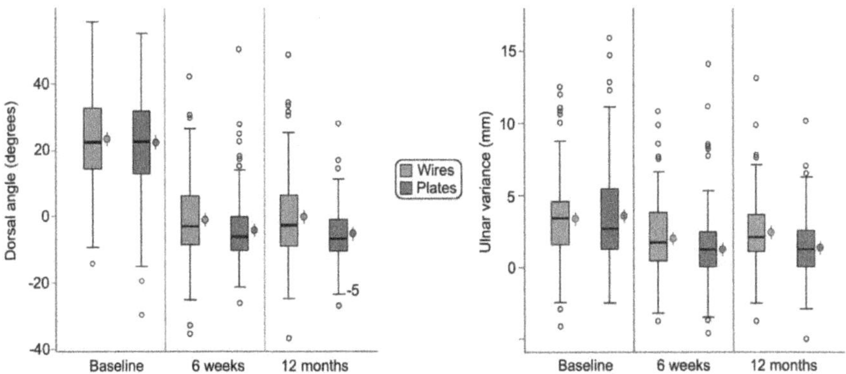

Figure 6.2. Box plots of baseline and postoperative scores and trends in means (filled circles) with 95% CI for dorsal angle and ulnar variance.

Criticisms and Limitations: Although over 12 000 patients were screened, only 461 (3.8%) were included in the study. As such, the cohorts in this study represent a small proportion of distal radius fractures. Seventy-one percent of operations were performed by nonconsultant/attending surgeons (specialist trainees 45%, staff grade 13%, other 12%). A significant number of surgeons had low prior operative experience (13% performed < 10 platings, 26% performed < 20 platings).

Other Relevant Studies and Information:

- 5-year F/U[5] of the DRAFFT trial again demonstrated no clinically or statistically significant difference between treatment groups in functional outcomes. However, there was a loss to F/U, with only 194 (44%) patients submitting scores. Only 3 (0.7%) patients had further surgery in the 5 years postinjury.
- Meta-analysis[6] in 2015 found a clinically insignificant improvement in functional outcomes with distal radius fractures managed with open reduction and internal fixation (ORIF) compared to K-wires.
- The British Society for Surgery on the Hand (BSSH)[7] recommends that dorsally displaced distal radius fractures that require surgery but can be reduced closed should be treated with K-wire fixation and casting. This is in keeping with the recommendations of the DRAFFT trial.
- The next stage of the trial is DRAFFT 2,[8] which is a randomized controlled trial (RCT) observing for manipulation and surgical fixation with K-wires vs. manipulation and casting in the treatment of dorsally displaced distal radius fractures.

Summary and Implications: In the DRAFFT trial, there were no statistically significant functional differences between K-wire fixation and ORIF for dorsally displaced extra-articular distal radius fractures. A 5-year F/U study confirmed no clinically or statistically significant difference between both treatment groups. K-wire fixation is less expensive to perform. Guidelines from the BSSH recommend K-wire fixation and casting as the preferred treatment option for this fracture pattern if it can be reduced closed.

CLINICAL CASE: DISTAL RADIUS FRACTURE IN THEATRE

Case History

The first patient on the trauma list is a fit and well right-hand-dominant 45-year-old patient who consented to manipulation under anesthesia ± K-wire fixation ± ORIF of a dorsally displaced extra-articular right distal radius fracture. The patient is a hairdresser who socially drinks alcohol and smokes. She had a mechanical fall yesterday as she slipped on the wet pavement and landed on an outstretched hand (Figure 6.3). The supervising attending/consultant wants to know the plan for stabilizing this fracture and if there is any evidence to support the surgical decision-making. What are the treatment options for this patient?

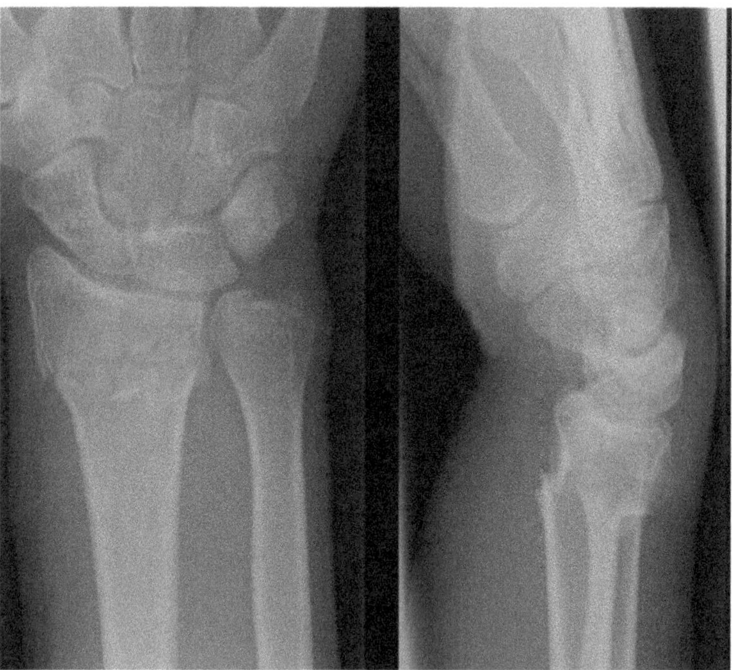

Figure 6.3. Anteroposterior and lateral plain radiograph of the right wrist demonstrating a dorsally displaced extraarticular distal radius fracture.

Suggested Answer

In this dorsally displaced extra-articular distal radius fracture, closed reduction is necessary as the initial step to ensure that it is reducible prior to fixation. If the fracture is reducible and stable, the fracture can be managed in a well-molded cast. If this is reducible and unstable, then the fracture should be stabilized with 2–3 K-wires and immobilized in plaster for 6 weeks. If this is not reducible or there is any intra-articular extension, one should proceed with ORIF using a flexor carpi radialis approach with a volar locking plate and early mobilization. Consider performing a computed axial tomography scan for complex fracture patterns to assist in surgical planning. There is good RCT evidence (DRAFFT and BSSH guidelines) that demonstrates that the long-term functional outcomes are similar regardless of which method of fixation is used as long as the fracture is appropriately reduced and stabilized.

References

1. Costa et al. UK DRAFFT: a randomised controlled trial of percutaneous fixation with Kirschner wires versus volar locking-plate fixation in the treatment of adult patients with a dorsally displaced fracture of the distal radius. Health Technol Assess. 2015;19(17):1–vi.
2. MacDermid et al. Patient rating of wrist pain and disability: a reliable and valid measurement tool. J Orthop Trauma. 1998;12(8):577–86.
3. Hudak et al. Development of an upper extremity outcome measure: the DASH (disabilities of the arm, shoulder and hand) [corrected]. The Upper Extremity Collaborative Group (UECG). Am J Ind Med. 1996;29(6):602–8. Erratum in: Am J Ind Med. 1996 Sep;30(3):372.
4. EuroQol Research Foundation. EQ-5D-5L user guide. 2019. https://euroqol.org/publications/user-guides.
5. Costa et al. Percutaneous fixation with Kirschner wires versus volar locking-plate fixation in adults with dorsally displaced fracture of distal radius: five-year follow-up of a randomized controlled trial. Bone Joint J. 2019 Aug;101-B(8):978–83.
6. Chaudhry et al. Are volar locking plates superior to percutaneous K-wires for distal radius fractures? A meta-analysis. Clin Orthop Relat Res. 2015;473(9):3017–27.
7. British Society for Surgery of the Hand. Best Practice for Management of Distal Radius Fractures—Surgery. BSSH Best Practice for Management of Distal Radius Fractures. 2018.
8. Achten et al. Surgical fixation with K-wires versus plaster casting in the treatment of dorsally displaced distal radius fractures: protocol for Distal Radius Acute Fracture Fixation Trial 2 (DRAFFT 2). BMJ Open. 2019;9:e028474.

7

Fracture Fixation in the Operative Management of Hip Fracture (FAITH)

An International, Multicenter, Randomized Controlled Trial

JAMES DALRYMPLE AND SANJAY SINHA

Study Nickname: FAITH trial

> We have shown a similar risk of hip reoperation in patient with low-energy femoral neck fractures randomly assigned to sliding hip screw as in those assigned to cancellous screws at 24 months; avascular necrosis occurred more frequently in patients allocated to sliding hip screw.
>
> —FAITH Investigators[1]

Citation: Fixation using Alternative Implants for the Treatment of Hip fractures (FAITH) Investigators. Fracture fixation in the operative management of hip fractures (FAITH): an international, multicentre, randomised controlled trial. Lancet. 2017;389:1519–27.

Research Question: Are sliding hip screws (SHSs) or cancellous screws (CSs) more effective at reducing the reoperation risk in patients with hip fractures?

Funding: National Institute of Health, Canadian Institutes of Health Research, Stichting NutsOhra, Netherlands Organisation for Health Research and Development, Physicians' Services Inc.

Year Study Began: 2008

Year Study Published: 2017

Study Location: 81 clinical centers in 8 countries: USA, Canada, Australia, Netherlands, Norway, Germany, UK, and India

Who Was Studied: Consenting patients > 50 years of age with a low-energy, isolated, and radiologically confirmed neck of femur (NOF) fracture suitable for fixation.

Who Was Excluded: Those with significant dementia or unlikely to comply with follow-up (F/U).

How Many Patients: 1108 randomized after screening

Study Overview: See Figure 7.1.

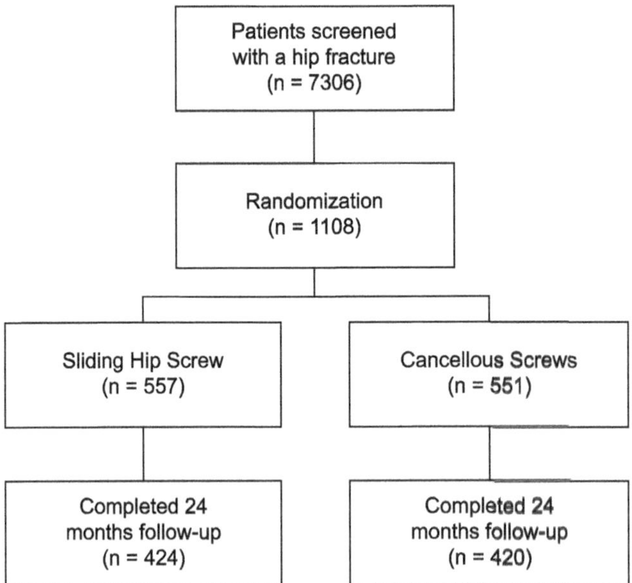

Figure 7.1. Overview of the study design.

Study Intervention: Patients allocated to the SHS group received a single 8-mm partially threaded screw fixed to the proximal femur with a side plate. The side plate consisted of 2–4 holes, and no supplemental fixation was used. The patients allocated to the CS group underwent fixation with multiple threaded screws.

A minimum of 2 screws with a diameter of at least 6.5 mm were used. The operating surgeons performing the fixation were required to have done at least 25 hip fracture fixations in their career and 5 in the year before participation. Surgeons were given criteria for acceptable postfixation fracture alignment on fluoroscopy and plain radiography.

Follow-Up: The mean length was 633 days.

Endpoints: Primary outcome was hip reoperation rate within 2 years to promote fracture healing, relieve pain, treat infection, or improve function. Secondary outcomes were mortality, fracture healing and fracture complications, avascular necrosis, medical adverse events, and health-related quality of life.

RESULTS

- *Protocol adherence:*
  - 844 (91%) patients completed the 24-month F/U period (Table 7.1).
  - Acceptable fracture reduction was achieved in 99% of patients with displaced fractures.
  - Surgeon compliance with the initially allocated surgical fixation technique was 97% for SHSs and 99% for CSs.
- *Reoperation rates* (*Figures* 7.2 and 7.3): The overall rate was 21% (20% SHSs vs. 22% CSs) with no significant difference between treatment groups ($p = 0.18$).
- *Avascular necrosis:* This was more prominent in the SHS group (50 vs. 28; $p = 0.03$).
- *Adverse events:* There was no significant difference in its rate between both treatments ($p = 0.82$).
- Subgroup analysis displayed more favorable results for the SHS in patients with a displaced fracture or basicervical fractures and in current smokers.

Table 7.1 Summary of Key Results

Outcome	**SHS Group**	**CS Group**	***p* Value**
Any reoperation	107 (20%)	117 (22%)	0.18
Avascular necrosis	50 (9%)	28 (5%)	0.03
Implant failure	42 (8%)	45 (8%)	0.81
Fracture healed by 2 years	262/398 (66%)	270/397 (68%)	0.71
Fracture NOT healed by 2 years	2/398 (1%)	1/397 (< 1%)	0.85
Mortality	72 (13%)	83 (15%)	0.21

100
90
80
70
0
0
180
360
540
730
Cancellous screws
Sliding hip screws
++ Censored results

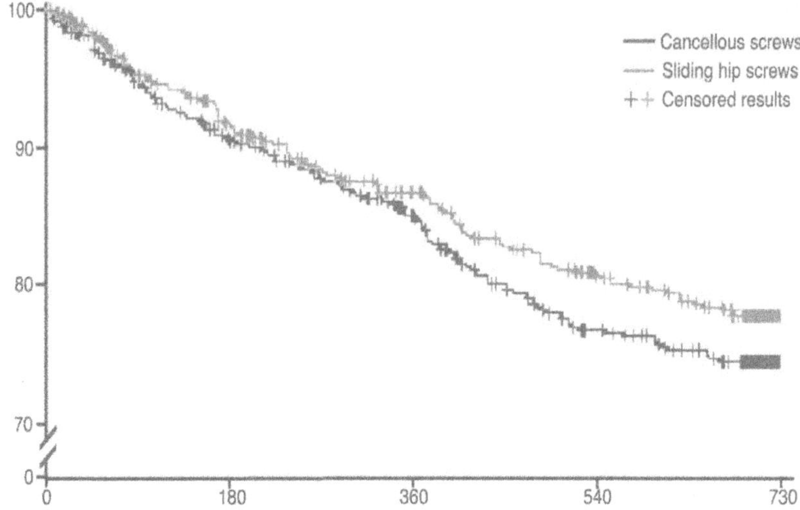

Figure 7.2. Kaplan-Meier curves for reoperation.

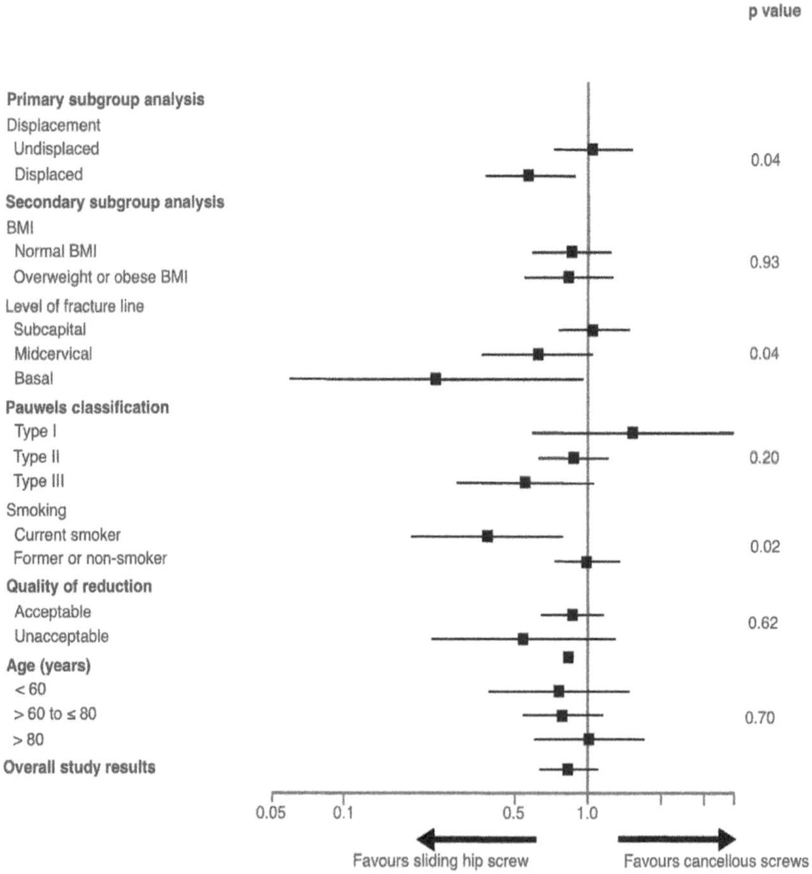

p value
Primary subgroup analysis
Displacement
Undisplaced
Displaced
0.04
Secondary subgroup analysis
BMI
Normal BMI
Overweight or obese BMI
0.93
Level of fracture line
Subcapital
Midcervical
Basal
0.04
Pauwels classification
Type I
Type II
Type III
0.20
Smoking
Current smoker
Former or non-smoker
0.02
Quality of reduction
Acceptable
Unacceptable
0.62
Age (years)
< 60
> 60 to ≤ 80
> 80
0.70
Overall study results
0.05
0.1
0.5
1.0
Favours sliding hip screw
Favours cancellous screws

Figure 7.3. Subgroup analyses of surgical fixation primary endpoint (reoperation).

Criticisms and Limitations: The surgeons, patients, and outcome adjudicators were not blinded. The primary endpoint was the reoperation rate, which is a subjective trigger and measure. Unavoidable variables that were not standardized included patient positioning, fracture reduction, surgical exposure, use of traction, surgical delay, type of anesthetic, physiotherapy, and rehabilitation programs.

Other Relevant Studies and Information:

- Significant data has been published that has established both the SHS and CS as acceptable techniques for the fixation of hip fractures.[2,3]
- SHSs have been shown to have a 2.6% reoperation rate across a sample size of 1024 subjects. This study, unlike the FAITH trial, did not require the operating surgeon to have performed a minimum number of such operations. This may explain the increased incidence of screw cutout and subsequent high rate of reoperation observed.[2]
- CSs have been shown to be an effective fixation device for NOF fractures with no difference in outcomes shown between the use of long (32-mm) or short (16-mm) threaded ones. However, CSs displayed a significantly higher reoperation rate of 25.2% in the short-thread group and 22.5% in the long-thread group.[3]

Summary and Implications: The FAITH trial showed that both the CS and SHS techniques are acceptable for use in the surgical fixation of intracapsular NOF fractures. The trial failed to show any significant difference in reoperation rate between SHSs and CSs. Both groups had similar fracture complication statistics (though patients with displaced or basicervical fractures and smokers did have a nonsignificant trend towards improved outcomes with the use of an SHS fixation technique).

CLINICAL CASE: SHS OR CS FIXATION FOR HIP FRACTURE FIXATION?

Case History

An independent 75-year-old woman with a low-energy fall at home presented to the Emergency Department complaining of left hip pain and being unable to bear weight. She has a past medical history including hypertension, chronic obstructive pulmonary disease, and ischemic heart disease. She usually walks without aids and assistance, and lives alone. Radiographs identify an isolated and displaced intracapsular left NOF fracture. The fracture pattern is reviewed by the attending and deemed suitable for fixation. The patient has been optimized for theatre by the geriatric team. Just before the operation the attending asks which fixation technique should be utilized for this patient based on currently available evidence.

Suggested Answer

There are various surgical techniques that could be used. The two most commonly used techniques are the SHS and the CS. The most recent evidence published in the FAITH trial failed to determine any statistically significant difference in outcomes between the SHS or multiple CSs for surgical fixation of a hip fracture. The reoperation rate was 21% overall, with subgroup analysis showing that patients with displaced or basicervical fractures as well as smokers may have improved outcomes with an SHS, but this had no effect on quality of life. In summary, the decision regarding the fixation technique to be used, based on current evidence, should be left to the operating surgeon based on their surgical expertise.

References

1. Fixation using Alternative Implants for the Treatment of Hip fractures (FAITH) Investigators. Fracture fixation in the operative management of hip fractures (FAITH): an international, multicentre, randomised controlled trial. Lancet. 2017;389:1519–27.
2. Chirodian et al. Sliding hip screw fixation of trochanteric hip fractures: outcome of 1024 procedures. Injury. 2005;36:793–800.
3. Parker et al. Short versus long thread cannulated cancellous screws for intracapsular hip fractures: a randomised trial of 432 patients. Injury. 2010;41(4):382–4.

8

Functional Outcomes Following Internal Fixation versus Hemiarthroplasty for Displaced Intracapsular Neck of Femur Fractures

ALI Z. NAQVI AND MICHAEL PEARSE

> Hemiarthroplasty gave better functional results, higher health related quality of life, and more independence than internal fixation. . . . Better results were found for hemiarthroplasty even when compared with patients with internal fixation that healed without complications.
>
> —Frihagen et al.[1]

Citation: Frihagen F, Nordsletten L, Madsen JE. Hemiarthroplasty or internal fixation for intracapsular displaced femoral neck fractures: randomised controlled trial. BMJ. 2007;335(7632):1251–4.

Research Question: Should patients with displaced intracapsular neck of femur (NOF) fractures be treated with a hemiarthroplasty (HA) or closed reduction and internal fixation (CRIF)?

Funding: Norwegian Foundation for Health and Rehabilitation through the Norwegian Osteoporosis Society and the Norwegian Research Council, Nycomed, Smith and Nephew, and OrtoMedic AS

Year Study Began: September 2002–March 2004

Year Study Published: 2007

Study Location: University Hospital, Norway

Who Was Studied: Premorbid ambulant patients age ≥ 60 years with radiographic evidence of angulation in either anteroposterior or lateral views.

Who Was Excluded: Medical comorbidities preventing safe anesthetic, patients with fractures > 96 hours, previous hip pathology.

How Many Patients: 222 patients

Study Design: See Figure 8.1.

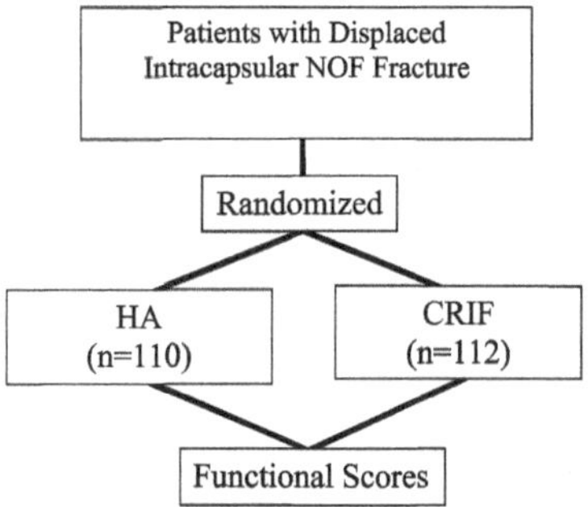

Figure 8.1. Overview of the study design.

Study Intervention: In this single-blinded and prospective randomized controlled trial, patients with a displaced intracapsular NOF fracture were randomized to receive HA vs. CRIF. Patients in the HA group underwent a Charnley-Hastings bipolar cemented HA, and those in the CRIF group underwent closed reduction followed by two parallel cancellous screws. Patients with irreducible fractures and those with poor screw purchase were changed to HA intraoperatively.

Follow-Up: 4, 12, and 24 months

Endpoints: Primary outcome was functional scores using the following:

- Hip function using Harris Hip Score[2] (HHS; instrument is used by the clinician to rate the patient's pain, function, and joint mobility, with scores ranging from 0 to 100 and higher scores indicating better outcomes)
- Health-related quality of life (QOL) using EQ-5D[3] (comprises 5 questions on mobility, self-care, pain, usual activities, and psychological status with 3 possible answers for each item [1 = no problem, 2 = moderate problem, 3 = severe problem])
- Ability to perform activities of daily living (ADLs) using Barthel index[4] (measures the extent to which somebody can function independently and has mobility in their ADLs, i.e., feeding, bathing, grooming, dressing, bowel control, bladder control, toileting, chair transfer, ambulation, and stair climbing; scores of < 20 indicate total dependency, scores of > 80 indicate independence, and scores in between signify varying degrees of dependency)

For all of these measures a higher score represents a better functional outcome. Secondary outcome was complications and reoperations.

RESULTS

- *Time:* Time to surgery and intraoperative time were significantly less with CRIF.
- *Function:* There were significantly lower Barthel index scores at both 12 and 24 months and poorer functional scores with CRIF (even in the presence of healed fractures without complications).
- *Complications/reoperations*: CRIF had 35% more complications (50% vs. 15%) and a significantly increased risk of reoperation.
- *Blood loss:* HA on average resulted in more blood loss by 10× and was more likely to require a blood transfusion (both $p = 0.001$).
- *EQ-5D:* HA patients had a higher visual analog score at 4 months by 8.7 points ($p = 0.01$) and index score at 24 months ($p = 0.03$).
- *HHS*: Mean scores improved in those with HA, significantly at 4 and 12 months and then insignificantly at 2 years (Table 8.1).
- *Mortality:* 2-year mortality was similar for both groups at 35%.

Table 8.1 Comparison of Functional Outcomes Following Fixation or Hemiarthroplasty

Harris Hip Score at X Months	HA Mean (SD)	CRIF Mean (SD)	*p* Value
4	67.7 (15.8) (n = 84)	59.6 (19.5) (n = 89)	0.003
12	72.6 (17.5) (n = 74)	65.8 (15.9) (n = 87)	0.001
24	70.6 (19.1) (n = 68)	67.3 (15.5) (n = 71)	0.26

Criticisms and Limitations: There is limited clinical application especially as the frail population was excluded and a younger population included in whom other options may be more appropriate (e.g., CRIF to preserve the native femoral head). Hip surgeons may also prefer to carry out a total hip arthroplasty rather than an HA, which was not discussed in the study. The authors discuss the use of a large number of surgeons with varying amounts of experience, which can introduce variations in operative technique and outcomes.

Other Relevant Studies and Information:

- A 2015 meta-analysis comparing CRIF vs. HA demonstrated improved functional outcomes in the HA group until the 6-year mark but no difference in function seen at 6–10 years postoperatively.[2]
- A similar study conducted in 2013 found that beyond the 2-year F/U period patients had similar outcomes when comparing CRIF vs. HA. Although complications and reoperations with CRIF remained high, the results demonstrated that outcomes were similar after 6 years postoperatively. Reoperations for CRIF again were higher, and most of these occurred in the first 2 years postoperatively.[3]
- Other studies agree that mortality rates did not differ between either intervention but either agree[4,5] or disagree[6] (especially in context of uncemented HA) as the treatment of choice.

Summary and Implications: The authors recommended the use of HA, which overall outperformed CRIF in displaced intracapsular NOF fractures with regard to patient-reported outcome measures and complications at all stages postoperatively. HA is a more invasive operation with increased intraoperative risks. Yet,

CRIF performed poorly in comparison to HA when functional outcomes and health-related QOL were compared over a 2-year period.

CLINICAL CASE: HA VERSUS CRIF FOR A DISPLACED INTRACAPSULAR NOF FRACTURE

Case History

An 84-year-old retired policeman is seen in the Emergency Department after falling in his kitchen. He has hypertension, hypothyroidism, and diabetes mellitus but remains relatively independent with his wife. On clinical examination he has a shortened and externally rotated right lower limb, which is neurovascularly intact. His abbreviated mental test score is 9/10. He is not on any anticoagulation medication and does not have antiplatelet therapy. Plain radiographs demonstrated a displaced intracapsular NOF fracture. He has been starved in preparation for surgery and the anesthetic team are planning a spinal block. As the operating surgeon, what is the surgical intervention of choice and how would one consent the patient and his wife?

Suggested Answer

Surgical intervention for this patient can be in the form of either fixation with parallel screws or arthroplasty. Given his functional status, it would be appropriate to discuss the risks and benefits of both surgical options with the patient but ultimately offer him an HA. Functional outcomes and patient-reported outcome measures were reported as being superior over a 24-month postoperative period in the study by Frihagen et al.[1] There was an increased risk of reoperation in the CRIF group and the possibility that the fracture would not reduce by closed technique, thus necessitating an HA. With his comorbidities, it would be beneficial to achieve the best result with a single and definitive operation to restore his QOL and reduce the risk of reoperation.

References

1. Frihagen et al. Hemiarthroplasty or internal fixation for intracapsular displaced femoral neck fractures: Randomised controlled trial. Br Med J. 2007;335(7632):1251–4.
2. Harris. Traumatic arthritis of the hip after dislocation and acetabular fractures: treatment by mold arthroplasty: an end-result study using a new method of result evaluation. J Bone Joint Surg Am. 1969;51(4):737–55.
3. Dolan P. Modeling valuations for EuroQol health states. Med Care. 1997;35(11): 1095–108.

4. Mahoney et al. Functional evaluation: the Barthel index. Md State Med J. 1965;14: 61–5.
5. Jiang et al. Does arthroplasty provide better outcomes than internal fixation at mid- and long-term followup? A meta-analysis. Clin Orthop Relat Res. 2015;473(8):2672–9.
6. Støen et al. Randomized trial of hemiarthroplasty versus internal fixation for femoral neck fractures: no differences at 6 years hip. Clin Orthop Relat Res. 2014;472(1):360–7.
7. Rezaie et al. Internal fixation versus hemiarthroplasty for displaced intra-capsular femoral neck fractures in ASA 3-5 geriatric patients. Open Orthop J. 2016;10:765–71.
8. Hedbeck et al. Internal fixation versus cemented hemiarthroplasty for displaced femoral neck fractures in patients with severe cognitive dysfunction: a randomized controlled trial. J Orthop Trauma. 2013;27(12):690–5.
9. Blomfeldt et al. Internal fixation versus hemiarthroplasty for displaced fractures of the femoral neck in elderly patients with severe cognitive impairment. J Bone Joint Surg Br. 2005;87(4):523–9. Erratum in J Bone Joint Surg Br. 2005;87(8):1166.

9

Surgical versus Nonsurgical Treatment of Adults with Displaced Fractures of the Proximal Humerus

The PROFHER Randomized Clinical Trial

SANJEEVE SABHARWAL AND PETER REILLY

Study Nickname: PROFHER

> Among patients with displaced proximal humeral fractures involving the surgical neck, there was no significant difference between surgical treatment compared with nonsurgical treatment.
>
> —PROFHER Trial Collaborators[1]

Citation: Rangan et al. Surgical vs nonsurgical treatment of adults with displaced fractures of the proximal humerus: the PROFHER randomized clinical trial. JAMA. 2015;313(10):1037–47.

Research Question: Does surgical management of displaced proximal humerus fractures result in better clinical outcomes than nonsurgical management?

Funding: National Institute for Health Research

Year Study Began: 2008

Year Study Published: 2015

Study Location: 32 UK National Health Service Hospitals

Who Was Studied: Patients aged > 16 years who had sustained a displaced proximal humerus fracture and were < 3 weeks of their injury date. Neer type 2, 3, and 4 fractures were included but the displacement criteria were relaxed (i.e., to the standard 1-cm displacement and 45-degree angulation).

Who Was Excluded: Patients with an associated dislocation, an open fracture, or a pathological fracture; patients with cognitive impairment, medical comorbidities that precluded having surgery, other musculoskeletal injuries, and neurovascular injuries, and those not within the hospital catchment area.

How Many Patients: 250

Study Overview: See Figure 9.1.

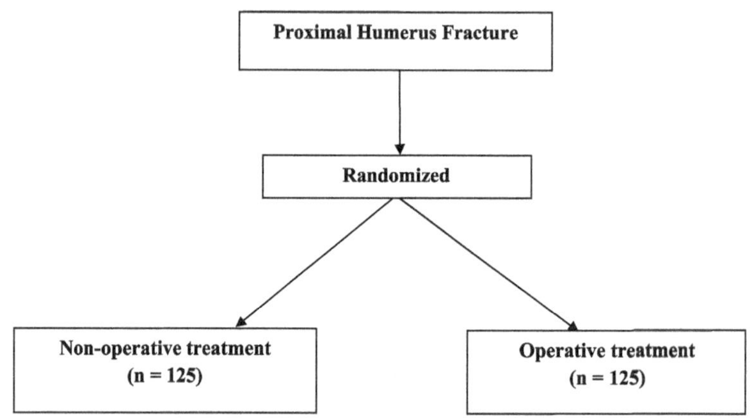

Figure 9.1. Study overview.

Study Intervention: Nonoperative and operative management were performed according to the normal practice of each hospital involved in the study. This was done to simulate real-world practices and to ensure that surgeons and physiotherapists were delivering the care pathways they were familiar with. Nonoperative patients were managed in a sling for 3 weeks, and surgically managed patients underwent either fixation or a shoulder hemiarthroplasty (HA). Internal fixation included nailing, plating, suture, or screw fixation procedures. Patients in both arms of the trial received physiotherapy and were also given information leaflets on self-care and home exercise programs. The timing at which physiotherapy was commenced was based on local hospital practices.

Follow-Up: At intervals up to 2 years

Endpoints: The primary outcome was the Oxford Shoulder Score[2] (OSS; 12-item patient-report questionnaire developed to evaluate the outcome of shoulder surgery, excluding surgery for instability. It contains 2 subscales, pain (20 points) and activities of daily living (ADLs; 40 points). Scores range from 0 to 60, with a higher score being consistent with increased disability. Secondary outcome measures included the Short Form-12[3] (SF-12; a survey evaluating health-related quality of life by measuring 8 scales: physical functioning, role physical, bodily pain, general health, vitality, social functioning, role emotional, and mental health), complications, secondary operations, and deaths.

RESULTS (TABLE 9.1)

- *Scores*:
  - *OSS*: There was no significant difference between the groups at 6 months, 12 months, and 24 months postinjury (Figure 9.2).
  - *SF-12*: There was no significant difference between the groups in both the physical and mental components at 6 months, 12 months, and 24 months postinjury.
- *Complications*: 30 (24%) patients in the surgical group had a complication at 2-year follow-up, and 23 (18.4%) patients in the nonsurgical group suffered a complication, though this difference did not reach statistical significance. Complications following surgery included problems with metalwork, surgical site infection, and nerve injury. Complications following nonsurgical treatment included symptomatic malunion and nonunion.
- *Reoperations*: There were 11 (8.8%) reoperations in each group.
- *Mortality:* There were 9 (7.2%) deaths in the surgical group at 2 years compared to 5 (4%) in the nonsurgical group; this difference was not statistically significant.

Table 9.1 Outcome Measures of the PROFHER Study

Outcome	Surgical Group	Nonsurgical Group	Difference	*p* Value
Mean age	65.4	66.6	—	—
OSS at 12 months	39.23	38.80	0.43	0.71
OSS at 24 months	40.11	40.40	0.29	0.80
12-month SF-12 physical component	45.51	44.22	1.29	0.36
24-month SF-12 physical component	45.68	44.20	1.48	0.33
12-month SF-12 mental component	48.24	50.20	1.96	0.17
24-month SF-12 mental component	49.30	50.69	1.39	0.35
Complications	30	23	7	0.28

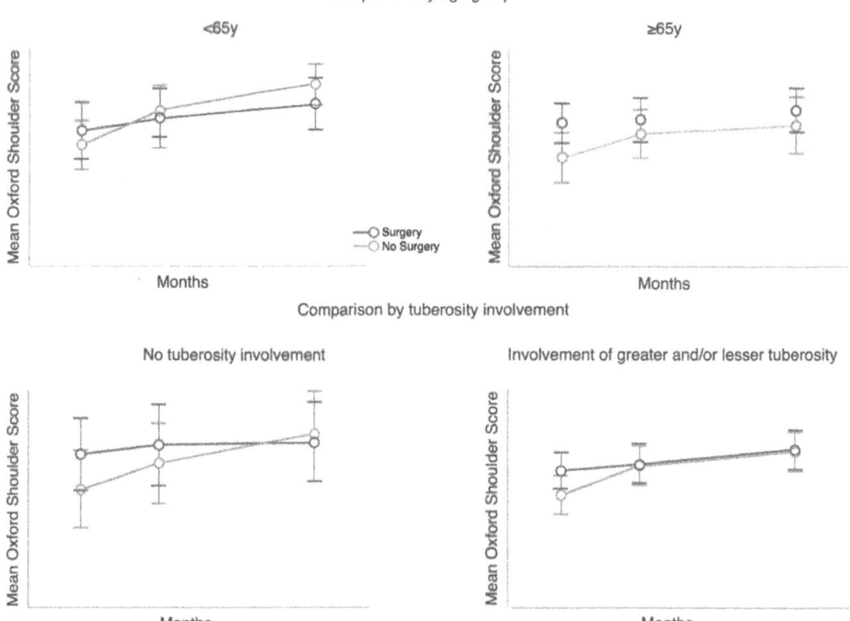

Figure 9.2. Comparison for Oxford Shoulder Score by age group and tuberosity involvement (error bars indicate 95% CI).

Criticisms and Limitations: The classification of fractures according to Neer's criteria[4] was adopted, but the threshold for displacement was relaxed, confounding study interpretation. Furthermore, the vast majority of included fractures were 2 and 3 part, with 4 parts accounting for < 5% in each group. It is possible that benefits of a surgical approach would have been apparent had there been greater inclusion of patients with more complex fractures.[5]

Other Relevant Studies and Information:

- Several other randomized trials have compared operative vs. nonoperative treatment of proximal humerus fractures (albeit with methodological limitations including single-center studies and fewer patients with specific treatment options and fracture types). These studies found no advantage in surgery over nonsurgical management[5,6] except for less pain with HA.[7]
- The PROFHER-2 trial[8,9] is now underway. It includes patients with 3- and 4-part fractures and compares nonoperative treatment vs. HA vs. reverse total shoulder arthroplasty as a 3-armed study.
- There is evidence to suggest that clinical practice has evolved due to the findings of the PROFHER trial, with most proximal humerus fractures being managed nonoperatively.[10]

Summary and Implications: The PROFHER trial found that for patients with a proximal humerus fracture involving the surgical neck, there was no difference between surgical vs. nonsurgical treatment in patient-reported clinical outcomes over 2 years. Studies evaluating nonoperative management among patients with the most complex humerus fractures are ongoing.

CLINICAL CASE: SURGERY OR NONOPERATIVE MANAGEMENT FOR A PROXIMAL HUMERUS FRACTURE

Case History

An 80-year-old man falls at home and sustains a left-sided 2-part proximal humerus fracture. This is an isolated injury without any associated neurovascular compromise. He is right-hand dominant and has a background history of hypertension and gout. He lives alone and is independently mobile. He has no cognitive impairment and enjoys fishing. Two years prior to this injury he underwent a total knee arthroplasty and had an uncomplicated recovery with a good functional outcome. He expresses that he wishes to have the treatment that gives him the best chance of functional recovery. Based on the results of the PROFHER trial, how would you manage this patient?

Suggested Answer

The PROFHER trial found that nonoperative and operative treatment had equivalent functional outcomes for patients with proximal humerus fractures. Although there are some criticisms of the study design because the proportion of patients who had a 4-part fracture was very small, for patients with a 2-part fracture who met the inclusion criteria of the trial, nonoperative treatment would be the preferred strategy for management. PROFHER is a useful part of the scientific armamentarium that informs clinical decision-making; however, it is important to consider the degree of displacement of the fracture, patient factors, and surgical expertise.

References

1. Rangan et al. Surgical vs nonsurgical treatment of adults with displaced fractures of the proximal humerus: the PROFHER randomized clinical trial. JAMA. 2015;313(10):1037–47.
2. Dawson et al. Questionnaire on the perceptions of patients about shoulder surgery. J Bone Joint Surg Br. 1996;78(4):593–600.
3. Ware et al. A 12-Item Short-Form Health Survey: construction of scales and preliminary tests of reliability and validity. Med Care. 1996;3:220–33.
4. Neer. Displaced proximal humeral fractures. I. Classification and evaluation. J Bone Joint Surg Am. 1970;52(6):1077–89.
5. Boons et al. Hemiarthroplasty for humeral four-part fractures for patients 65 years and older: a randomized controlled trial. Clin Orthop Relat Res. 2012;470(12):3483–91.
6. Fjalestad et al. Displaced proximal humeral fractures: operative versus non-operative treatment—a 2-year extension of a randomized controlled trial. Eur J Orthop Surg Traumatol. 2014;24(7):1067–73.
7. Olerud et al. Hemiarthroplasty versus nonoperative treatment of displaced 4-part proximal humeral fractures in elderly patients: a randomized controlled trial. J Shoulder Elbow Surg. 2011;20(7):1025–33.
8. Rangan et al. Effectiveness and cost-effectiveness of reverse shoulder arthroplasty versus hemiarthroplasty versus non-surgical care for acute 3 and 4 part fractures of the proximal humerus in patients aged over 65 years—the PROFHER-2 randomised trial. 2018. www.isrctn.com/ISRCTN76296703
9. Sabharwal et al. Trials based on specific fracture configuration and surgical procedures likely to be more relevant for decision making in the management of fractures of the proximal humerus: findings of a meta-analysis. Bone Joint Res. 2016;5(10):470–80.
10. Jefferson et al. Impact of the PROFHER trial findings on surgeons' clinical practice: an online questionnaire survey. Bone Joint Res. 2017;6(10):590–9.

10

A Critical Analysis of Prospective Randomized Controlled Trial of an Intramedullary Nail versus Dynamic Hip Screw and Plate Fixation for Intertrochanteric Fractures of the Femur

SHALIN SHAUNAK, KAPIL SUGAND, AND BARRY ROSE

> The use of an intramedullary device in the treatment of intertrochanteric femoral fractures is still associated with a higher but nonsignificant risk of postoperative complications. Routine use of the Gamma nail in this type of fracture cannot be recommended over the current standard treatment of dynamic hip screw and plate.
>
> —Adams et al.[1]

Citation: Adams et al. Prospective randomized controlled trial of an intramedullary nail versus dynamic screw and plate for intertrochanteric fractures of the femur. J Orthop Trauma. 2001;15(6):394–400.

Research Question: Should either the dynamic hip screw (DHS) and plate fixation (i.e., Richards device) or the intramedullary nail (IMN; i.e., Stryker Gamma nail) for intertrochanteric neck of femur fractures be used and why?

Funding: Not disclosed

Year Study Began: 1994

Year Study Published: 2001

Study Location: Orthopaedic Trauma Unit, The Royal Infirmary of Edinburgh, Scotland

Who Was Studied: Patients admitted to the unit with intertrochanteric fractures of the femur.

Who Was Excluded: Inability to give informed consent, patients too frail for any operative intervention, and residence outside the region of the hospital.

How Many Patients: 400

Study Overview: See Figure 10.1.

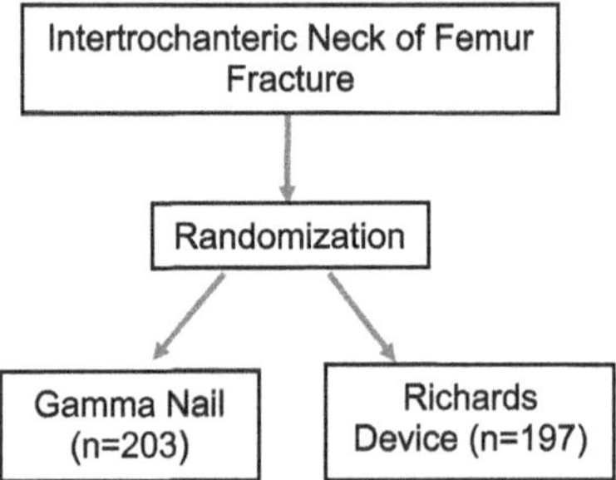

Figure 10.1. Study overview.

Study Intervention: All 400 patients were randomized using a double-blinded technique to either arm (Gamma nail vs. Richards device). Each fracture was recorded and classified using both the Evans-Jensen[2] and AO Foundation/Orthopaedic Trauma Association (AO/OTA) classifications. Patients were matched for sex, age, preadmission residence, cognitive scores, and premorbid mobility. The fracture patterns across both groups were similar, spanning all categories of both classifications.

Follow-Up: 1 year or until death; daily follow-up during inpatient stays, outpatient follow-up at 3, 6, and 12 months postoperatively

Endpoints: These were divided into the following:

(i) *Intraoperative parameters* (mean preoperative delay, mean surgical time, blood loss, postoperative hemoglobin, transfusion requirement)
(ii) *Complications* (superficial and deep infection, deep venous thrombosis [DVT])
(iii) *Reoperation* (numbers and reasons for reoperations, tip-apex distance [TAD])
(iv) *Functional Outcomes* (Harris Hip Score [HHS], type of residence, mobility, reoperation, readmission to hospital)

RESULTS

- Both treatment modalities had similar rates (Table 10.1) of:
  - *Mean follow-up (F/U)*: Between 35 and 36 weeks (range 1 day to 52 weeks) for both cohorts
  - *HHS*: Similar at 3, 6, and 12 months without statistical significance
  - No patient was withdrawn
  - Reoperation rates (Richards device 4% vs. Gamma nail 6% without statistical significance)
  - Functional outcomes
  - Preoperative delays
  - Postoperative hemoglobin
  - Postoperative complication rates (superficial and deep infections, DVT)
- Differences between both modalities were as follows:

Factors Favoring Gamma Nails	Factors Favoring Richards Device
Slightly less intraoperative blood loss	Shorter operative time
Lower TAD (Figures 10.2 and 10.3)	Lower transfusion rates

Table 10.1 Summary of Results between Gamma Nail and Richards Device (mean [95% CI])

Outcome	Gamma Nail (n = 203)	Richards Device (n = 197)
	Demographics	
Mean age (y; range)	81.2 (48–99)	80.7 (32–102)
M:F	39:164	49:148
Complete F/U at 1 year	126 (62.1%)	121 (61.4%)
	Intraoperative outcomes	
Mean preoperative delay (d)	1.7 (1.5–1.9)	1.8 (1.6–2.1)
Mean surgical time (min)	55.4 (52.7–58.2)[a]	61.3 (58.2–64.4)[a]
Mean blood loss (ml)	244.4 (191.4–297.3)	260.4 (215.0–305.9)

Outcome	Gamma Nail (n = 203)	Richards Device (n = 197)
Mean postoperative hemoglobin (g/l)	101.2 (98.6–104.8)	100.9 (97.4–102.9)
No. needing transfusion	108[b]	88[b]
	Complications (%)	
Superficial infection	2.9%	2%
Deep infection	1.4%	1%
DVT	4.4%	5.1%
	Reoperation (n =) due to:	
Postoperative femoral fracture	3 (shaft)	1 (subcapital)
Cutout of lag screw	6	3
Plate pull-off	0	2
Local tenderness	2	0
Elective removal	1	2
Total reoperations	12 (6%)	8 (4%)
	Functional outcomes	
Harris Hip Scores	"Similar"	"Similar"
Deaths within 1 year	59 (29.2%)	61 (31%)
Staying in own home	75	76
Independently mobile	56	55

[a] Signifies $p = 0.008$.
[b] Not significant.

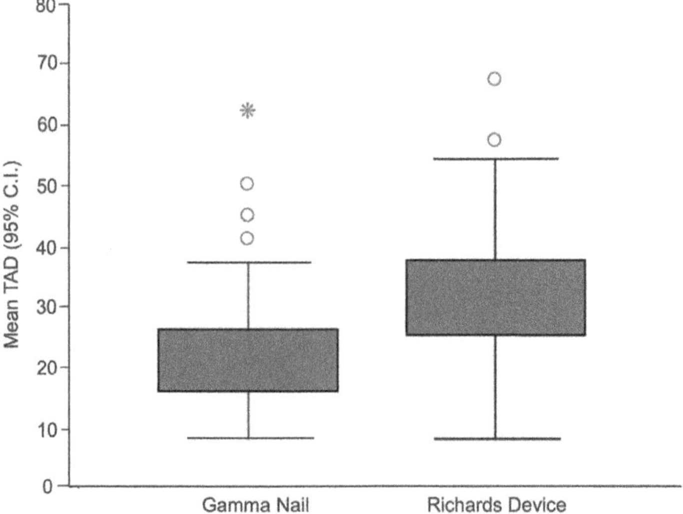

Figure 10.2. Mean TAD for all patients.

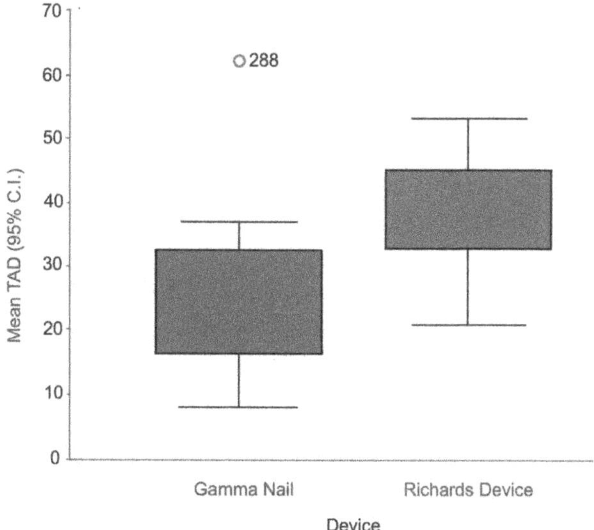

Figure 10.3. Mean TAD for patients with fixation failure.

Criticisms and Limitations: There was no mention of the seniority of the surgeon performing the interventions (i.e., if attending or other). Additionally, there was no mention of which technique was the most commonly carried out prior to the intervention (i.e., the center's "gold standard") and no mention of economic/cost factors. Thirty-one patients were unable to visit the outpatient department for functional assessment and were contacted by telephone with limited information collected.

Other Relevant Studies and Information:

- Barton et al.[3] demonstrated similar results for both DHS and IMN. This led them to surmise that sliding hip screws were superior as they provided similar outcomes at less expense.
- A review analysis by Parker et al.[4] involving 20 trials and 3646 patients found that IMNs were associated with higher complication rates and consequent reoperation rates vs. the Richards device. There were no major differences with respect to infection, mortality, or complications.
- National Institute for Health and Care Excellence (NICE)[5] guidelines recommend "using extramedullary implants such as a sliding hip screw in preference to an intramedullary nail in patients with trochanteric fractures above and including the lesser trochanter (AO classification

types A1 and A2)" and "using an intramedullary nail to treat patients with a subtrochanteric fracture." These principles are also supported by the Getting It Right First Time (GIRFT) initiative.[6,7]

Summary and Implications: For intertrochanteric fractures of the femur, both the intramedullary Gamma nail and Richards device were associated with similar overall outcomes; however, each treatment was associated with distinct complications (i.e., femoral fractures in Gamma nail and plate pull-off in Richards device). Based on this and other studies, NICE guidelines recommend extramedullary implants in preference to IMN in patients with trochanteric fractures above and including the lesser trochanter, but IMN to treat patients with a subtrochanteric fracture.

CLINICAL CASE: INTERTROCHANTERIC NECK OF FEMUR FRACTURE—HOW TO FIX IT?

Case History

A 90-year-old lady sustains a mechanical fall at home and denies any prodromal symptoms. She was unable to weight bear afterwards and presented to the Emergency Department with a shortened and externally rotated left lower limb. She complains of groin pain and inability to move. Her past medical history consists of hypothyroidism, obesity, hypertension, and chronic renal disease. She has a care package at home, is an ex-smoker, and drinks a glass of wine every day. A plain pelvic radiograph confirms a left 2-part intertrochanteric neck of femur fracture. According to this study, which surgical option should be offered to the patient?

Suggested Answer

This patient is in need of fixation of her intertrochanteric neck of femur fracture. The surgical options depend on several circumstances. It would be helpful to classify the fracture configuration based on Evans-Jensen[2] classification. As long as there is no absolute indication to commit to IMN (i.e., reverse oblique fracture configuration) or any subtrochanteric extension of the fracture, then DHS ought to be considered. There is evidence to suggest that an IMN device should not be favored over DHS, especially in this case. There is also an operator-dependent factor whereby it is easier to gain access to DHS devices globally, which additionally offers a more economically viable option.

References

1. Adams et al. Prospective randomized controlled trial of an intramedullary nail versus dynamic screw and plate for intertrochanteric fractures of the femur. J Orthop Trauma. 2001;15(6):394–400.
2. Jensen. Classification of trochanteric fractures. Acta Orthop Scand. 1980;51(5): 803–10.
3. Barton et al. Comparison of the long gamma nail with the sliding hip screw for the treatment of AO/OTA 31-A2 fractures of the proximal part of the femur: a prospective randomized trial. J Bone Joint Surg Am. 2010;92(4):792–8.
4. Parker et al. Gamma and other cephalocondylic intramedullary nails versus extramedullary implants for extracapsular hip fractures in adults. Cochrane Database Syst Rev. 2005;(4):CD000093. Review. Update in Cochrane Database Syst Rev. 2008;(3):CD000093.
5. National Institute for Health and Care Excellence. Hip fracture: management. Clinical guideline (CG124). May 2017. www.nice.org.uk/guidance/cg124/chapter/recommendations
6. Getting It Right First Time. A national review of adult elective orthopaedic services in England. March 2015. www.gettingitrightfirsttime.co.uk/wp-content/uploads/2017/06/GIRFT-National-Report-Mar15-Web.pdf
7. Getting It Right First Time. Getting it right in orthopaedics. Reflecting on success and reinforcing improvement. A follow-up on the GIRFT national specialty report on orthopaedics. February 2020. www.gettingitrightfirsttime.co.uk/wp-content/uploads/2020/02/GIRFT-orthopaedics-follow-up-report-February-2020.pdf

11

Nonoperative Treatment versus Plate Fixation of Displaced Midshaft Clavicle Fractures

ANDREW DAVIES AND PETER REILLY

> Operative fixation of a displaced fracture of the clavicular shaft results in improved functional outcome and a lower rate of malunion and nonunion compared with nonoperative treatment at one year of follow-up. Hardware removal remains the most common reason for repeat intervention in the operative group.
>
> —Canadian Clavicle Trial Investigators[1]

Citation: Canadian Orthopaedic Trauma Society. Nonoperative treatment compared with plate fixation of displaced midshaft clavicular fractures. A multicenter, randomized clinical trial. J Bone Joint Surg Am. 2007;89(1):1–10.

Research Question: Does nonoperative treatment or plate fixation of displaced fractures of the clavicular shaft lead to superior shoulder function, patient satisfaction, and fracture union?

Funding: Orthopaedic Trauma Association and Zimmer Inc.

Year Study Began: 2001

Year Study Published: 2007

Study Location: 8 hospitals across Canada

Who Was Studied: Adult patients aged 16–60 years with completely displaced midshaft clavicle fractures, where a minimum of 3 screws could be placed in the proximal and distal fragments.

Who Was Excluded: Open fractures, pathological fractures, delayed presentation > 28 days, or fractures associated with neurovascular deficit. Although patients with an upper limb injury distal to the shoulder were excluded, those with concomitant shoulder girdle fractures were included.

How Many Patients: 132

Study Overview: See Figure 11.1.

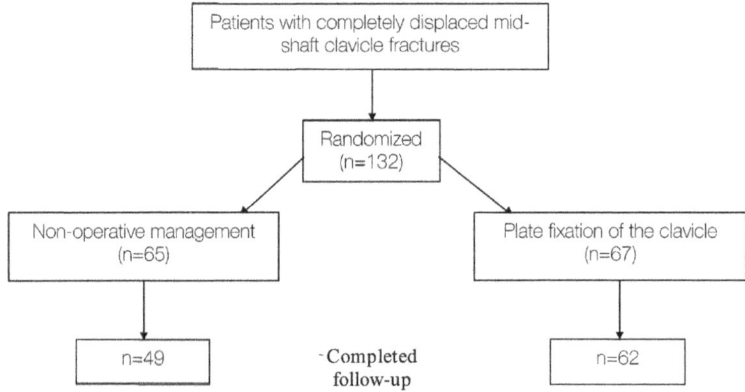

Figure 11.1. Study overview.

Study Intervention: The nonoperative group received a sling for 6 weeks followed by physiotherapy when the fracture had united. The operative group underwent fixation with a small fragment plate on the superior clavicle with a minimum of 3 screws in the proximal and distal fragments. Comminuted fragments were fixed with a lag screw or held with a suture. No bone graft was used. Postoperative management included a sling for 7–10 days followed by range of motion (ROM) exercises and strengthening exercises when the fracture had reached union.

Follow-Up: 12 months

Endpoints: Outcomes consisted of Constant shoulder scores[2] (a 100-point scale composed of a number of parameters that define the level of pain and the ability to carry out the normal daily activities); Disabilities of the Arm, Shoulder, and Hand (DASH; a disability score where a "perfect" extremity would typically score 0 [range 4–8])[3] scores; patient satisfaction; fracture union; ROM; and complications.

RESULTS (TABLE 11.1)

- The Constant shoulder and DASH scores were superior in the operative group at each time point of 6, 12, 26, and 52 weeks ($p < 0.01$). The difference was approximately 6–12 points for the Constant score and 7–20 points for the DASH score (Figure 11.2).

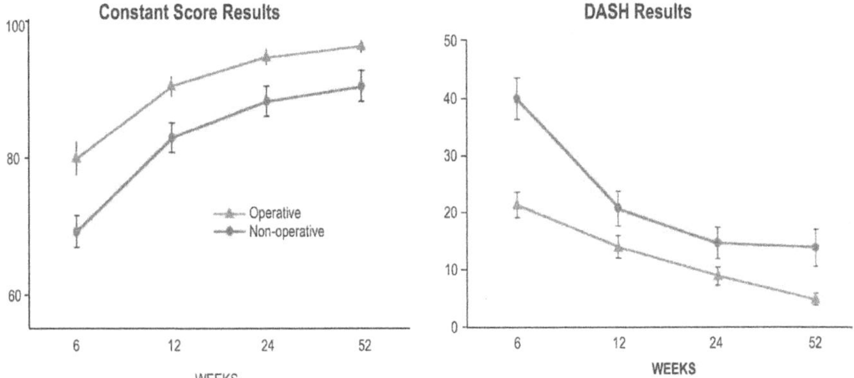

Figure 11.2. Graphic analysis comparing the mean Constant shoulder and DASH scores in the operative and nonoperative groups at 6, 12, 24, and 52 weeks of follow-up. A higher Constant and lower DASH scores indicate better scoring.

- *Patient satisfaction:* Patients in the operative group were more likely to reply "yes" to the question "are you satisfied with your shoulder?" at all time points. The odds ratio was 3.5 at 52 weeks ($p = 0.002$). Patients in the operative group were more likely to be satisfied with the appearance of the shoulder.
- *ROM:* There were no significant differences in ROM.
- *Metalwork issues:* Metalwork irritation and prominence occurred in 11 (17.7%) of the operative group, of which 5 (8.1%) underwent plate removal.

Table 11.1 Summary of the Key Findings

Outcome	**Operative Group ($n = 62$)**	**Nonoperative Group ($n = 49$)**	***p* Value**
Constant score at 1 year	96	90	< 0.01
DASH score at 1 year	5	14	< 0.01
Nonunion at 1 year	2 (3%)	7 (14%)	0.042
Malunion requiring further treatment	0	9 (18%)	0.001
Hardware irritation ± prominence	11 (18%)	0	0.001
Wound infection ± dehiscence	3 (5%)	0	0.253
Satisfaction with appearance	52 (84%)	26 (53%)	0.001

Criticisms and Limitations: A large proportion of patients in the nonoperative group did not complete follow-up (F/U) (25%); patients may not have attended F/U due to satisfactory recovery. A higher proportion of the patients in the nonoperative group were female (15/49) compared to the operative group (9/53). The intended sample size of 60 was not reached, which undermines the validity of the results. The assessors were not blinded to the group allocation, which may have introduced detection bias.

Other Relevant Studies and Information:

- Ahrens et al.[4] randomized 301 patients with displaced midshaft clavicle fractures to nonoperative management or fixation. The nonunion rate was higher in the nonoperative group (11% vs. 0.8%) at 9 months. In the operative group further surgery was necessary to remove the plate in 5 (7.5%) patients, and 1 required a revision. The Constant and DASH scores were superior in the operative group at 6 and 12 weeks. There was no difference at 9 months.
- A further study by Robinson et al.[5] found a higher number of nonunions in the nonoperative group (15% vs. 1%). Operative intervention led to superior Constant and DASH scores at 1 year; however, the difference was of < 5 points and of uncertain clinical significance. When those with nonunions were excluded, there was no significant difference in function between both groups. Twelve percent of patients in the operative group required plate removal.

Summary and Implications: In this trial, plate fixation was associated with fewer nonunions and malunions at 1 year vs. nonoperative management. Fixation resulted in superior shoulder function at 6, 12, 26, and 52 weeks, although the difference was small. Thirteen percent of patients required reoperation due to metalwork irritation or surgical site infection. Patients with midshaft clavicular fractures should be counseled regarding the advantages and disadvantages of each management option.

CLINICAL CASE: ACUTE CLAVICLE FRACTURE IN A YOUNG AND ACTIVE PATIENT

Case History

A 26-year-old male accountant attends the fracture clinic with a completely displaced and shortened right midshaft clavicle fracture (Figure 11.3) sustained during a rugby tackle 5 days ago. This is an isolated, closed injury without any associated neurovascular deficit. The overlying skin is neither tented nor threatened. He is otherwise fit and well, is right-hand dominant. and does not smoke. He has suffered no previous injuries to this clavicle. He is keen to return to sport as soon as possible. His friend had a similar injury last year and was managed conservatively, and the patient wishes to consider his treatment options. Based on the Canadian Clavicle Trial, what treatment would one recommend?

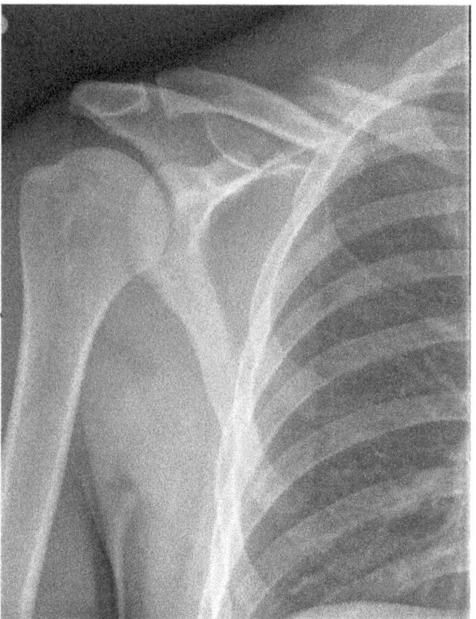

Figure 11.3. Plain radiograph of clavicle.

Suggested Answer

This trial highlights the need for adequate patient counseling regarding management options. An early return to activities and optimization of postoperative function are the priorities for both the patient and his surgeon. The results of this trial would support surgical intervention in these circumstances, given the increased risk of nonunion and malunion with conservative management. However, he should be made aware of the risks of metalwork irritation (18%) and the risk of reoperation due to metalwork irritation or surgical site infection (13%). It is important to consider appropriate patient selection and this patient is classified as a low-risk stratification.

References

1. Canadian Orthopaedic Trauma Society. Nonoperative treatment compared with plate fixation of displaced midshaft clavicular fractures. J Bone Joint Surg Am. 2007;89:1–10.
2. Constant et al. A clinical method of functional assessment of the shoulder. Clin Orthop Relat Res. 1987;(214):160–4.
3. Beaton et al. Measuring the whole or the parts? Validity, reliability, and responsiveness of the Disabilities of the Arm, Shoulder and Hand outcome measure in different regions of the upper extremity. J Hand Ther. 2001;14(2):128–46.
4. Ahrens et al. The Clavicle Trial: a multicenter randomized controlled trial comparing operative with nonoperative treatment of displaced midshaft clavicle fractures. J Bone Joint Surg Am. 2017;99:1345–54.
5. Robinson et al. Open reduction and plate fixation versus nonoperative treatment for displaced midshaft clavicular fractures. J Bone Joint Surg Am. 2013; 95:1576–84.

12

Treating Acute Achilles Tendon Ruptures

HENRY MAGILL AND TIM SINNETT

> Open operative treatment of acute Achilles tendon ruptures significantly reduces the risk of re-rupture compared with non-operative treatment, but operative treatment is associated with a significantly higher risk of other complications.
>
> —KHAN ET AL.[1]

Citation: Khan RJ, Fick D, Keogh A, Crawford J, Brammar T, Parker M. Treatment of acute Achilles tendon ruptures. A meta-analysis of randomized, controlled trials. J Bone Joint Surg Am. 2005;87(10):2202–10.

Research Question: Is surgery (open and percutaneous) more effective than non-surgical (casting and early mobilization) management for acute Achilles tendon rupture?

Funding: None

Year Study Began: 2005

Year Study Published: 2005

Study Location: University of Western Australia, Perth, Australia

Who Was Studied: All subjects with acute Achilles rupture who were randomized to operative (open or minimally invasive) and nonoperative (casting or functional bracing) interventions were included.

Who Was Excluded: All retrospective studies, randomized controlled trials (RCTs) with insufficient primary outcome data, and trials with poor randomization methodology. Any data involving delayed presentation (beyond 3 weeks) or rerupture were also excluded.

How Many Patients: 800

Study Overview: See Figure 12.1.

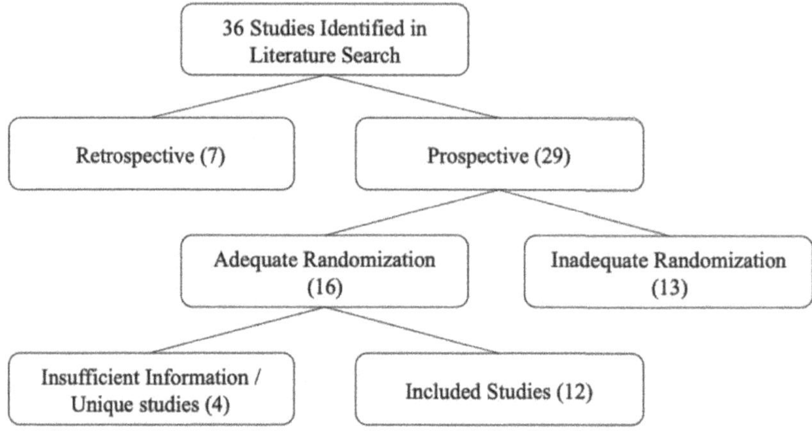

Figure 12.1. Study overview to determine relevant studies included in the meta-analysis.

Study Interventions: A total of 12 RCTs were included (n = 800); 4 studies (n = 356) compared open repair vs. nonoperative management,[2–5] 5 studies (n = 273) compared postoperative cast immobilization alone vs. cast immobilization with early mobilization,[6–11] 2 studies (n = 94) compared percutaneous vs. open Achilles repair,[5,11] and 2 studies (n = 99) compared postoperative cast immobilization vs. functional bracing.[12,13] Data from 1 study was used in 2 sections of the meta-analysis, hence the discrepancy in the overall number of patients and studies mentioned.[5] Methodological rigor and bias were variable across all studies. A 12-point quality assessment score was calculated for each to quantify bias in selection, performance, detection, and attrition.

Follow-Up: This was divided into the following 4 categories:

(i) Open repair vs. nonoperative management: 8-30 months
(ii) Cast immobilization alone vs. cast immobilization with early mobilization: 5–80.4 months

(iii) Percutaneous vs. open Achilles repair: 6–8 months
(iv) Postoperative cast immobilization vs. functional bracing: 12 months

Endpoints: Rerupture and infection rates were determined individually as primary outcome measures. All other complications (including adhesions and disturbed sensibility) were then pooled. All dichotomous endpoints were assessed at varying follow-up intervals.

RESULTS

(1) *Open repair vs. nonoperative management (n = 356)*
The study with the highest methodological quality discovered a significant reduction in the rerupture rate[2] (Figure 12.2). Pooled data revealed a rerupture rate of 3.5% in the operative group and 12.6% in the nonoperative group (relative risk [RR] = 0.27; 95% CI: 0.11–0.64, $p = 0.0003$). This may suggest an advantage associated with surgical repair when compared to nonoperative management. However, overall pooled complications (other than rerupture) were 34.1% in the operative group compared to 2.7% in the nonoperative group (RR = 10.6; 95% CI: 4.82–23.28, $p < 0.00001$). Infection rates were 4% in the operative group and none were reported in the nonoperative group (RR = 4.89; 95% CI: 1.09–21.91, $p = 0.04$).

(2) *Postoperative cast immobilization alone vs. cast immobilization with early mobilization (n = 273)*
No study determined a significant difference in rate of rerupture between these groups. Overall pooled complications (excluding rerupture) were reported as 35.7% in the cast immobilization group compared to 19.5% in the early mobilization group (RR = 1.88).

(3) *Percutaneous vs. open Achilles repair (n = 94)*
No significant difference was demonstrated between these groups in terms of rerupture rate. Pooled data revealed a complication rate (other than rerupture) of 26.1% in the open group compared to 8.3% in the percutaneous group (RR = 2.84). Interestingly, pooled infection rates were reported as 19.6% in the open group and none in the percutaneous group.

(4) *Postoperative cast immobilization vs. functional bracing (n = 99)*

No significant difference was demonstrated between these groups in terms of rerupture rate.

Postoperative functional bracing was associated with a lower complication rate (excluding rerupture) when compared to cast immobilization (19.5% vs. 35.7%, RR = 1.88).

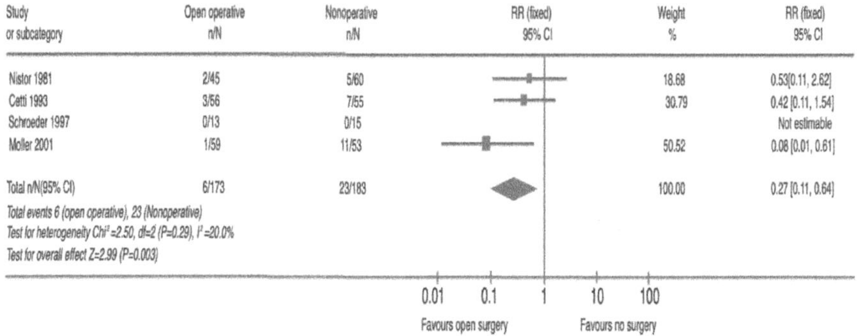

Figure 12.2. Prevalence of rerupture associated with open operative and nonoperative treatment. Values are given as the number of patients with a rerupture (n)/number of patients in the group (N), with a summation of the totals, RR, and 95% CI.

Criticisms and Limitations: Overall complication rates in the percutaneous group are based on pooled data from a small study population with a degree of inconsistency between studies. Additionally, "early mobilization" involved a large variety of regimens and therefore conclusions must be interpreted with caution.

Other Relevant Studies and Information:

- Other meta-analyses have highlighted similar findings, suggesting that operative treatment is associated with a significantly lower rerupture rate, varying from 5% to 7%.[14–17]
- Jiang et al. also demonstrated a significant increase in all other pooled complications with surgery (varying between 16% and 21%).[14]
- A further meta-analysis agreed with the findings of this study; however, it demonstrated no statistical difference with respect to return to function between operative and nonoperative groups.[18]
- Yet, further large studies have determined an earlier return to work in the operative group.[14]
- Only a few, smaller studies have suggested no statistically significant difference between operative and nonoperative groups with regard to rerupture and long-term function.[19–21]

- American Association of Orthopaedic Surgeons[22] recommendations for surgical and nonsurgical management are both weak but have demonstrated satisfactory results. Whereas nonsurgical management has resulted in lower complication rates, surgical repair has demonstrated a faster recovery time, quicker return to sports, and a lower rerupture rate.
- When taking into consideration the current evidence and the opinion of the expert panel members of the American College of Foot and Ankle Surgeons, a consensus was achieved that Achilles tendon ruptures should not always be treated with operative intervention,[23] even when the ratio of operative to nonoperative treatment increased from 1.41 to 1.65, suggesting that surgeons in the United States have been slower to adopt nonoperative treatment than their European counterparts.[21]

CLINICAL CASE: ACUTE ACHILLES RUPTURE IN A YOUNG ADULT

Case History

A 30-year-old male "weekend warrior" presents to the Emergency Department following a sudden and forced plantar flexion injury to his right foot during a tennis match. He is otherwise fit, well, and active. Clinical examination revealed a tender and palpable gap of the Achilles tendon with a positive Simmonds-Thompson test (i.e., no dorsiflexion of the foot with squeezing the calf). Ultrasound imaging showed a complete Achilles tendon rupture 6 cm from the calcaneal insertion and a gap of 8 mm (in equinus). He has performed an online search and is currently fearful of complications such as infection and nerve damage. Based on the evidence of this meta-analysis, how should this patient be treated?

Suggested Answer

The results from Khan et al.[1] would suggest that patients like this would benefit from surgical repair as it will significantly reduce the rate of rerupture. He should be offered and appropriately counseled for both operative and nonoperative treatments. This study highlights the importance of a patient-specific approach and a shared decision-making model, where he should be made aware of the increased risk of other complications associated with surgery. If surgery were opted for, this study would suggest a percutaneous approach and early mobilization for optimal operative outcomes.

References

1. Khan et al. Treatment of acute Achilles tendon ruptures: a meta-analysis of randomized, controlled trials. J Bone Joint Surg Am. 2005;87(10):2202–10.
2. Möller et al. Acute rupture of tendo Achillis between surgical and non-surgical treatment. J Bone Joint Surg Am. 2001;83(6):843–8.
3. Cetti et al. Operative versus nonoperative treatment of Achilles tendon rupture. Am J Sports Med. 1993;21(6):791–9.
4. Nistor et al. Surgical and non-surgical treatment of Achilles tendon rupture. A prospective randomized study. J Bone Joint Surg Am. 1981;63(3):394–9.
5. Schroeder et al. Treatment of acute Achilles tendon ruptures: open vs. percutaneous repair vs. conservative treatment. Orthop Trans. 1997;21(4):1228.
6. Cetti et al. A new treatment of ruptured Achilles tendons. A prospective randomized study. Clin Orthop Relat Res. 1994;(308):155–65.
7. Kerkhoffs et al. Functional treatment after surgical repair of acute Achilles tendon rupture: wrap vs walking cast. Arch Orthop Trauma Surg. 2002;122(2):102–5.
8. Mortensen et al. Early motion of the ankle after operative treatment of a rupture of the Achilles tendon. A prospective, randomized clinical and radiographic study. J Bone Joint Surg Am. 1999;81(7):983–90.
9. Maffulli et al. Early weightbearing and ankle mobilization after open repair of acute midsubstance tears of the Achilles tendon. Am J Sports Med. 2003;31(5):692–700.
10. Kangas et al. Early functional treatment versus early immobilization in tension of the musculotendinous unit after Achilles rupture repair: a prospective, randomized, clinical study. J Trauma. 2003;54(6):1171–80.
11. Lim et al. Percutaneous vs. open repair of the ruptured Achilles tendon - a prospective randomized controlled study. Foot Ankle Int. 2001;22(7):559–68.
12. Saleh et al. The Sheffield splint for controlled early mobilisation after rupture of the calcaneal tendon. A prospective, randomised comparison with plaster treatment. J Bone Joint Surg Am. 1992;74(2):206–9.
13. Petersen et al. Randomized comparison of CAM walker and light-weight plaster cast in the treatment of first-time Achilles tendon rupture. Ugeskr Laeger. 2002;164(33):3852–5.
14. Jiang et al. Operative versus nonoperative treatment for acute Achilles tendon rupture: a meta-analysis based on current evidence. Int Orthop. 2012;36(4):765–73.
15. Wilkins et al. Operative versus nonoperative management of acute Achilles tendon ruptures: a quantitative systematic review of randomized controlled trials. Am J Sports Med. 2012;40(9):2154–60.
16. Soroceanu et al. Surgical versus nonsurgical treatment of acute Achilles tendon rupture: a meta-analysis of randomized trials. J Bone Joint Surg Am. 2012;94(23):2136–43.
17. Ochen et al. Operative treatment versus nonoperative treatment of Achilles tendon ruptures: systematic review and meta-analysis. BMJ. 2019;364:k5120.
18. Bhandari et al. Treatment of acute Achilles tendon ruptures a systematic overview and metaanalysis. Clin Orthop Relat Res. 2002;(400):190–200.
19. Willits et al. Operative versus nonoperative treatment of acute Achilles tendon ruptures. J Bone Joint Surg Am. 2010;92(17):2767–75.

20. Nilsson-Helander et al. Acute Achilles tendon rupture: a randomized, controlled study comparing surgical and nonsurgical treatments using validated outcome measures. Am J Sports Med. 2010;38(11):2186–93.
21. Wang et al. Operative versus nonoperative treatment of acute Achilles tendon rupture: an analysis of 12,570 patients in a large healthcare database. Foot Ankle Surg. 2015;21(4):250–3.
22. Kou J. AAOS Clinical Practice Guideline: acute Achilles tendon rupture. J Am Acad Orthop Surg. 2010;18(8):511–13.
23. Naldo et al. ACFAS Clinical Consensus Statement: acute Achilles tendon pathology. J Foot Ankle Surg. 2021;60(1):93–101.

13

Close Contact Casting versus Surgery for Initial Treatment of Unstable Ankle Fractures in Older Adults

JOHN HARDMAN AND MICHAEL PEARSE

Study Nickname: Ankle Injury Management (AIM) trial

> Among older adults with unstable ankle fracture, the use of close contact casting compared with surgery resulted in similar functional outcomes at 6 months. Close contact casting may be an appropriate treatment for such patients.
>
> —AIM Trial Collaborators[1]

Citation: Willett K, Keene DJ, Mistry D, Nam J, Tutton E, Handley R, Morgan L, Roberts E, Briggs A, Lall R, Chesser TJS, Pallister I, Lamb SE, Ankle Injury Management (AIM) Trial Collaborators. Close contact casting vs surgery for initial treatment of unstable ankle fractures in older adults. JAMA. 2016;316(14):1455–63.

Research Question: Does close contact casting (CCC) offer comparable outcomes to surgical management in the definitive treatment of unstable ankle fractures in the elderly, whilst avoiding both the complications and healthcare resource use associated with open surgery?

Funding:
Pilot Phase: AO Research Foundation
AIM trial: National Institute of Health Research (NIHR)
Report: NIHR Oxford Biomedical Research Unit funding scheme

Year Study Began: 2010

Year Study Published: 2016

Study Location: 24 UK hospitals

Who Was Studied: Adults aged > 60 years presenting with overtly unstable acute malleolar fractures. Patients were required to be ambulatory prior to injury.

Who Was Excluded: Patients with critical limb ischemia, insulin-dependent diabetes mellitus, and active leg ulceration—all of which are risk factors for wound healing complications. Preexisting ankle arthritis, cognitive impairment, and those considered high anesthetic risk were also excluded.

How Many Patients: 620

Study Overview: See Figure 13.1.

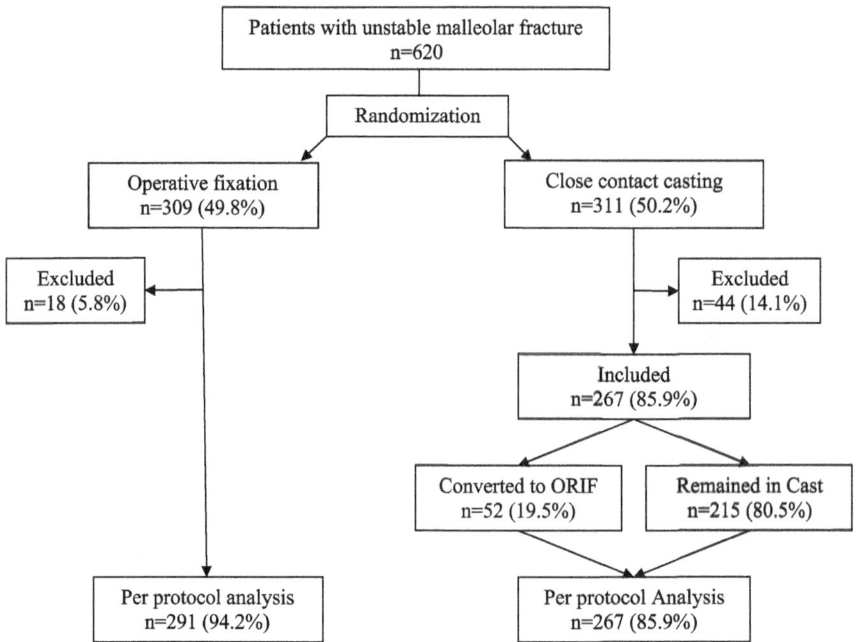

Figure 13.1. Study overview.

Study Intervention: Operative fixation was carried out in accordance with AO principles. Implant selection, weight-bearing status, and postoperative immobilization were according to preference of the treating surgeon. In the casting group, plaster of Paris was applied directly to a single layer of synthetic wool over a stockinette bandage. Foam padding was used to protect pressure areas. Surgeons received standardized training in closed reduction and casting techniques. The procedure was performed under spinal or general anesthesia with fluoroscopic guidance. Weightbearing was restricted for a minimum of 4 weeks from cast application. Reduction was monitored with serial plain radiographs, and loss of reduction led to remanipulation or conversion to fixation. Perioperative antibiotics and thromboprophylaxis in both groups was adhered to as per local policy.

Follow-Up: At 6 weeks and 6 months

Endpoints: Primary outcome included ankle function using the Olerud-Molander Ankle Score (OMAS; a functional rating scale from 0 [totally impaired] to 100 [completely unimpaired] and based on 9 items: pain, stiffness, swelling, stair climbing, running, jumping, squatting, supports, and activities of daily living). Secondary outcomes included quality of life scores (SF-12 [self-reported outcome measure assessing the impact of health on everyday life] and EQ-5D-3L [questionnaire for patient-reported outcome measure on quality of life consisting of 5 dimensions with each having 3 response levels of severity]), pain scores (subsections of OMAS and EQ-5D), and patient satisfaction (rated 1–5). Resource use, complications, and radiographic evidence of nonunion or malunion were also recorded.

RESULTS (TABLE 13.1)

- *Scores:*
  - No significant difference in ankle function (OMAS) was reported at 6 months.
  - Quality of life, pain, and patient satisfaction were equivalent at both 6 weeks and 6 months.
- *Complications:* Fewer treatment-related complications were observed in the casting group including infection and wound breakdown.
- *Conversion:* 23% of the casting group experienced loss of reduction requiring further intervention, of which 84% underwent internal fixation.
- *Inpatient stay:* Length of stay was equivalent between both groups.
- *Theater time:* Overall theater time was significantly reduced in the casting group.
- *Imaging:* Radiographic nonunion and malunion were both significantly higher in the casting group.

Table 13.1 SUMMARY OF THE AIM TRIAL KEY FINDINGS AT 6 MONTHS

Outcome	Surgery	Casting	*p* Value[a]
Olerud-Molander Ankle Score	64.5	66.0	0.74
EQ-5D	0.76	0.76	0.97
Infection/wound breakdown	10%	1%	< 0.001
Theater time (min)	85	44	< 0.001
Radiographic nonunion	1%	10%	0.045
Radiographic malunion	3%	15%	< 0.001

[a] Derived from quoted 95% CI.

Criticisms and Limitations: The analysis of the casting group includes the outcomes of the 19% who underwent internal fixation. This is statistically valid but indicates that a similar portion of patients initially treated with casting may go on to require surgery to achieve equivalence to early fixation. Patients at increased risk for wound complications, such as those with insulin-dependent diabetes or active leg ulcers, were not included in the study but may also be at greater risk of postoperative complications. The results should be extrapolated with caution in this group. Participating surgeons received standardized training as part of the trial protocol. Those looking to replicate results must ensure they have a standardized skillset in CCC.

Other Relevant Studies and Information:

- The AIM trial group published follow-up data at 3 years[2] to establish whether radiological nonunion or malunion would result in loss of equivalence between the 2 groups should symptoms of posttraumatic arthritis manifest later. The study demonstrated equivalent OMAS scores at 3 years. Post hoc analysis of nonunions and malunions did demonstrate significantly reduced OMAS scores in these groups, regardless of treatment modality.
- Several recent publications also report favorable results with conservative management of minimally displaced medial malleolar fracture, either as an isolated injury[3,4] or in combination with operative reduction of the lateral malleolus.[5]
- BOAST guidelines recommend CCC as an option in patients aged > 60 years provided that reduction can be maintained.[6]

Summary and Implications: The AIM trial demonstrates equivalent functional outcomes for either CCC or surgical fixation in the management of unstable ankle fractures in patients > 60 years. Casting is also associated with reduced resource use and lower rates of postoperative complications. CCC may be considered as an alternative to surgery in this patient group. This should be carried out under formal anesthesia and patients should be monitored for loss of reduction. Patients should also be aware that operative fixation may ultimately prove necessary.

CLINICAL CASE: UNSTABLE ANKLE FRACTURE IN THE ELDERLY

Case History

A 72-year-old lady presents acutely following a fall. She gives a clear history of catching her shoe on a step and reports pain in her ankle. It is an isolated injury. Her medical history includes only hypertension, which is well controlled. She lives alone and is independent. On examination there is diffuse swelling around the ankle. But the skin is intact, with no blistering or areas of compromise. There is no neurovascular deficit. Plain radiograph demonstrates a displaced bimalleolar ankle fracture. She is advised that her ankle is broken and may require surgery. However, she recently lost her husband when he had a pulmonary embolism following hip fracture surgery. She is keen to avoid any surgery to treat her fracture. Based on this evidence, how should the patient be counseled?

Suggested Answer

The patient is typical of the AIM trial study population. She has no physiological impairment that might preclude general anesthesia. Her soft tissues are not compromised, and she has no history of diabetes mellitus. Either treatment option would therefore be technically possible.

The study supports the use of CCC to provide similar functional outcomes to early operative fixation. There would also be a reduced risk for postoperative complications. In counseling this patient, it would be important to explain that treatment with a cast will still require spinal/general anesthesia and would be performed in an operating theater. There is also a 1 in 5 chance that the cast will not control the reduction and open surgery will be required to achieve the same functional outcome.

References

1. Willett et al. Close contact casting vs surgery for initial treatment of unstable ankle fractures in older adults. JAMA. 2016;316(14):1455–63.
2. Keene et al. Three-year follow-up of a trial of close contact casting vs surgery for initial treatment of unstable ankle fractures in older adults. JAMA. 2018 Mar 27;319(12):1274–76.
3. Herscovici et al. Conservative treatment of isolated fractures of the medial malleolus. J Bone Joint Surg Br. 2007;89-B:89–93.
4. Hanhisuanto et al. The functional outcome and quality of life after treatment of isolated medial malleolar fractures. Foot Ankle Surg. 2017;23:225–29.
5. Hoelsbrekken et al. Nonoperative treatment of the medial malleolus in bimalleolar and trimalleolar ankle fractures: a randomized controlled trial. J Orthop Trauma. 2013;27:633–7.
6. British Orthopaedic Association and British Association of Foot and Ankle Surgeons. The management of ankle fractures. August 2016. https://www.boa.ac.uk/resource/boast-12-pdf.html

14

Open Reduction and Internal Fixation versus Primary Arthrodesis for Primarily Ligamentous Lisfranc Joint Injuries

MICHAEL RAFFERTY, EDMUND IEONG, AND IAN GILL

> A primary stable arthrodesis of the medial two or three rays appears to have a better short and medium term outcome than open reduction and internal fixation of ligamentous Lisfranc joint injuries.
>
> —Ly et al.[1]

Citation: Treatment of primarily ligamentous Lisfranc joint injuries: primary arthrodesis compared with open reduction and internal fixation. A prospective, randomized study. J Bone Joint Surg Am. 2006;88(3):514–20.

Research Question: Are the short- and medium-term outcomes of primary partial arthrodesis comparable to open reduction and internal fixation (ORIF) of ligamentous Lisfranc joint injuries?

Funding: None

Year Study Began: 1998

Year Study Published: 2006

Study Location: Department of Orthopaedic Surgery, University of Minnesota, Minneapolis, Minnesota

Who Was Studied: Patients with an acute or subacute (< 1 month old) primarily ligamentous Lisfranc injury with no major (i.e., comminuted or intra-articular) fractures; those with a "fleck sign" indicating avulsion fractures of the Lisfranc ligament were also included.

Who Was Excluded: Patients were excluded if there was a fracture at the first or second metatarsal; other substantial foot, ankle, or leg injuries; any previous surgery for their injury; insulin-dependent diabetes mellitus; ipsilateral ankle fusion; peripheral vascular disease; peripheral neuropathy; and rheumatoid arthritis.

How Many Patients: 41

Study Overview: See Figure 14.1.

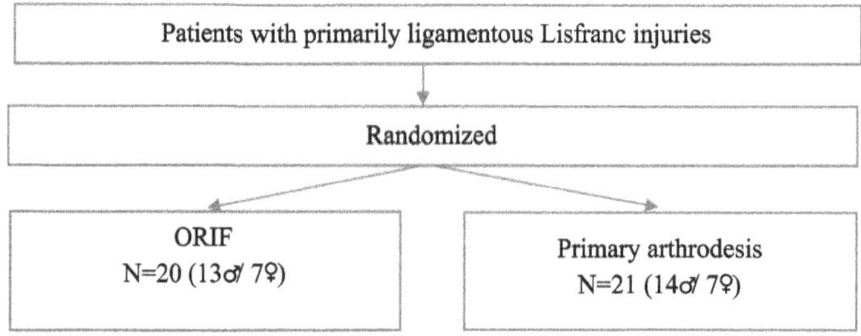

Figure 14.1. Summary of study design.

Study Intervention: The arthrodesis group underwent resection of the cartilage and fibrous tissue, then reduction and screw fixation of the first and second rays. The third ray was fused if there was clinical or radiological evidence of instability. If the lateral rays were unstable, then these were stabilized with temporary Kirschner wire (K-wire) fixation for 6 weeks. If patients had intercuneiform instability, then the joint was also included in the fusion.

The open reduction group involved internal screw fixation of the medial two or three rays. The indication for K-wire fixation for the lateral rays was the same as the arthrodesis group.

All patients underwent two dorsal incisions. All patients were immobilized in a non-weight-bearing cast for 6–8 weeks, followed by full weight bearing for 4 weeks in a fracture boot. Physiotherapy commenced at 6–10 weeks and patients were prescribed orthotics as required.

Follow-Up: Postoperatively, patients had follow-up (F/U) at 2 weeks, 6 weeks, 3 months, 6 months, and then yearly. The average duration of F/U was 42 months (range 25–60 months) in the open reduction group and 43.4 months (range 25–60 months) in the arthrodesis group.

Endpoints: Outcome measures included patient satisfaction, return to their previous level of physical activity prior to the injury (functional questionnaire), complications including the need for a second surgery, the patient's visual analog scale (VAS) pain scores (0–10), and the American Orthopaedic Foot and Ankle Society (AOFAS) Midfoot scale[2] (standardized evaluation incorporating both subjective and objective information with patients reporting on their pain and physicians assessing alignment; scores range from 0 to 100 [i.e., healthy] points).

RESULTS

Complications:

- *In the open reduction group*:
  - 16/20 (80%) patients underwent secondary surgery to remove screws that were prominent or painful at an average of 6.75 months (range 3–16 months).
  - 15/20 (75%) patients had loss of correction, deformity, or degenerative joint disease on F/U radiographs; of these 5 required conversion to arthrodesis.
- *In the arthrodesis group, there were 7 reoperations*:
  - 2 patients had a delayed or nonunion, requiring adjuvant therapy or further surgery. All patients eventually achieved union. The average time to union was 10.6 weeks.
  - 1 required percutaneous flexor tendon release for claw toes secondary to posttraumatic compartment syndrome.
  - 4 required removal of screws at an average of 6.5 months but never done before 3 months postoperatively.
- *Functional questionnaire*: Patients were more satisfied in the arthrodesis group than in the open reduction group, as seen in Table 14.1.
- *Return to preinjury levels*: The percentage of patients who were able to return to their preinjury level of physical activity in the arthrodesis group was 62%, 86%, and 92%, vs. 44%, 61%, and 65% in the open reduction group, at 6 months, 12 months, and 24 months respectively.
- *AOFAS midfoot scale*: At 2 years the average AOFAS midfoot score was 88.0 points in the arthrodesis group vs. 68.6 points in the open reduction group ($p = 0.005$). After exclusion of the 5 patients in the open

reduction group who underwent conversion to arthrodesis, the average AOFAS score in the open reduction group was 62.5 points, which was significantly lower than in the arthrodesis group ($p < 0.0024$).
- *VAS score*: At 2 years, the average VAS score was 1.2 in the arthrodesis group vs. 4.1 in the open reduction group ($p = 0.0002$).

Table 14.1 SUMMARY OF KEY FINDINGS

Outcome	**Open Reduction Group ($n = 20$)**	**Arthrodesis Group ($n = 21$)**	**p Value**
	Satisfaction		
Very satisfied	8 (40%)	16 (76%)	
Somewhat satisfied	3 (15%)	5 (24%)	
Neutral	3 (15%)	—	
Dissatisfied	6 (30%)	—	
	Complication		
Loss of correction	15 (75%)	N/A	
Second surgery needed			
Remove hardware	16 (80%)	4 (19%)	
Convert arthrodesis	5 (25%)	n/a	
Other	—	3[a] (14%)	
	AOFAS Midfoot score		
At 2 years	68.6	88.0	0.005
At final follow-up	57.1	86.9	< 0.0001
VAS score at 2 years	4.2	1.2	0.0002
Anatomical alignment	5	20	

[a] 1 patient required a bone graft, 1 patient a bone stimulator, and 1 a flexor tendon release.

Criticisms and Limitations: Allocation of treatment with open randomization, odd or even format, may have introduced a selection bias. High numbers of hardware removal in the open reduction group may be a confounder to the second operation. These results are only applicable to patients with primarily ligamentous injuries and cannot be extrapolated for Lisfranc injuries with major fractures.

Other Relevant Studies and Information:

- Kuo et al.[3] described the finding that not all the patients healed following ORIF and also that 6/15 (40%) patients developed osteoarthritis.
- Mulier et al.[4] compared 16 patients with ORIF vs. 6 patients with partial arthrodesis vs. 6 with complete arthrodesis of all 5 tarsometatarsal joints. The complete fusion group had the worst functional outcome. In

addition, 94% of patients in the open reduction group had radiographic degenerative changes at the tarsometatarsal joints at final F/U.

- Sheibani-Rad et al.[5] performed a systematic review to compare primary arthrodesis and ORIF for Lisfranc fractures. Six studies with a total of 193 patients met the inclusion criteria. At 1-year F/U, they found no statistical difference in AOFAS scores in patients who had an anatomical reduction.
- Henning et al.[6] prospectively randomized 40 patients with acute tarsometatarsal fractures or fracture dislocations to either primary arthrodesis or ORIF. They found a significantly higher rate of secondary surgeries in the ORIF group, but insignificant differences in SF-36 scores and satisfaction rates.

Summary and Implications: In primarily ligamentous Lisfranc injuries, this study demonstrates significantly better VAS, AOFAS, and satisfaction rates in the arthrodesis group compared to the ORIF group at final F/U. The return to preinjury levels of physical and sports activities was higher in the arthrodesis group at 6, 12, and 24 months, but was only significantly higher at 2 years. The arthrodesis group also had fewer complications and fewer secondary operations compared to the open reduction group. These results suggest that patients with a primarily ligamentous Lisfranc injury should be treated with primary arthrodesis instead of traditional ORIF.

CLINICAL CASE: SURGICAL OPTIONS ON LIGAMENTOUS LISFRANC INJURY

Case History

A 54-year-old male sustained an isolated foot injury while cycling. His past medical history includes hypertension. He is taking antihypertensive medication and he is a nonsmoker. Clinical examination elicited midfoot swelling and plantar ecchymosis. Piano key test was positive with hypermobility between the first and second rays. He is unable to fully weight-bear due to pain. Standard weight-bearing plain radiograph showed divergence of the first and second metatarsals with no fractures seen. Based on the results of this randomized trial, how should one proceed?

Suggested Answer

All clinical signs are also indicative of the injury. This patient is typical of a patient in this trial as he had no major comorbidities and sustained a purely ligamentous Lisfranc injury without fractures. This trial suggests that he would benefit more with primary arthrodesis of the involved tarsometatarsal joints rather than ORIF of the Lisfranc injury. The results of the trial suggest that arthrodesis is associated with better AOFAS scores, better VAS scores, fewer complications, and fewer secondary operations.

References

1. Ly et al. Treatment of primarily ligamentous Lisfranc joint injuries: primary arthrodesis compared with open reduction and internal fixation. A prospective, randomized study. J Bone Joint Surg Am. 2006;88(3):514–20.
2. Kitaoka et al. Clinical rating systems for the ankle-hindfoot, midfoot, hallux, and lesser toes. Foot Ankle Int. 1994;15(7):349–53.
3. Kuo et al. Outcome after open reduction and internal fixation of Lisfranc joint injuries. J Bone Joint S Am. 2000;82:1609–18.
4. Mulier et al. Severe Lisfranc injuries: primary arthrodesis or ORIF? Foot Ankle Int. 2002;23:902–5.
5. Sheibani-Rad et al. Arthrodesis versus ORIF for Lisfranc fractures. Orthopedics. 2012;35(6):e868–73.
6. Henning et al. Open reduction internal fixation versus primary arthrodesis for Lisfranc injuries: a prospective randomized study. Foot Ankle Int. 2009;30(10):913–22.

15

Highly Cross-Linked Polyethylene Reduces Wear and Revision Rates in Total Hip Arthroplasty

MOHAMMED MONEM, KAPIL SUGAND, AND MICHAEL PEARSE

> XLPE liners have significantly reduced wear and are associated with a greater implant survival rate at 10 years compared with conventional UHMWPE liners.
>
> —Devane et al.[1]

Citation: Devane PA, Horne JG, Ashmore A, Mutimer J, Kim W, Stanley J. Highly cross-linked polyethylene reduces wear and revision rates in total hip arthroplasty: a 10-year double-blinded randomized controlled trial. J Bone Joint Surg Am. 2017;99(20):1703–14.

Research Question: Do the wear rates of highly cross-linked polyethylene (XLPE) liners outperform the current conventional ultra-high-molecular-weight polyethylene (UHMWPE) liners in patients with total hip replacements (THRs) and their subsequent clinical outcomes in a double-blinded 10-year study?

Funding: DePuy grant for extra radiographs required over and above routine radiographs. DePuy had no input into study design or analysis on their disclosure.

Year Study Began: 2001

Year Study Published: 2017

Study Location: Wellington, New Zealand

Who Was Studied: Patients aged 45–75 years with noninflammatory arthritis requiring a THR.

Who Was Excluded: Patients declining to participate, patients who were pregnant, patients who had medical comorbidities that impaired ability to walk (i.e., Charnley C classification), and patients with inflammatory arthritis.

How Many Patients: 91

Study Overview: See Figure 15.1.

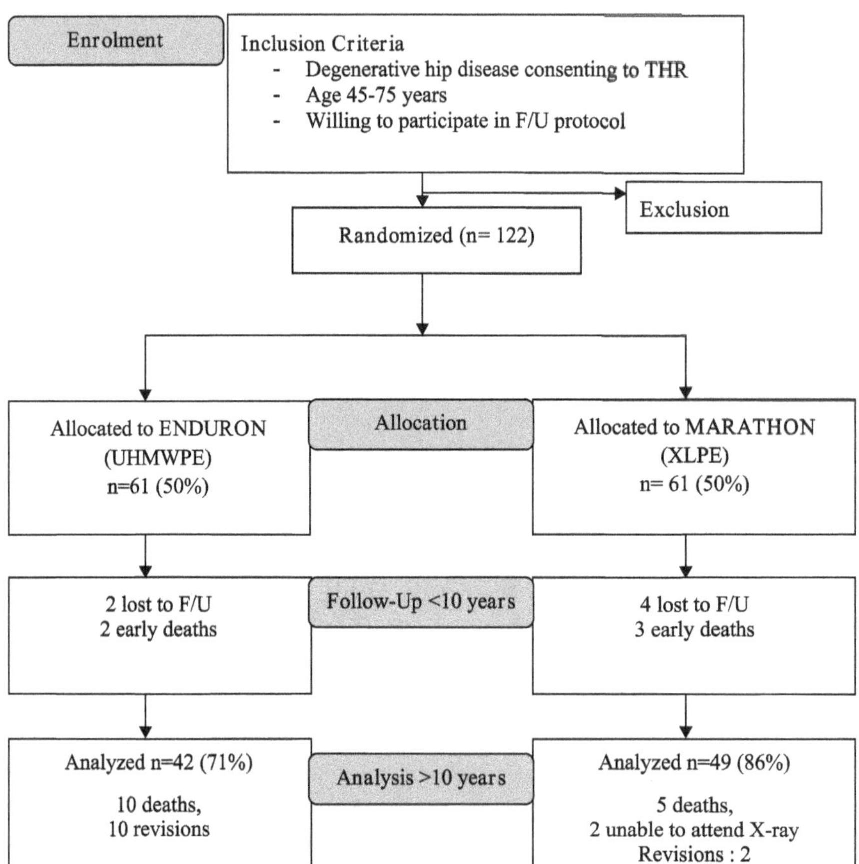

Figure 15.1. Study overview and a summary of the CONSORT diagram.

Study Intervention: This was a single-center double-blinded study comparing 2 different acetabular polyethylene liners in patients with noninflammatory arthritis who were randomized. The THRs were inserted by 2 senior surgeons, each using either a posterior or a direct lateral approach. All patients received a Charnley Elite size 2 femoral stem (DePuy, Warsaw, Indiana, USA), a 28-mm cobalt/chromium femoral head, and a 29-mm inner diameter polyethylene liner. Ninety-one patients were followed up in intervals for a period of at least 10 years. During this period, the patients were clinically monitored using the Oxford Hip Score[2] (OHS; joint-specific patient-reported outcome measure designed to assess disability in patients undergoing THR with score ranging from 12 to 60, where higher score equates to a better perception) and the Short Form (SF)-12[3] for patient-reported outcomes. Patients had anteroposterior and lateral plain radiographs that were periodically analyzed for wear, osteolysis, and loosening of components. Other adverse outcomes including dislocations were analyzed. The rate of wear and clinical outcomes of both cohorts with different acetabular liners were reported.

Follow-Up:

- 6 weeks
- 6 months
- 12 months
- 2 years
- 5 years
- 10 years

Endpoints: Clinical outcomes included patient-reported outcomes with SF-12 and OHS. Radiological outcomes included wear rates (Figure 15.2) with 2D and 3D analysis of plain radiographs using specialist software (Rev 7 and PolyWare).

RESULTS

- *Patient demographics:*
  - All 122 patients recruited were accounted for at 10 years.
  - 116 (95%) patients were included for radiological analysis. The remaining patients had either died of causes unrelated to the index surgery, moved out of the area within 2 years of surgery, or did not have sufficient radiographs for analysis.

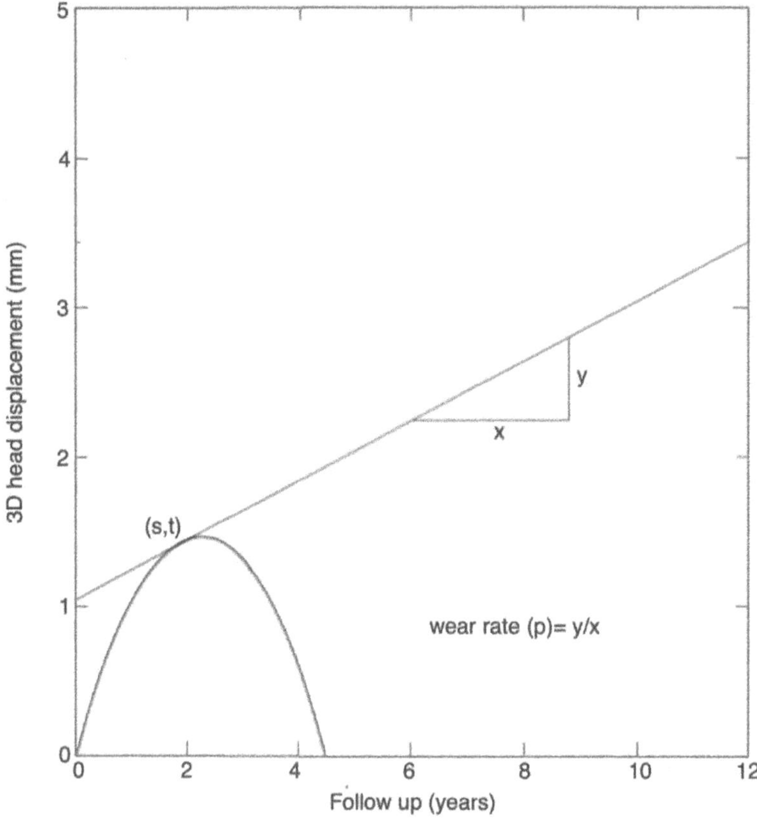

Figure 15.2. Two functions representing 3D femoral head displacement. The straight line represents polyethylene wear whereby the slope represents its rate (p). The intersection of the straight line with the y-axis indicates the true polyethylene creep.

- 91 (74.5%) patients had adequate clinical and radiological analysis at the end of the 10-year period.
  - Of the remaining patients, 9 (10%) had revision surgery, 21 (23%) had died, 2 (2%) had developed dementia, and 1 (1%) was housebound due to inclusion body myositis and could not return for follow-up (F/U).
- *Acetabular liner*: The Marathon (XLPE) had a significantly reduced 2D, 3D, and volumetric wear compared to the Enduron (UHMWPE).
- *Mean wear rate (95% CI; mm/year)*: 2D wear rate was 0.03 (0.01–0.04) in the Marathon (XLPE) vs. a much higher wear rate of 0.27 (0.23–0.29) in the Enduron (UHMWPE) liners. Similarly, volumetric wear was 10.25 (1.5–18) in the Marathon (XLPE) vs. 139.9 (130–148) in the Enduron liner group (Figure 15.3, Tables 15.1 and 15.2).

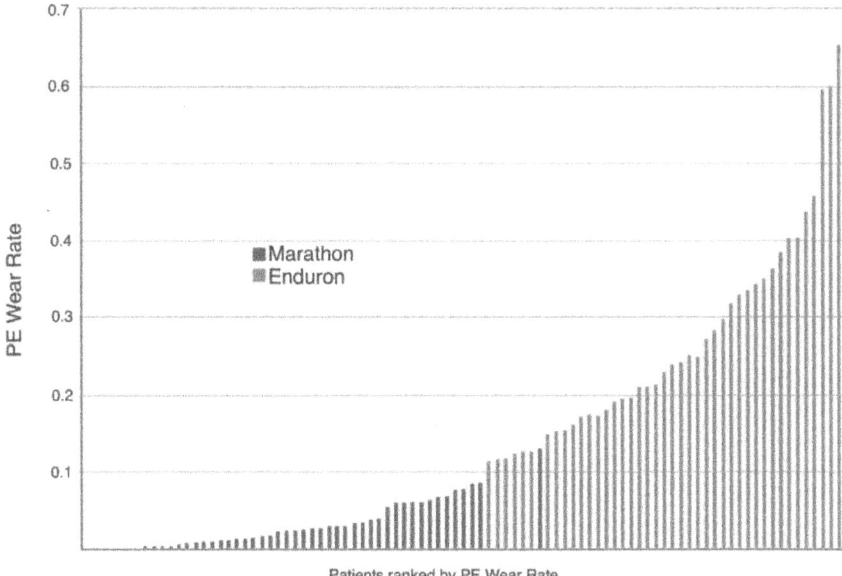

Figure 15.3. Rate of polyethylene wear for the 91 patients with a minimum 10-year F/U.

Table 15.1 Summary of Key Findings for Wear Rates

Wear rates (n = 116 with sufficient radiological data for analysis)				
		Mean		***p* Value**
		Enduron (n = 59)	**Marathon (n = 57)**	
2D wear	mm/year	0.27	0.03	< 0.001
3D wear	mm/year	0.28	0.03	
Volumetric wear	mm^3/year	139.9	19.25	

Table 15.2 Summary of Regression Values of Individual Patients with at Least 10-Year F/U (N = 91)

Regression values after at least 10 years postoperatively (n = 91)		
Mean Outcome	**Enduron**	**Marathon**
N (%)	42 (46%)	49 (54%)
Follow-up (y)	11	
Wear rate (mm/y)	0.27	0.03
Bedding-in time (y)	1.7	0.7
Creep + wear (mm)	0.62	0.42
Creep (mm)	0.2	0.4

- *Thickness of liner:* This had no effect on wear rate on either liner when compared to themselves, but there was a notable difference between them (Table 15.3).

Table 15.3 Liner Thickness vs. Mean Wear for Patients with Minimum 10-Year F/U ($N = 91$)

Relation between liner thickness and mean wear after 10 years postoperatively ($n = 91$)

	Liner	**Liner Thickness (mm)**			
		< 8	**8–10**	**> 10**	**All (range)**
N implants	*Marathon*	18	24	7	49
	Enduron	20	17	5	42
Wear rate (mm/y)	*Marathon*	0.03	0.03	0.04	0.03 (0–0.13)
	Enduron	0.26	0.26	0.32	0.27 (0.12–0.65)
Time until wear-through (y)	*Marathon*	762	657	1329	791 (81.4–5479)
	Enduron	36	43	43.6	39.7 (13.5–85.4)

- *OHS:* This was slightly lower in the Enduron (41) vs. the Marathon (44) but not significant ($p = 0.06$).
- *SF-12:* Similarly, there was no difference in SF-12 scores between the Enduron and Marathon acetabular liners for both mental and physical health.
- *Group allocation, implant sizes, and positioning:* Age, number of patients, and cup size were very similar in both the Enduron and Marathon liners, as outlined in Table 15.4. The average cup size in both groups was 54 mm with an anteversion of 12 and 13 degrees respectively.

Table 15.4 Baseline Characteristics in Cohort with XLPE vs. UHMWPE

Demographics ($n = 116$)	**Enduron ($n = 59$)**	**Marathon ($n = 57$)**
Number of patients	59	57
Age (range in y)	61 (49–75)	61 (46–75)
Male:female	31:28	31:21
Left:right	30:29	19:38
Surgeon (JH:PD)	39:20	34:23
Cup size (mm)	54 (48–60)	54 (48–60)
Abduction angle (°)	47.7 (29.4–61)	48.8 (31–66.7)
Anteversion (°)	12.8	13.8

- *Gender allocation:* There was a higher male-to-female ratio in both the Enduron (52.5% male: 47.5% female) and Marathon (59.6% male: 40.4% female) groups respectively.
- *Osteolysis:* This was seen in 20 (22%) patients with 80% ($n = 16$) in the Enduron group vs. 20% ($n = 4$) in the Marathon group.

- *Dislocations*: This was seen in 6 (6.6%) patients. All had a posterior approach. Of these, 4 (66.6%) had Enduron liners and 2 (33.3%) had Marathon liners.
- *Revisions (%, 95% CI):* Of the 12 (13.2%) revisions, 3 were due to liner wear. The liners were revised at 8.1, 9.6, and 12 years postoperatively. Six revisions were due to aseptic loosening/osteolysis of the femoral stem and 3 due to stem fracture. There were 10 (83%) revisions in the Enduron group. The remaining 2 revisions were in the Marathon group. Of these 2, 1 was for stem fracture and the other for cement mantle failure. At 10 years postoperatively, those with the Enduron liners (14.6%, 2.7–23.4) had a significantly higher revision rate than those with Marathon liners (1.9%, 0–5.4).
- *Survival rate:* Kaplan-Meier survival curves for both options are depicted in Figure 15.4.

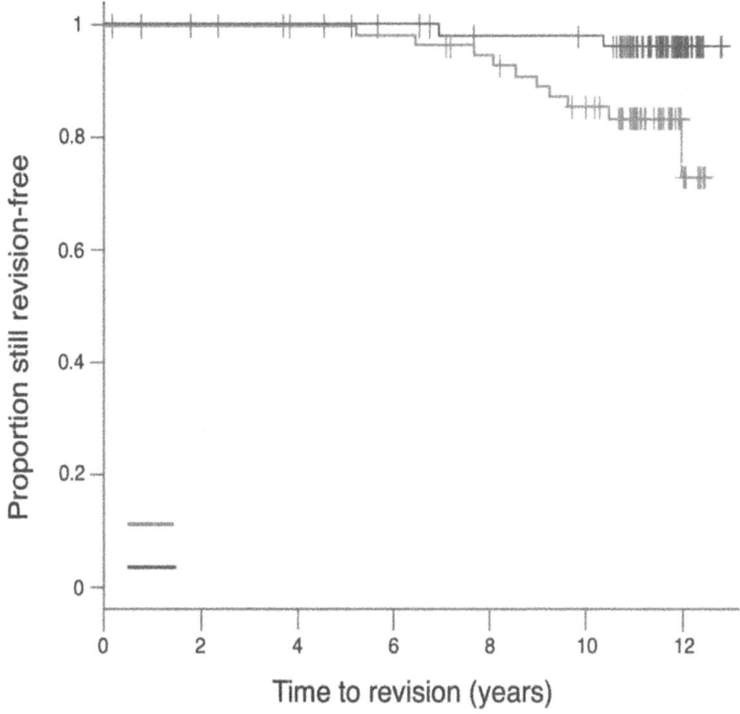

Figure 15.4. Kaplan-Meier survival curve for the Enduron and Marathon groups. At 10 years postoperatively, the revision rate was 14.6% (95% CI: 47–23.4) in the Enduron group and 1.9% (95% CI: 0–5.4) in the Marathon group. At 12 years postoperatively, the revision rate was 27.0% (95% CI: 2.7–45.3) in the Enduron group and 3.8% (95% CI: 0–8.8) in the Marathon group.

Criticisms and Limitations: This is a single-center study with liners from a single manufacturer. There were 2 senior surgeons using lateral and posterior approaches. Ideally more surgeons would have been used from more centers in numerous countries to add further weight to the findings. The F/U period could have been extended to observe the natural history of this prosthesis and bearing combination chosen. There was no computed tomography imaging to measure wear.

Other Relevant Studies and Information:

- It is widely known that THRs eventually become loose, which is explained by debris-related osteolysis requiring revision arthroplasty. This applies to all debris-forming surfaces. Other bearings such as metal on metal have their established side effect profile including pseudotumors and metallosis, which led to soft tissue destruction and need for revision surgery. Ceramic-on-ceramic surfaces face the commonly described squeak but also could develop the risk of "catastrophic" fracture and debris formation.[2–4]
- Other studies confirmed that cross-linking of polyethylene has shown to have a lower rate of volumetric wear and hence will last longer before requiring revision for wear.[5–7]
- The lower rate of wear on highly cross-linked polymer applies to all surfaces of the femoral head including ceramic and chrome.
- The lower wear rate also applies to younger patients who have had their primary arthroplasty surgery at < 50 years of age. This effect has also been reproduced in multicenter cohort studies.[8,9]

Summary and Implications: UHMWPE (Enduron) liners are among the most widely available liners used for THR. The most common reason for revision is aseptic loosening. In an aim to reduce debris-related osteolysis, XLPE (Marathon) acetabular liners have reduced wear rates compared to UHMWPE liners. The revision rate was significantly greater in the Enduron liners compared to the Marathon liners. The 10-year survival rate of the cohort with XLPE liners was higher than in those with conventional UHMWPE liners despite similar baseline characteristics. Orthopaedic surgeons need to consider XLPE as their first choice for acetabular liners for their hip arthroplasty as their outcomes are superior to the UHMWPE acetabular liners.

CLINICAL CASE: DECISION-MAKING IN CHOOSING YOUR THR LINER

Case History

A 70-year-old female patient presents to the clinic with severe chronic right hip pain. Severe osteoarthritis was confirmed with both clinical examination and plain radiographs. She has been listed for an elective THR. On the day of the operation, 2 acetabular liners are presented by the brand-new scrub nurse. The options of liner include metal-on-XLPE vs. UHMWPE. Which liner should be utilized based on this study? Does the thickness of the liner affect the wear rate? Which liner has an associated higher rate of dislocations and osteolysis and a higher revision rate after a decade of F/U?

Suggested Answer

The preferred option for this patient would be a liner that is durable and avoids the need for early revision. After choosing to use a metal head, the option to pick between a UHMWPE and an XLPE liner arises. The evidence thus far has shown that the XLPE liner bearing has a superior performance over its counterpart UHMWPE in regard to wear rates. The XLPE liner has shown to be superior in clinical outcome with reduced rates of revisions, osteolysis, and dislocations. Interestingly, both liners whilst in situ have similar patient-reported outcomes. The XLPE also has a superior outcome radiologically in 2D and 3D wear analysis. The thickness of the liner has a theoretically longer duration of wear, but the wear rate is similar and, more importantly, implant survival is higher with XLPE.

References

1. Devane et al. Highly cross-linked polyethylene reduces wear and revision rates in total hip arthroplasty: a 10-year double-blinded randomized controlled trial. J Bone Joint Surg Am. 2017;99(20):1703–14.
2. Wylde et al. The Oxford hip score: the patient's perspective. Health Qual Life Outcomes. 2005;3(1):66.
3. Ware et al. A 12-Item Short-Form Health Survey: construction of scales and preliminary tests of reliability and validity. Med Care. 1996;3:220–33.
4. Yin et al. Is there any difference in survivorship of total hip arthroplasty with different bearing surfaces? A systematic review and network meta-analysis. Int J Clin Exp Med. 2015;8(11):21871–85.

5. Ha et al. Ceramic liner fracture after cementless alumina-on-alumina total hip arthroplasty. Clin Orthop Relat Res. 2007;458 (458):106–10.
6. Glyn-Jones et al. Risk factors for inflammatory pseudotumour formation following hip resurfacing. J Bone Joint Surg Br. 2009;91(12):1566–74.
7. Röhrl et al. No adverse effects of submelt-annealed highly crosslinked polyethylene in cemented cups: an RSA study of 8 patients 10 years after surgery. Acta Orthop. 2012;83(2):148–52.
8. Greiner et al. Fixation and wear with contemporary acetabular components and cross-linked polyethylene at 10-years in patients aged 50 and under. J Arthroplasty. 2015;30(9):1577–85.
9. Lachiewicz et al. Wear and osteolysis of highly crosslinked polyethylene at 10 to 14 years: the effect of femoral head size. Clin Orthop Relat Res. 2016;474(2):365–71.
10. Garvin et al. Low wear rates seen in THAs with highly crosslinked polyethylene at 9 to 14 years in patients younger than age 50 years. Clin Orthop Relat Res. 2015;473(12):3829–35.
11. Bragdon et al. The 2012 John Charnley Award. Clinical multicenter studies of the wear performance of highly crosslinked remelted polyethylene in THA. Clin Orthop Relat Res. 2013;471:393–402.

16

Hemiarthroplasty or Total Hip Arthroplasty for the Treatment of a Displaced Intracapsular Fracture in Active Elderly Patients

ANTHONY JANAHAN THAYAPARAN, ASHOK SINGH, BILAL AL-OBAIDI, ROBIN K. STRACHAN, AND DOMINIC SPICER

Study's Nickname: ARTHRO trial

> We found no difference in the outcome after treatment with either a hemiarthroplasty or [total hip arthroplasty, THA] in active elderly patients with an intracapsular fracture of the hip, 12 years post-operatively.
>
> —Tol et al.[1]

Citation: Tol MC, van den Bekerom MP, Sierevelt IN, Hilverdink EF, Raaymakers EL, Goslings JC. Hemiarthroplasty or total hip arthroplasty for the treatment of a displaced intracapsular fracture in active elderly patients: 12-year follow-up of randomised trial. Bone Joint J. 2017;99-B(2):250–4.

Research Question: In active elderly patients with intracapsular neck of femur (NOF) fractures, which prosthesis is superior in the long term, hemiarthroplasty (HA) or total hip arthroplasty (THA)?

Funding: No funding received

Year Study Began: 1995 (original study)

Year Study Published: 2017

Study Location: Academic Medical Center, Amsterdam, The Netherlands

Who Was Studied: All patients aged > 70 years admitted between January 1995 and January 2002 with displaced intracapsular NOF fractures. They had to provide informed consent, understand written Dutch, and have no contraindication to anesthesia or metastatic disease.

Who Was Excluded: Those who did not meet the above inclusion criteria (including refusal to consent), those had advanced radiological osteoarthritis or rheumatoid arthritis, bed bound patients (or those barely mobile from bed to chair), and those who did not receive the prosthesis to which they were randomized.

How Many Patients: 281

Study Overview: See Figure 16.1.

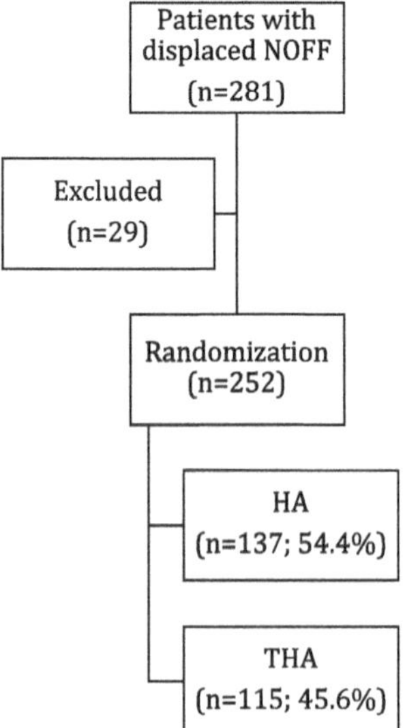

Figure 16.1. Study overview.

Study Intervention: Patients admitted with displaced intracapsular NOF fractures were recruited. The patients were then randomized to receive either a cemented THA or HA. Patients were followed up at 1 and 5 years (reported and published) and at 12 years. Evaluation of patients at each point in time was conducted via telephone interviews. Other patient demographics were obtained from family members, family physicians, and other healthcare professionals. Plain film pelvic radiography was sought in those who reported symptoms during their assessment.

Follow-Up: 1, 5, and 12 years postoperatively

Endpoints: Primary outcome was the modified Harris Hip Score (HHS),[2] which evaluates various hip disabilities and methods of treatment in an adult population on a scale of 1–100. Secondary outcomes were rate of revision, mortality, and prosthesis-related or general complications.

RESULTS

- *Demographics:*
  - At 12 years, 50 (19.8%) patients were still alive to follow-up (F/U), with 47 (94%) being female; 32 (64%) were from the HA group and 18 (36%) from the THA group.
  - The mean age at the time of injury was 77.2 years in the HA group vs. 78.5 years in the THA group. Fracture laterality was evenly distributed between the 2 groups (Table 16.1).
- *Score:* The mean modified HHSs were 70.3 and 69.3 ($p = 0.85$) in the HA and THA groups respectively, at 12 years.
- *Complication:* There were no dislocations in either group and no revisions.
- *Mortality:* The mortality rate was 77% in the HA group vs. 84% in the THA group, but statistically insignificant ($p = 0.13$).

Table 16.1 Results of the 12-Year Follow-Up (N = x [%])

	Original Population		**12 Year Follow-Up**	
	HA (*n* = 137)	**THA (*n* = 115)**	**HA (*n* = 32)**	**THA (*n* = 18)**
	Demographics, *n* (%)			
Female	115 (84)	90 (78)	30 (94)	17 (94)
Male	22 (16)	25 (22)	2 (6)	1 (6)
Mean age of trauma (SD)	80.3 (6.2)	82.1 (6.3)	77.2	78.5
Mean follow-up years (SD)			12.4	11.3

	Original Population		12 Year Follow-Up	
	HA (n = 137)	THA (n = 115)	HA (n = 32)	THA (n = 18)
Fracture side, n (%)				
Left	78 (57)	74 (64)	15 (47)	11 (61)
Right	59 (43)	41 (36)	17 (53)	7 (39)
Comorbidities, n (%)				
Malignancy	11 (8)	6 (5)	1 (3)	0 (0)
Cardiovascular	34 (25)	38 (33)	4 (13)	7 (39)
Respiratory	16 (12)	18 (16)	1 (3)	1 (5)
Neurological	26 (19)	33 (29)	2 (6)	3 (17)
Diabetes mellitus	19 (14)	11 (10)	3 (9)	0 (0)
Musculoskeletal	22 (16)	31 (27)	4 (13)	7 (39)
American Society of Anesthesiologists grade, n (%)				
I	19 (14)	11 (9)	9 (28)	4 (22)
II	77 (56)	48 (42)	19 (59)	9 (50)
III	33 (24)	44 (38)	4 (13)	4 (22)
IV	5 (4)	10 (9)	0 (0)	1 (6)
V	0 (0)	0 (0)	0 (0)	0 (0)
Unknown	3 (2)	2 (2)	0 (0)	0 (0)

Outcome Measures at Follow-Up	HA n = 32	THA n = 18	p Value
Mean modified HHS (SD)	70.3 (16.3)	69.3 (20.0)	0.85
Mean HHS pain (SD)	39.8 (9.1)	37.2 (10.0)	0.44
Mean HHS function (SD)	16.4 (8.8)	18.3 (7.4)	0.34
Satisfaction of treatment, n (%)	27 (84)	11 (61)	0.47
Revision operation, n (%)	0 (0)	0 (0)	N/A
Dislocation of prosthesis, n (%)	0 (0)	0 (0)	N/A

Criticisms and Limitations: Investigators were not blinded to the type of operation. The only complications recorded after discharge were dislocation and revision surgery. Telephone interviews were the only method utilized for F/U. At 12 years, only 20% of patients from the original study were available for F/U.

Other Relevant Studies and Information:

- Another randomized controlled trial (RCT)[3] confirmed superior short-term clinical results (mean F/U of 3 years) and fewer complications with THA vs. HA (*n* = 81). As a F/U study,[4] THA resulted in lower mortality but also superior level of function after a mean F/U of 9 years, despite increased dislocation rate compared to HA. This was corroborated by another RCT demonstrating improved function and quality of life in patients with THA at 48 months.[5]

- Keating et al.[6] studied reduction and fixation vs. HA and THA, finding fixation to be the least favorable option and THA displaying significantly improved functional outcome scores at 2 years than the other groups.
- Systematic review and meta-analyses[7,8] confirmed that THA (as opposed to HA) benefitted patients with displaced NOF fractures, conferring a lower rate of reoperation and higher functional scores (despite higher dislocation rate).
- The Hip Fracture Evaluation with Alternatives of Total Hip Arthroplasty versus Hemi-Arthroplasty (HEALTH)[9] study is the most recent international multicenter RCT that randomly assigned 1495 patients aged > 50 years with displaced NOF fractures into either HA or THA. Incidence of secondary procedures did not differ between both groups over 24 months of F/U; yet THA offered a clinically unimportant improvement in function and quality of life.
- National Institute for Health and Care Excellence guidelines[10] recommend to "offer replacement arthroplasty (THA or HA) to patients with a displaced intracapsular hip fracture." Furthermore, it is advised to "offer THA rather than HA to patients with a displaced intracapsular hip fracture who: (i) were able to walk independently out of doors with no more than the use of a stick and, (ii) are not cognitively impaired and (iii) are medically fit for anesthesia and the procedure."
- THA ought to be performed by hip specialists, as opposed to HA, which can be performed by trauma-trained orthopaedic surgeons as recommended by the Getting It Right First Time initiative.[11,12]

Summary and Implications: This trial involving patients with displaced intracapsular NOF fractures found that at 12 years postoperatively, there was no significant difference in the rate of complications, revision surgery, or mortality between THA and HA. In light of these findings, the authors concluded that patients > 70 years should generally undergo a faster cemented hip HA rather than THA.

CLINICAL CASE: TOTAL HIP ARTHROPLASTY VERSUS HEMIARTHROPLASTY FOR DISPLACED NECK OF FEMUR FRACTURES

Case History

A 75-year-old gentleman slips inside his kitchen and falls onto his right hip. He was brought into the Emergency Department by ambulance. The plain radiographs confirm a displaced subcapital NOF fracture. He suffers from moderately severe Parkinson's disorder, which is visibly progressing according to his wife in spite of the patient being compliant with his treatment. He furniture walks and has already fallen twice this year. He denies any other significant past medical history. He is also starting to be more forgetful and finding it difficult to find his words. According to this study, what management options should be offered to this patient?

Suggested Answer

The optimal treatment for displaced subcapital NOF fracture in this patient is HA, as it reduces the risk of postoperative dislocations. Arthroplasty is often the preferred option for a displaced (intracapsular) NOF fracture. In active elderly patients and those with preexisting arthritic hip pain, THA is the treatment of choice. As a long-term solution, it has equivalent functional outcome if not better compared to HA, but lower risk of reoperation. There is no difference in mortality, infection, or complication rates. However, the risk of dislocation compared to HA is greater. Hence, in patients who are at risk of recurrent falls and demonstrate cognitive decline, HA is a safer option. Another option to consider for this patient would be a constrained THA (i.e., dual mobility) if he was more independently mobile and did not have cognitive dysfunction. Another factor to consider for THA is that unlike HA, it ought to be performed by hip specialists (so their availability and resources must be factored in).

References

1. Tol et al. Hemiarthroplasty or total hip arthroplasty for the treatment of a displaced intracapsular fracture in active elderly patients: 12-year follow-up of randomised trial. Bone Joint J. 2017;99-B(2):250–4.
2. Harris. Traumatic arthritis of the hip after dislocation and acetabular fractures: treatment by mold arthroplasty. An end-result study using a new method of result evaluation. J Bone Joint Surg Am. 1969;51(4):737–55.
3. Baker et al. Total hip arthroplasty and hemiarthroplasty in mobile, independent patients with a displaced intracapsular fracture of the femoral neck. A randomized, controlled trial. J Bone Joint Surg Am. 2006;88(12):2583–9.
4. Avery et al. Total hip replacement and hemiarthroplasty in mobile, independent patients with a displaced intracapsular fracture of the femoral neck. J Bone Joint Surg Br. 2011;93-B(8):1045–8.
5. Hedbeck et al. Comparison of bipolar hemiarthroplasty with total hip arthroplasty for displaced femoral neck fractures. J Bone Joint Surg. 2011;93(5):445–50.
6. Keating et al. Randomized comparison of reduction and fixation, bipolar hemiarthroplasty, and total hip arthroplasty. J Bone Joint Surg. 2006;88(2):249–60.
7. Yu et al. Total hip arthroplasty versus hemiarthroplasty for displaced femoral neck fractures: meta-analysis of randomized trials. Clin Orthop Relat Res. 2012;470(8): 2235–43.

8. Burgers et al. Total hip arthroplasty versus hemiarthroplasty for displaced femoral neck fractures in the healthy elderly: a meta-analysis and systematic review of randomized trials. Int Orthop. 2012;36(8):1549–60.
9. HEALTH Investigators. Total hip arthroplasty or hemiarthroplasty for hip fracture. N Engl J Med. 2019;381(23):2199–208.
10. National Institute for Health and Care Excellence. Hip fracture: management. Clinical guideline (CG124). May 2017. www.nice.org.uk/guidance/cg124/chapter/recommendations
11. Getting It Right First Time. A national review of adult elective orthopaedic services in England. March 2015. www.gettingitrightfirsttime.co.uk/wp-content/uploads/2017/06/GIRFT-National-Report-Mar15-Web.pdf
12. Getting It Right First Time. Getting It Right in Orthopaedics. Reflecting on success and reinforcing improvement. A follow-up on the GIRFT national specialty report on orthopaedics. February 2020. www.gettingitrightfirsttime.co.uk/wp-content/uploads/2020/02/GIRFT-orthopaedics-follow-up-report-February-2020.pdf

17

Alignment in Total Knee Arthroplasty

A Comparison of Computer-Assisted Surgery with the Conventional Technique

PIYUSH MAHAPATRA AND DINESH NATHWANI

> Computer-assisted Total Knee Arthroplasty gives a better correction of alignment of the leg and orientation of the components compared with the conventional technique.
>
> —Bäthis et al.[1]

Citation: Bäthis H, Perlick L, Tingart M, Lüring C, Zurakowski D, Grifka J. Alignment in total knee arthroplasty. A comparison of computer-assisted surgery with the conventional technique. J Bone Joint Surg Br. 2004;86-B:682–7.

Research Question: Does computer-assisted surgery yield better correction of limb alignment and improve component position in total knee arthroplasty (TKA)?

Funding: Funding source not reported. Navigation system provided by BrainLAB, Heimsteten, Germany. No other commercial funding or benefits declared.

Year Study Began: August 2002

Year Study Published: 2004

Study Location: Department of Orthopaedics, University of Regensburg, Germany

Who Was Studied: 2 unselected groups of 80 consecutive patients undergoing primary TKA. Patients were allocated to either the computer-assisted or conventional group based on scheduled date of surgery. This was arranged independently by a hospital secretary.

Who Was Excluded: No exclusion criteria were defined with regard to age, gender, the degree of deviation of the axis of the leg, or previous surgery.

How Many Patients: 160

Study Overview: See Figure 17.1.

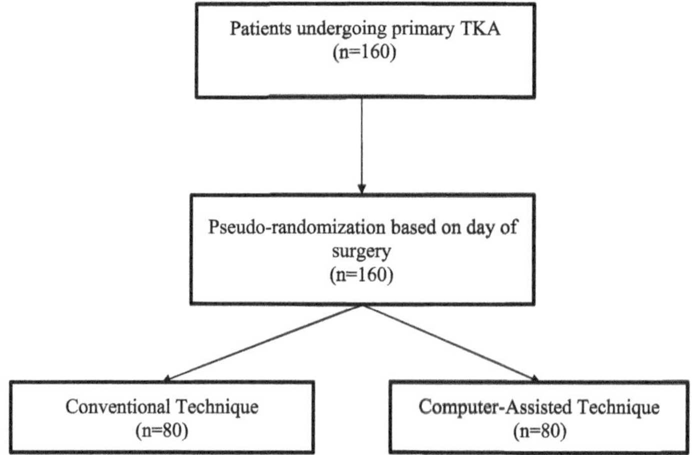

Figure 17.1. Patient allocation.

Study Intervention: The computer-assisted technique was performed with the use of a navigation system (VectorVision CT-free Knee; BrainLAB, Munich, Germany). Key points were registered into the system including hip center, medial and lateral malleoli, and key knee landmarks. Bone surface information was also collected and an adapted bone model was created. The software suggested a proposal for component position based on preset preferences, but adjustments could be made by the surgeon. The navigation system allowed continuous assessment of the limb axis and ligamentous laxity throughout the range of motion (ROM).

In the conventional group, extramedullary instrumentation was used for the tibial component and intramedullary instrumentation for the femoral component. The femoral valgus angle was determined on preoperative long leg weight-bearing radiographs.

Follow-Up: Not clearly defined but outcomes were early postoperative radiographic measures.

Endpoints: Primary outcome was mechanical axis of the leg. Secondary outcomes included femoral and tibial component alignment in both coronal and sagittal views. Outcomes were measured using full length weight-bearing radiographs by 2 independent reviewers.

RESULTS (TABLE 17.1)

- Median deviation in postoperative mechanical axis was 0 degrees in the computer-assisted group vs. 1 degree in the conventional group.
- 96% of TKAs in the computer-assisted group (vs. 78% in the conventional group) had a postoperative mechanical axis within a range of ± 3 degrees.
- Maximum deviation in mechanical axis in the computer-assisted group was 5 degrees vs. 8 degrees in the conventional group.
- Mean deviation in the frontal femoral component angle from the neutral axis was 1.5 degrees in the computer-assisted group and 2.1 degrees in the conventional group. There was a maximum deviation of 4 degrees in the computer-assisted group vs. 8 degrees in the conventional group.
- Mean deviation in the frontal tibial component angle from the neutral axis was 1.2 degrees in the computer-assisted group and 1.5 degrees in the conventional group.
- There was a 2.2-degree mean difference in the lateral femoral component angle and a 2-degree mean difference in the lateral tibial component angle between the 2 groups.
- No conversions from computer-assisted to conventional technique was observed during the study.

Table 17.1 SUMMARY OF RESULTS[a]

Measure	Computer-Assisted Technique	Conventional Technique	*p* Value
Postoperative mechanical axis	0° Interquartile range (−1° to + 1°)	1° Interquartile range (−2° to + 2°)	0.016
Frontal femoral component angle[b]	1.5° (95% CI: 1.2–1.7)	2.1° (95% CI: 1.7–2.4)	< 0.01

Measure	Computer-Assisted Technique	Conventional Technique	*p* Value
Frontal tibial component angle[b]	1.2° (95% CI: 1.0–1.5)	1.5° (95% CI: 1.2–1.7)	0.20
Lateral femoral component angle	7.3° (95% CI: 6.6–8.1)	9.5° (95% CI: 8.5–10.4)	< 0.001
Lateral tibial component angle	2.5° (95% CI: 1.9–3.1)	4.5° (95% CI: 4.0–5.2)	< 0.001
Operating time (min)	78 ± 12	64 ± 11	< 0.01

[a] All angles are measured in degrees. Median values used for postoperative mechanical axis. Mean values used for component alignment.
[b] Measured as deviation from neutral axis.

Criticisms and Limitations: The study did not have true randomization. Patients were allocated to a treatment arm based on the day of the week of surgery, which may introduce selection bias and other confounding factors. Mixed reporting of measures was used (mean and median) without clear reporting of normality of the data set. No patient-reported outcome measure (PROM) data was recorded to reflect on patient satisfaction and preference of technique.

Other Relevant Studies and Information:

- There have been randomized controlled trials that have demonstrated that computer-assisted TKA improves component position and limb alignment[2,3] when compared to conventional techniques
- A large meta-analysis[4] has corroborated the findings of this study that computer-assisted surgery does improve the accuracy and reproducibility of component positioning in TKA. In particular, it reduces the number of patients who are outliers (i.e., outside ± 3 degrees from the mechanical axis).
- Registry data has shown some improvement in revision rates with computer-assisted surgery, with particular revisions for malalignment,[5] and in patients < 65 years.[6] However, there has not been any convincing evidence of improved functional outcomes in patients undergoing computer-assisted TKA.[7]

Summary and Implications: This prospective pseudo-randomized study suggested that there is an improvement in mechanical alignment of the limb after TKA when using a computer-assisted technique. There is an improvement in accuracy and reliability of component positioning (i.e., fewer patients have components positioned outside ± 3 degrees from the mechanical axis). There is an 11–18-minute increase in overall surgical time. It still remains to be seen whether improvements in component positioning lead to improvements in clinical outcomes, pain, PROMs, functionality, loosening, and revision rates.

CLINICAL CASE: ALIGNMENT IN TOTAL KNEE ARTHROPLASTY—A COMPARISON OF COMPUTER-ASSISTED SURGERY WITH THE CONVENTIONAL TECHNIQUE

Case History

A 55-year-old previously active gentleman comes to see you with severe left knee pain secondary to severe tricompartmental knee osteoarthritis as demonstrated on imaging (Figure 17.2). He is keen to return to playing golf on a social level. He has come to see you because he has read that you work in a center that offers computer-assisted knee surgery and he is interested in finding out more. He has seen that cost of the computer-assisted option is higher and wants to speak to you about which option you think is best for him. What will you tell him based on this study?

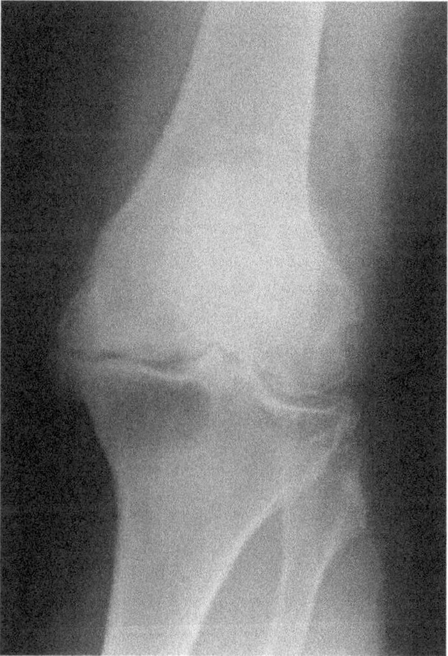

Figure 17.2. Plain anteroposterior radiograph of left knee demonstrating radiological features of severe degenerative joint disease.

Suggested Answer

A recent study comparing computer-assisted TKA with a conventional technique has shown that computer-assisted surgery is more likely to lead to a better-aligned knee joint. There is also a smaller chance of the implant being positioned outside of the normally accepted safe window. There are lots of other studies that report similar results. The surgery itself does take slightly longer, but in experienced hands this is only approximately 15 minutes longer.

There is evidence from the Australian Joint Registry[5] that in his age group (< 65 years), the TKA may last longer if computer-assisted surgery is used. However, it is still not clear if the knee replacement will function any better compared to conventional technique. Overall, computer-assisted surgery allows surgeons to place components more accurately and reliably, which may be of some benefit. However, the conventional technique also has a proven track record.

References

1. Bäthis et al. Alignment in total knee arthroplasty. A comparison of computer-assisted surgery with the conventional technique. J Bone Joint Surg Br. 2004;86(5):682–87.
2. Chauhan et al. Computer-assisted knee arthroplasty versus a conventional jig-based technique. A randomised, prospective trial. J Bone Joint Surg Br. 2004;86(3):372–77.
3. Choong et al. Does accurate anatomical alignment result in better function and quality of life? Comparing conventional and computer-assisted total knee arthroplasty. J Arthroplasty. 2009;24(4):560–69.
4. Mason et al. Meta-analysis of alignment outcomes in computer-assisted total knee arthroplasty surgery. J Arthroplasty. 2007;22(8):1097–106.
5. Dyrhovden et al. Survivorship and relative risk of revision in computer-navigated versus conventional total knee replacement at 8-year follow-up. Acta Orthop. 2016;87(6):592–99.
6. de Steiger et al. Computer navigation for total knee arthroplasty reduces revision rate for patients less than sixty-five years of Age. J Bone Joint Surg Am. 2015;97(8):635–42.
7. Burnett et al. Computer-assisted total knee arthroplasty is currently of no proven clinical benefit: a systematic review. Clin Orthop Relat Res. 2013;471(1):264–76.

18

Reverse Shoulder Arthroplasty versus Hemiarthroplasty for Acute Proximal Humeral Fractures

A Blinded, Randomized, Controlled, Prospective Study

PIERS PAGE, KAPIL SUGAND, AND RISHI DHIR

> The findings of this study indicated that reverse shoulder arthroplasty (RSA) was superior to hemiarthroplasty (HA) with respect to pain, functional outcome, and revision rate.
>
> —Sebastiá-Forcada et al.[1]

Citation: Sebastiá-Forcada E, Cebrián-Gómez R, Lizaur-Utrilla A, Gil-Guillén V. Reverse shoulder arthroplasty versus hemiarthroplasty for acute proximal humeral fractures. A blinded, randomized, controlled, prospective study. J Shoulder Elbow Surg. 2014;23(10):1419–26.

Research Question: Does performing a reverse total shoulder arthroplasty (RTSA) instead of the traditional hemiarthroplasty (HA) for complex proximal humeral fractures in the elderly yield superior outcomes?

Funding: No funding statement provided

Year Study Began: 2009

Year Study Published: 2014

Study Location: Alicante, Spain

Who Was Studied: Patients > 70 years with acute, complex proximal humeral fractures and who were candidates for shoulder arthroplasty. Displaced 4-part fractures, 3-part fracture-dislocations, and head-split fractures with more than 40% joint surface involvement were considered complex. Patients with apparent rotator cuff injuries identified intraoperatively were not excluded.

Who Was Excluded: Patients with contraindication to surgery, previous shoulder surgery, ipsilateral upper limb fracture, or neurological disorders were excluded.

How Many Patients: 62

Study Overview: See Figure 18.1.

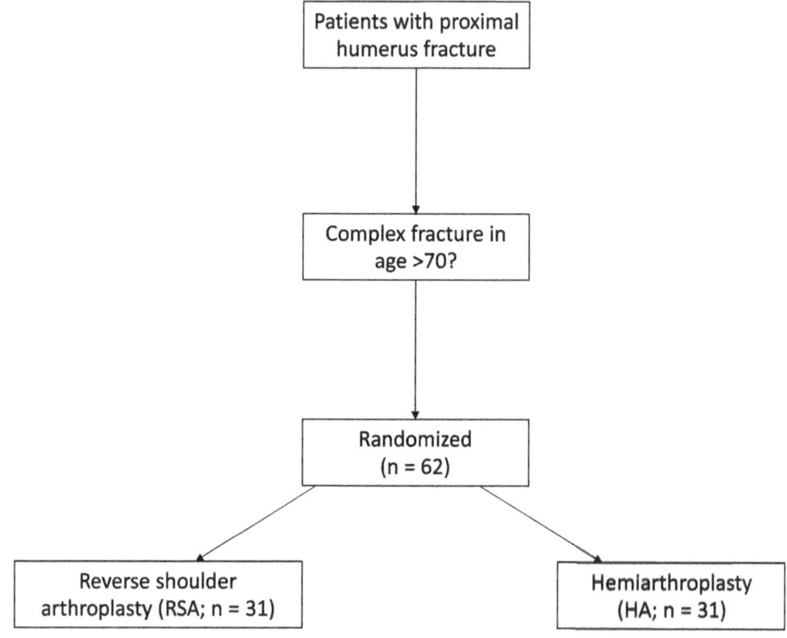

Figure 18.1. Study overview.

Study Intervention: A standard surgical technique and protocol were used for this study, with all procedures performed by 2 surgeons experienced in shoulder surgery with a standardized technique and setup. Patients in the HA group underwent surgery using the SMR modular system (Lima, Italy) with a deltopectoral approach, preservation of deltoid insertion, and biceps tenodesis, and implanted in 30-degree retroversion. Those in the RTSA group underwent surgery again through the deltopectoral approach using the SMR modular system with a titanium alloy, hydroxyapatite-coated glenosphere implanted with 10 degrees of inferior inclination and neutral version using 2 screws, and the humeral component implanted with 20 degrees of retroversion using a chamfered cross-linked polyethylene liner. Both groups were immobilized in a sling for 2 weeks postoperatively.

Follow-Up: Mean 28.5 (24–49) months

Endpoints: The primary outcome measure was the Constant-Murley (CM) shoulder outcome score,[2] which is a multi-item functional scale assessing pain severity, function (e.g., activities of daily living), range of motion (ROM), and strength of the affected shoulder. Secondary outcomes were University of California—Los Angeles (UCLA;[3] a shoulder rating scale encompassing pain, function, ROM, strength and satisfaction) and Disabilities of the Arm, Shoulder, and Hand (QuickDASH;[4] a 30-item questionnaire quantifying physical function and symptoms in musculoskeletal upper limb disorders) scores.

RESULTS (TABLE 18.1)

- *Timing:* Mean time interval between trauma and surgery was 5.1 days (range 1–12 days). Mean operative time was 90.4 (range 80–120) minutes for the RTSA group and 80.2 (range 57–110) minutes for the HA group ($p = 0.001$). Mean postoperative follow-up (F/U) was 29.4 months (range 24–44 months) in the RTSA group and 27.7 months (range 24–49 months) in the HA group ($p = 0.279$).
- *Baseline:* There were no significant preoperative differences between the groups.
- *Pain*: The RTSA group had no or mild/occasional pain compared to 10 (32%) HA patients with moderate or severe pain ($p = 0.002$).
- *Clinical failure:* 8 (26%) RTSA patients were considered to have a clinical failure (i.e., nonadjusted CM score < 50) compared to 17 (57%) HA patients ($p = 0.013$).
- *Patient-reported outcome measures (PROMs):* The RTSA group had significantly higher CM and UCLA scores, but the HA group had higher DASH scores.
- *Function*: The RTSA group had significantly improved forward elevation, abduction, and external rotation, but there was no difference in internal rotation between groups.
- *Radiological evidence*: There was no significant evidence of loosening of any component in both groups.
- *Role of tuberosity healing:* Failure of the tuberosity to heal in the HA group led to a significantly worse mean CM score and ROM except for rotation. In the RTSA group, the results were irrespective of tuberosities healing.

- *Effect of irreparable cuff tear:* 3 (10%) HA patients had proximal migration with a significantly lower CM score than those without an irreparable cuff tear ($p = 0.001$). However, the mean CM score of the 5 (16%) RTSA patients with an irreparable tear was not significantly different from that of the remaining patients of the HA group ($p = 0.072$). When patients with an irreparable tear were excluded from both groups, the mean CM score was significantly higher in the RTSA group than in the HA group (57.2 vs. 41.4; $p = 0.001$).
- *Revision surgery*: 6 patients (19.4%) in the HA group required revision to RTSA for proximal migration (i.e., massive cuff tear or deficit); 1 patient (3.2%) in the RTSA group required 2-stage revision for deep infection.
- *Complications and revisions*:
- HA group:
  - 1 intraoperative humeral fracture
  - 1 superficial infection
  - 1 manipulation under anesthesia secondary to postoperative stiffness
  - 6 patients with proximal migration requiring revision to RTSA at a mean of 15.6 months (range 11–20 months) because of severe pain and limited function. The CM scores of these patients after revision averaged 21.8 (range 8–51) due to decreased activity level, ROM, and arm positioning.
- RTSA group
  - 1 hematoma that resolved with conservative treatment
  - 1 deep wound infection (*Staphylococcus aureus*) at 13 months postoperatively that required a 2-stage revision
- *Arthroplasty survival: RTSA vs. HA (Figure 18.2)*
  - Considering only revision for any reason as an endpoint, the 40-month survival was 96.8% (95% CI: 90.5%–100%) and 80.0% (95% CI: 65.6%–94.3%; $p = 0.043$) respectively.
  - When revision or clinical failure was used as the endpoint, these were 71.0% (95% CI: 55.1%–86.9%) and 43.3% (95% CI: 25.6%–65.1%; $p = 0.029$) respectively.

Table 18.1 Summary of Key Findings

	RTSA Group	**HA Group**	***p* Value**
Constant score	56.1 (24–80)	40.0 (8–74)	0.001
UCLA score	29.1 (16–34)	21.1 (6–34)	0.001
DASH score	17.5 (12–30)	24.4 (13–41)	0.001
Forward elevation (o)	120.3 (40–180)	79.8 (20–180)	0.001
Abduction (o)	112.9 (50–170)	78.7 (30–150)	0.001
External rotation (o)	4.7 (0–10)	3.3 (0–10)	0.023
Internal rotation (o)	2.7 (0–6)	2.6 (0–6)	0.914
Revision no. (%)	1/31 (3.2)	6/31 (19.4)	

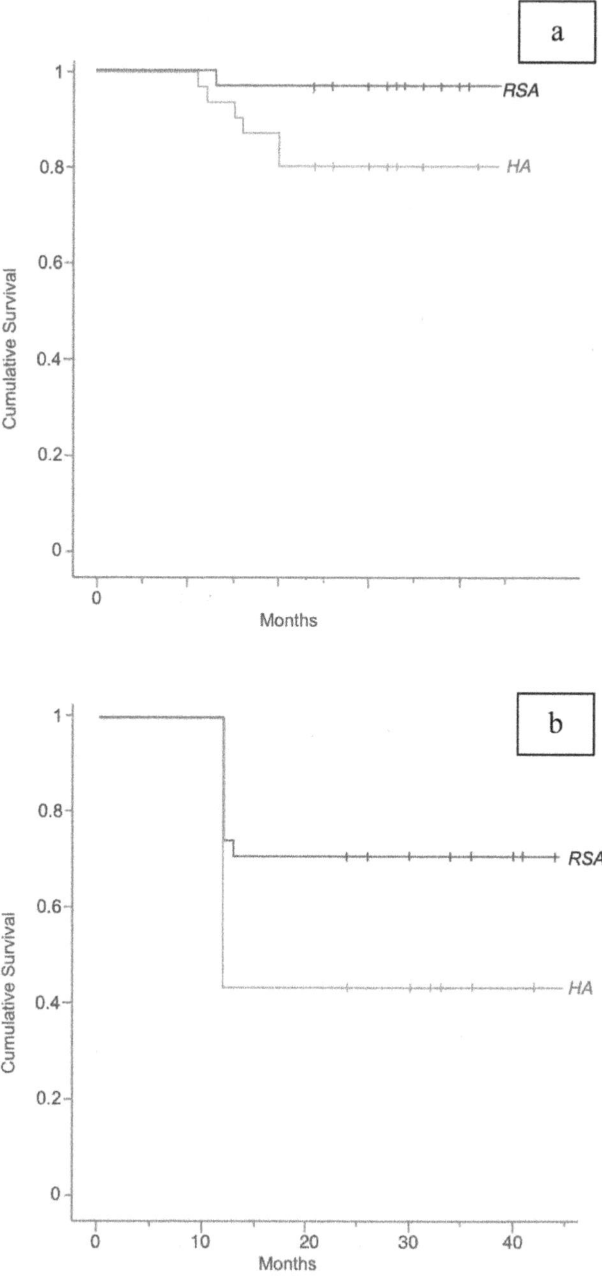

Figure 18.2. (a) Kaplan-Meier arthroplasty survival curves with revision for any reason as the endpoint. (b) Kaplan-Meier arthroplasty survival curves with revision or clinical failure as the endpoint.

Criticisms and Limitations: The study has a short F/U period with respect to arthroplasty, at a mean of over 2 years. Due to the small sample size, it was inadequately powered to compare each treatment option with respect to several key outcomes.

Other Relevant Studies and Information:

- Austin et al.[5] performed a systematic review and meta-analysis of RTSA and HA in proximal humeral fractures in older patients, finding that:
  - Functional outcomes and ROM were improved with lower revision rates in RTSA.
  - Caution should be exercised in interpretation of these results, because minimum F/U was 6 months and most common major complications of RTSA are unlikely to be evident so early.
- Ferrel et al.[6] performed a similar study, with no lower age limit but longer minimum F/U, finding:
  - There was no difference in functional outcome scores.
  - There were lower revision rates with improved forward elevation (118 degrees vs. 108 degrees) and abduction (98 degrees vs. 94 degrees) in the RTSA group compared to the HA group, but reduced external rotational ROM (20 degrees vs. 30 degrees).
  - Caution again is required because of only 1-year F/U.
- The Cochrane Collaborative[7] has deemed the quality of evidence on this topic as "low quality evidence from one trial" by Sebastiá-Forcada et al.[1]
- Jonsson et al.[8] conducted the latest related randomized controlled trial ($n = 84$, mean age 79.5 years, and 90% women). The mean CM score was greater in RTSA vs. HA (58.7 vs. 47.7 points; mean difference of 11.1 points [95% CI: 3.0–18.9; $p = 0.007$]). RTSA had fewer adverse events (3 vs. 4); but greater mean satisfaction (79 mm vs. 63 mm; $p = 0.011$), flexion (125 degrees vs. 90 degrees; $p < 0.001$), and abduction (112 degrees vs. 83 degrees; $p < 0.001$). However, there was no difference in Western Ontario Osteoarthritis of the Shoulder index, pain, or EQ-5D index scores. Among patients aged > 80 years ($n = 38$), there was no difference between RTSA and HA treatment in pain (17 mm vs. 9 mm; $p = 0.17$) or shoulder satisfaction (77 mm vs. 74 mm; $p = 0.73$).

Summary and Implications: This study randomized 62 patients aged > 70 years with complex proximal humeral fractures to either HA or RTSA. Patients in the RTSA group had better CM scores, forward elevation, and abduction but relatively short F/U for arthroplasty. Depending on the surgical skillset, availability of instrumentation, and patient's suitability as well as longer duration of surgery, RTSA ought to be considered compared to HA. Low revision rates were seen in both groups, but with a short F/U and a study design not equipped to detect this outcome.

CASE STUDY: COMPLEX PROXIMAL HUMERAL FRACTURE IN THE OLDER PATIENT

Case History

Mr. A is a right-hand-dominant 74-year-old retired headteacher who likes to spend time in his garden and workshop. He is the main carer for his wife, who has advanced Parkinson's disorder, and bowls in his spare time. He fell whilst out walking last week, sustaining an isolated injury seen in Figure 18.3. The patient is known to have hypertension, borderline diabetes mellitus, and hypercholesterolemia. He has had a history of vitamin D deficiency and has only been offered supplements by his doctor recently. Based on this study, how should this patient be managed?

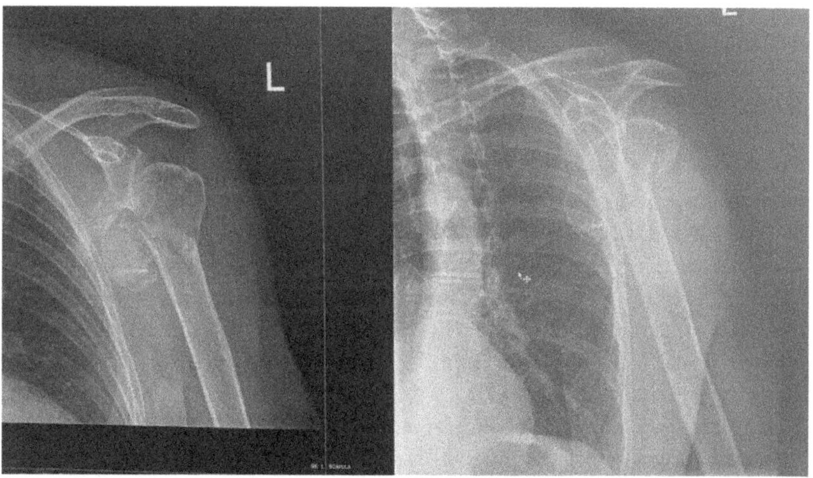

Figure 18.3. Plain radiographs of non-reconstructible proximal humeral fracture.

Suggested Answer

This is a challenging injury, as the fracture is highly comminuted, and both the age group and mechanism suggest that this is a fragility fracture. Hence, bone quality is likely to be suboptimal. Computed axial tomography imaging may better delineate the morphology of the fracture, but, assuming that this demonstrated the fracture to be as complex as appears here, the patient should be counseled about conservative vs. surgical options as well as secondary pharmacological prevention. Principally, there are concerns that fixation may fail and may also entail a prolonged period of reduced function in the immediate postoperative period. By contrast, some form of replacement surgery may permit earlier return to function. Primarily, it is worth considering whether the patient would benefit most from RTSA or HA. According to Sebastiá-Forcada et al.,[1] PROMs, forward elevation, and abduction were all improved in the RTSA group without an increase in revision rate. Nevertheless, with a short F/U period of over 2 years, other postoperative complications including notching and associated loosening may not have yet become apparent, which should be discussed and documented during the formal consenting process.

References

1. Sebastiá-Forcada et al. Reverse shoulder arthroplasty versus hemiarthroplasty for acute proximal humeral fractures. A blinded, randomized, controlled, prospective study. J Shoulder Elbow Surg. 2014;23(10):1419–26.
2. Constant et al. A clinical method of functional assessment of the shoulder. Clin Orthop Relat Res. 1987;214:160–4.
3. Amstutz et al. UCLA anatomic total shoulder arthroplasty. Clin Orthop Relat Res. 1981;155:7–20.
4. Beaton et al. Development of the QuickDASH. J Bone Joint Surg Am. 2005;87(5):1038–46.
5. Austin et al. Decreased reoperations and improved outcomes with reverse total shoulder arthroplasty in comparison to hemiarthroplasty for geriatric proximal humerus fractures. J Orthop Trauma. 2019;33(1):49–57.
6. Ferrel et al. Reverse total shoulder arthroplasty versus hemiarthroplasty for proximal humeral fractures: a systematic review. J Orthop Trauma. 2015;29(1):60–8.
7. Handoll et al. Interventions for treating proximal humeral fractures in adults. Cochrane Database Syst Rev. 2015;11:CD000434.
8. Jonsson et al.; Collaborators in the SAPF Study Group. Reverse total shoulder arthroplasty provides better shoulder function than hemiarthroplasty for displaced 3- and 4-part proximal humeral fractures in patients aged 70 years or older: a multicenter randomized controlled trial. J Shoulder Elbow Surg. 2021;30(5):994–1006.

19

Should Acute Scaphoid Fractures Be Fixed?

A Randomized Controlled Trial

ANNA PANAGIOTIDOU AND MIKE ELVEY

> Early internal fixation of minimally displaced fractures of the scaphoid waist, which would heal in a cast, could lead to overtreatment of a large proportion of such fractures. Thus, we recommend an alternative approach of "aggressive" conservative treatment. This involves identification of a delayed or a non-union at around six weeks and surgical stabilization of only these fractures.
>
> —Dias et al.[1]

Citation: Dias JJ, Wildin CJ, Bhowal B, Thompson JR. Should acute scaphoid fractures be fixed? A randomized controlled trial. J Bone Joint Surg Am. 2005;87(10):2160–8.

Research Question: How do the functional outcomes and union rates compare when acute scaphoid waist fractures are treated with open reduction and internal fixation (ORIF) vs. cast immobilization?

Funding: None

Year Study Began: Data collected from October 1996 to November 1999

Year Study Published: 2005

Study Location: Leicester Royal Infirmary, UK

Who Was Studied: All skeletally mature patients of working age with a clear, but minimally displaced or undisplaced, bicortical fracture through the scaphoid waist that were seen in the clinic within a week from the time of injury.

Who Was Excluded: Patients with preexisting upper limb symptoms, associated injuries, unicortical fractures, tuberosity fractures, and trans-scaphoid perilunate dislocations.

How Many Patients: 88

Study Overview: See Figure 19.1.

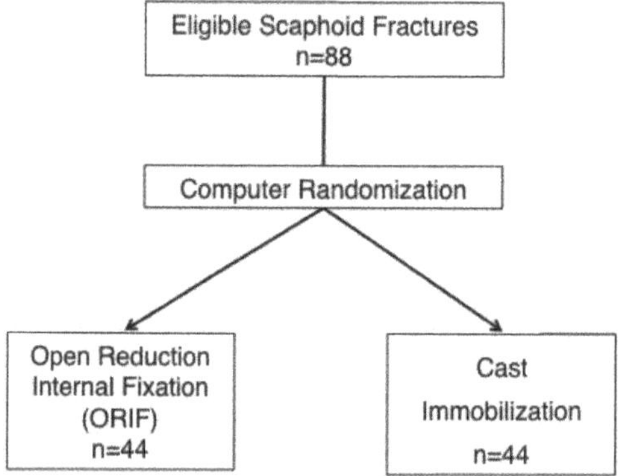

Figure 19.1. Summary of the study design.

Study Intervention: Patients randomized to the ORIF group underwent surgery at a mean of 9.2 days postinjury. A volar approach was utilized, allowing exposure of the fractured scaphoid. The fracture was then fixed with a Herbert headless compression screw. Patients were placed in a bulky dressing for 2 weeks postoperatively and were able to move the hand and wrist.

Patients randomized to nonoperative management were immobilized in a functional below-elbow cast for 8 weeks. This cast did not include the thumb, and the wrist was held in a slightly dorsiflexed position. After 8 weeks the patients were allowed to mobilize the hand and wrist.

Posttreatment all patients were encouraged to return to all activities that did not pose a risk of a fall or injury to the hand.

Follow-Up: All patients underwent clinical and radiographical assessment at 2, 8, 12, 26, and 52 weeks.

Endpoints: Outcome measures of pain, tenderness, range of motion (ROM), grip strength, and Patient Evaluation Measure (PEM) scores were assessed clinically, and time to union was assessed radiographically at each follow-up (F/U). Return to work and ability to perform work tasks comfortably were late outcome measures.

RESULTS (TABLE 19.1)

Data from both groups underwent repeated-measured analysis to determine the following:

i. Treatment effect (i.e., the overall difference between treatments)
ii. Treatment by visit interaction (i.e., the difference of treatment at each F/U visit)
   - *Overall*: Cast immobilization vs. ORIF showed no difference in the overall treatment effect or in the treatment-by-visit interaction for pain and tenderness.
   - *PEM score*: This was not calculated at baseline but F/U assessment from 2 weeks onward showed a significant treatment effect.
   - *Union*: 22.7% (n = 10) of fractures treated with cast immobilization did not show evidence of union on plain scaphoid radiographs at 12 weeks and showed persistence of a fracture gap on computed axial tomography (CAT) scanning at 16 weeks.
   - *Grip strength*: This showed a significant treatment effect for ORIF compared to cast immobilization. The increased grip strength was most marked at 8 and 12 weeks for the ORIF group and remained significant at 1 year.
   - *ROM*: ROM did not show an overall treatment effect. Patients who underwent ORIF had a significantly better ROM at 8 weeks F/U compared to cast immobilization. However, at 12 weeks this difference was no longer present.
   - *Return to work*: The ORIF group returned to work within 5 weeks and the cast immobilization group returned to work within 6 weeks. Both groups were able to perform work tasks comfortably within 2 weeks of return to work.
   - *Complications:* There were no complications in the cast immobilization group. There were no major complications in the ORIF group. There was a 30% incidence of minor complications, the majority of which were related to the scar, and none required further surgery.

Table 19.1 Summary of the Study's Key Findings

Outcomes	**ORIF vs. Cast Immobilization**			
	Overall Treatment Effect	***p* Value**	**Treatment by Visit (Follow-Ups)**	***p* Value**
Pain	No difference	$p = 0.75$	No difference	$p = 0.73$
Tenderness	No difference	$p = 0.57$	No difference	$p = 0.1$
ROM	No difference	$p = 0.24$	Improved ROM for ORIF only at week 8, no difference thereafter	$\mathbf{p = 0.001}$
Grip strength	Overall improved grip strength for ORIF group	$\mathbf{p = 0.006}$	Most significant improvement in grip strength for ORIF group seen at weeks 8 and 12	$\mathbf{p = 0.025}$
PEM score	Overall better PEM score for ORIF group	$\mathbf{p = 0.023}$	No difference	$p = 0.13$
Radiographic union	—	—	10 fractures treated with cast immobilization showed evidence of nonunion vs. 0 fractures treated with ORIF	$\mathbf{p = 0.001}$

Criticisms and Limitations: There was potential to bias in both clinical and radiological assessments as neither the authors nor the patients were blinded to the treatment allocation secondary to the presence of a scar and metalwork. The authors used an open volar approach (rather than a percutaneous approach, which has become a standard approach for un/minimally displaced scaphoid waist fractures). This is likely to be a key factor in their 30% complication rate, the majority of which were related to the scar.

Other Relevant Studies and Information:

- Davis et al.[2] published on the prediction of outcome of nonoperative management. Summarized from the results of a number of smaller studies, the key findings include:
  - Experts were unable to accurately predict union based on initial radiograph findings (pattern/comminution/classification).
  - Experts were unable to predict union based on initial CAT findings—all undisplaced fractures united, and one-third of displaced fractures failed to unite.

- Less than 50% of fractures with 2 mm or more dorsal displacement on a 4-week CAT scan progressed to union.
- Dias et al.[3] have recently presented the results of the Scaphoid Waist Internal Fixation for Fractures Trial (SWIFFT) study, a multicenter randomized controlled trial evaluating early surgical intervention of scaphoid waist fractures with cast immobilization and expedited fixation of nonunions. At 1 year there was no clinical difference between both groups, and cast treatment was significantly more cost effective without the risk of operative complications.

Summary and Implications: This study suggests that most of the benefits of early fixation of undisplaced/minimally displaced scaphoid waist fractures, including return of grip strength and ROM, are transient. Operative management did not significantly reduce the time to return to work. Surgery improved union rates; however, this was associated with a 30% (minor) complication rate and, if universally employed, would result in the operative management of a large number of fractures that would otherwise heal in a cast. Due to an inability to accurately predict which fractures will unite without intervention, the authors proposed "aggressive conservative treatment," reserving surgery for fractures with a clear gap on CAT after 6 weeks of cast immobilization.

CLINICAL CASE: ACUTE SCAPHOID FRACTURES: TO TREAT OR NOT TO TREAT?

Case History

A 29-year-old right-hand-dominant self-employed electrician is seen in the fracture clinic 5 days following a fall onto his dominant hand sustained on a night out. He is a fit and well nonsmoker with no previous injuries. Clinical examination reveals isolated midanatomical snuff box tenderness. A plain radiograph is suggestive of a scaphoid waist fracture. An urgent CAT scan confirms a minimally displaced waist fracture in the midthird. The patient is keen to return to work as soon as possible and is willing to undergo surgery if this would help. Based on the results of this study, how should the patient be counseled?

Suggested Answer

This study suggests that most of the benefits of early surgery are transient, and nonunion following cast immobilization can be successfully managed with delayed surgery. Predicting which fractures will not unite with a cast remains the main clinical challenge, and adopting a policy of early intervention for all scaphoid waist fractures would result in overmanagement of a large number of patients. For this patient, this study has shown that he is unlikely to be able to return to heavy manual work any quicker following surgery than cast immobilization providing that his fracture heals. He should be able to perform light tasks comfortably after 2 weeks of cast treatment. There is likely to be temporary stiffness for several weeks after the cast is removed, which will normalize by 3 months. Surgery is associated with improved healing rates; however, it has a high (minor) complication rate and may be unnecessary with no clear functional benefit.

References

1. Dias et al. Should acute scaphoid fractures be fixed? A randomized controlled trial. J Bone Joint Surg Am. 2005;87(10):2160–8.
2. Davis. Prediction of outcome of non-operative treatment of acute scaphoid waist fracture. Ann R Coll Surg Engl. 2013;95(3):171–6.
3. Dias et al. Scaphoid Waist Internal Fixation for Fractures Trial (SWIFFT) protocol: a pragmatic multi-centre randomised controlled trial of cast treatment versus surgical fixation for the treatment of bi-cortical, minimally displaced fractures of the scaphoid waist in adults. BMC Musculoskelet Disord. 2016;17:248.

20

Primary Arthroscopic Stabilization for a First-Time Anterior Dislocation of the Shoulder

A Randomized, Double-Blind Trial

ANGELOS ASSIOTIS AND HARPAL SINGH UPPAL

> Patients who are thirty-five years of age or younger and are treated by an anatomic arthroscopic repair of the anteroinferior aspect of the labrum after a first-time shoulder dislocation have a significantly reduced risk of recurrent instability compared with those who have an arthroscopic examination and lavage alone. . . . However, the benefits of primary stabilization must be considered together with its drawbacks.
>
> —Robinson et al.[1]

Citation: Robinson CM, Jenkins PJ, White TO, Ker A, Will E. Primary arthroscopic stabilization for a first-time anterior dislocation of the shoulder. A randomized, double-blind trial. J Bone Joint Surg Am. 2008;90(4):708–21.

Research Question: Should young adults under the age of 35 years with a first-time anterior shoulder dislocation be treated with an arthroscopic Bankart repair or with an arthroscopic examination and lavage of the glenohumeral joint?

Funding: None

Year Study Began: 2001

Year Study Published: 2008

Study Location: Royal Infirmary of Edinburgh, Scotland

Who Was Studied: Consecutive unselected patients between 15 and 35 years at the time of first-time anterior dislocation of the shoulder, presenting locally. They had radiographic confirmation of dislocation caused by an external force, presenting to the shoulder clinic within 2 weeks after the dislocation.

Who Was Excluded: The authors excluded patients who experienced anterior shoulder dislocations following seizures or with atraumatic instability, patients who declined participation in the study or randomization, and patients with associated fractures of the glenoid or proximal humerus or other concomitant musculoskeletal injury.

How Many Patients: 84

Study Overview: See Figure 20.1.

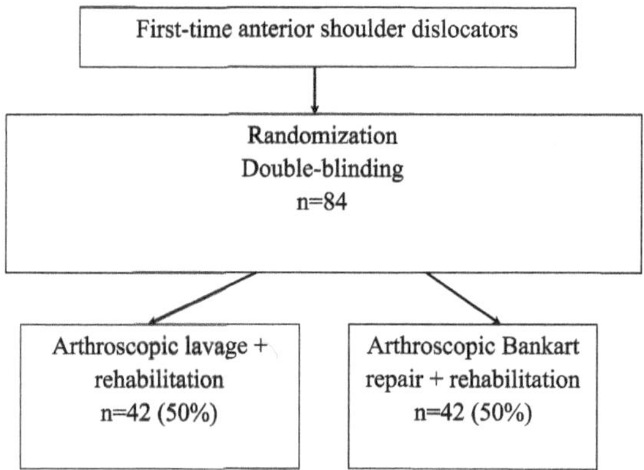

Figure 20.1. Summary of study design.

Study Intervention: All patients were operated on by the same surgeon. Patients in the lavage group underwent arthroscopic examination of the joint, evacuation of the hemarthrosis, and lavage with 3 liters of fluid. Patients in the Bankart repair group underwent irrigation as above and then went on to have their capsulolabral lesion repaired with absorbable suture anchors. If noted during the procedure, they also underwent repair of superior labral tear from anterior to posterior and osseous Bankart lesions, which were not initially noticed on plain radiographs at presentation. Both groups were subsequently treated in an identical manner, with a sling in internal rotation/neutral abduction for 6 weeks. Pendulum exercises commenced after the procedure, and following sling removal at 6 weeks all patients underwent a physiotherapist-supervised rehabilitation program. Unrestricted movement commenced at 12 weeks postoperatively.

Follow-Up: Final follow-up (F/U) at 2 years after primary dislocation. Patients were also followed up at 6 weeks, 3 months, 6 months, and 1 year after shoulder dislocation.

Endpoints: Primary endpoint was recurrent radiographic and/or clinical instability within 2 years after the primary shoulder dislocation. Secondary outcomes were functional outcome scores (Disabilities of the Arm, Shoulder, and Hand[2] [DASH; questionnaire quantifying physical function and symptoms in musculoskeletal upper limb disorders], SF-36[3] [outcome measure tool utilized for self-reported measure of health], Western Ontario Shoulder Instability Index[4] [WOSI; 21-item self-assessment of shoulder function for patients with instability problems]) at 6, 12, and 24 months, patient satisfaction, range of motion (ROM), and direct health service costs at 2 years after initial dislocation.

RESULTS (TABLE 20.1)

- *Complications:* The arthroscopic Bankart repair group, compared to the lavage group, had a significant reduction to the relative risk of a radiographically proven repeat dislocation (76%) and overall instability (82%) at 2 years. Survival analysis is depicted in Figure 20.2.

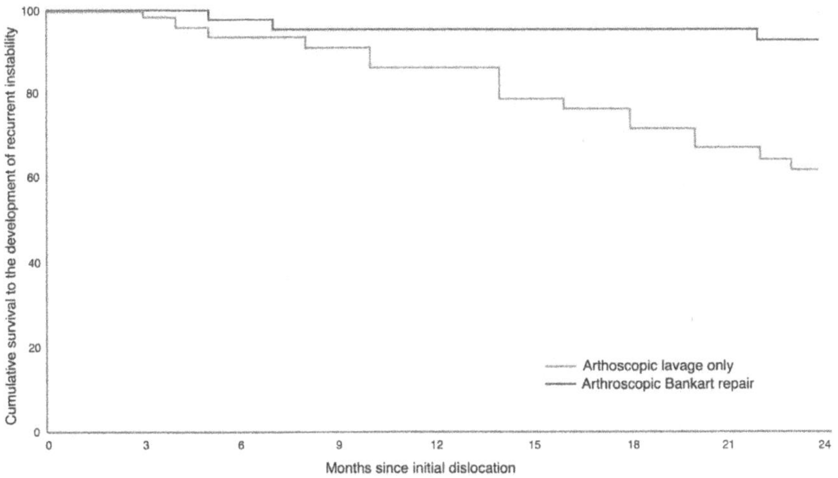

Figure 20.2. Survival analysis after the primary dislocation of both treatment cohorts, with development of all recurrent instability at the endpoint.

- *Instability:* Mean time to recurrent instability was 11.3 months for the Bankart repair group and 13.6 months for the lavage group.
- *Numbers needed to treat (NNT):* If all patients underwent primary arthroscopic Bankart repair, the NNT to prevent 1 patient from sustaining a further dislocation was 4.7 patients.
- *Scores (Figures 20.3a and b):*
  - The Bankart repair group had statistically significant better DASH and WOSI scores at 2 years, compared to the lavage group, but not at 6 or 12 months.
  - In patients with stable shoulders, between the 2 groups there was no difference in the DASH and WOSI scores at any time point.

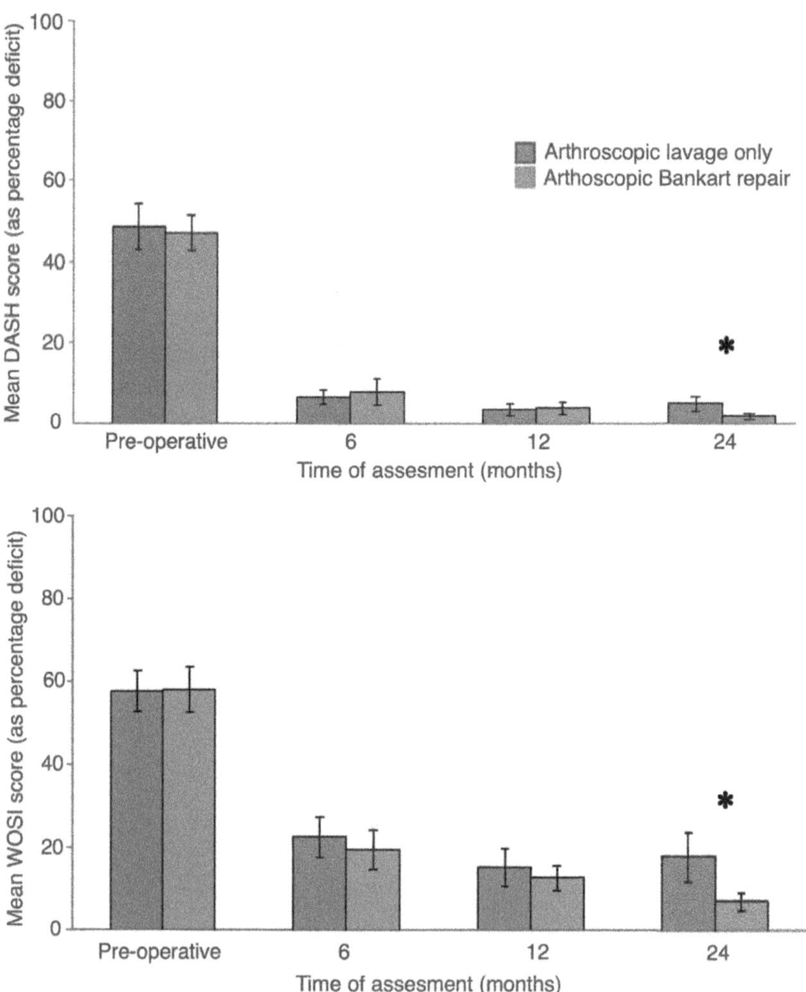

Figure 20.3. (a) Mean DASH scores and (b) mean WOSI scores: % deficit of the score for both cohorts during the 2 years after dislocation. Error bars indicate 95% CI of the mean. * signifies significant difference between cohorts ($p < 0.05$).

- *ROM:* There was no difference at any timepoint between both groups.
- *Cost:* The mean direct cost of treatment in the first 2 years after the primary dislocation was GBP £748.9 *less* for the Bankart repair group compared to the lavage group, despite the initial greater cost of an arthroscopic Bankart repair.

Table 20.1 SUMMARY OF KEY FINDINGS AT 2 YEARS AFTER PRIMARY DISLOCATION

Outcome	Arthroscopic Bankart Repair Group	Arthroscopic Lavage Group	*p* Value
Radiographic repeat dislocation	3/42 (7%)	12/42 (29%)	0.02
All recurrent instability	3/42 (7%)	16/42 (38%)	0.01
Satisfaction	94.1%	74.8%	< 0.001
Relative risk of discontinuing contact sport	—	3.4	0.007

Criticisms and Limitations: Although the primary outcome measure of recurrent instability is defined in the study, it still remains an endpoint that does not offer methodological robustness. It relies on patients' perception of their joint and clinical examination signs, which are examiner dependent. The study as constructed is designed to give an answer with regard to the primary outcome measure. Making multiple further assessments on other unpowered outcome measures increases the probability of the results being subject to type II error. Currently, preoperative investigations of such patients often include computed axial tomography or magnetic resonance imaging arthrogram; at the time of publishing this study these were not as widely available. This should be remembered when considering the pragmatic nature of this study in current practice. There is no conclusive evidence to support that arthroscopic stabilization of primary anterior shoulder dislocations leads to reduced revision rates compared to arthroscopic reconstruction for recurrent shoulder dislocation; one may consider treating specific patients nonoperatively initially, before selecting to operate on that subgroup of patients that go on to develop recurring instability.

Other Relevant Studies and Information:

- 2 other randomized clinical studies reported that primary arthroscopic repair in patients with first-time traumatic anterior shoulder dislocations is preferable compared to nonoperative management, especially in the younger and more active population group.[5,6]

- A level I trial with a considerable long-term F/U demonstrated that open Bankart repair confers improved functional outcomes at 10 years after the dislocation event compared to the group that did not undergo a repair.[7]
- When considering open or arthroscopic Bankart repair, a systematic review failed to demonstrate any significant difference in recurrence of instability or functional outcomes at a mean of 11 years of F/U. The majority of the studies included in this systematic review were level III or level IV, a fact demonstrating the relevant paucity of high-level studies with a long-term F/U.[8]

Summary and Implications: In a carefully designed study, the authors suggest that arthroscopic repair of a primary anterior traumatic shoulder dislocation confers improved functional outcomes and a reduced risk of recurrent instability when compared to arthroscopic lavage. This study helped to establish the significant role of arthroscopic Bankart repair in managing such patients. However, this procedure remains prophylactic and should not be generalized to all patients; there remains a need to consider individualized patient-specific factors when dealing with a first-time anterior shoulder dislocation. Finally, in the years since this study was published, surgical randomized controlled study design has improved, and this study has specific flaws that limit its relevance to the wider population.

CLINICAL CASE: PRIMARY ARTHROSCOPIC BANKART REPAIR IN A YOUNG MALE WITH A FIRST-TIME SHOULDER DISLOCATION

Case History

A 23-year-old, otherwise healthy, left-hand-dominant male patient presents with his first anterior left shoulder dislocation following a fall while playing semiprofessional football. He undergoes a successful reduction under conscious sedation in the Emergency Department and presents to the fracture clinic 10 days after the injury. A teammate of his with a similar injury in the past suggested that all young healthy patients with this injury should have urgent keyhole surgery to have better function and guarantee that the shoulder does not dislocate again. How should this patient be treated according to this study?

Suggested Answer

This study elegantly demonstrated that primary arthroscopic repair of a Bankart lesion confers improved functional outcomes and a reduced risk of recurrent instability at 2 years after surgery. However, it does not demonstrate any functional difference between patients in the 2 groups that have stable shoulders in that timeframe, and it does confirm that surgery is not without risks. A way to approach this case would be to explain that on this occasion, "one size does not fit all," and that any management decision should consider individual patient-specific factors. Although he is a patient at high risk of developing recurrent instability (62% risk at 2 years according to Brownson et al.[9]) and therefore a patient that could benefit from an acute repair according to this study, one would be reasonable to suggest cross-sectional imaging prior to embarking on surgery.[8] Finally, the patient should understand that arthroscopic Bankart repair does not negate the possibility of a future dislocation event.

References

1. Robinson et al. Primary arthroscopic stabilization for a first-time anterior dislocation of the shoulder. A randomized, double-blind trial. J Bone Joint Surg Am. 2008;90(4):708–21.
2. Hudak et al. Development of an upper extremity outcome measure: the DASH (Disabilities of the Arm, Shoulder, and Hand). Am J Indust Med. 1996;29(6):602–8.
3. Ware Jr. The MOS 36-Item Short-Form Health Survey (SF-36). I. Conceptual framework and item selection. Med Care. 1992;30:473–83.
4. Kirkley et al. The development and evaluation of a disease-specific quality of life measurement tool for shoulder instability. The Western Ontario Shoulder Instability Index (WOSI). Am J Sports Med. 1998;26(6):764–72.
5. Bottoni et al. Arthroscopic versus open shoulder stabilization for recurrent anterior instability: a prospective randomized clinical trial. Am J Sports Med. 2006;34(11):1730–7.
6. Kirkley et al. Prospective randomized clinical trial comparing the effectiveness of immediate arthroscopic stabilization versus immobilization and rehabilitation in first traumatic anterior dislocations of the shoulder: long-term evaluation. Arthroscopy. 2005;21(1):55–63.
7. Jakobsen et al. Primary repair versus conservative treatment of first-time traumatic anterior dislocation of the shoulder: a randomized study with 10-year follow-up. Arthroscopy. 2007;23(2):118–23.
8. Harris et al. Long-term outcomes after Bankart shoulder stabilization. Arthroscopy. 2013;29(5):920–33.
9. Brownson et al. BESS/BOA Patient Care Pathways: traumatic anterior shoulder instability. Shoulder Elbow. 2015;7(3):214–26.

21

A Controlled Trial of Arthroscopic Knee Surgery versus Placebo for Osteoarthritis

TIM MAHESWARAN, KAPIL SUGAND, AND KHALED M. SARRAF

Study's Nickname: The Moseley Trial

> In this controlled trial involving patients with osteoarthritis of the knee, the outcomes after arthroscopic lavage or arthroscopic debridement were no better than those after a placebo procedure.
>
> —MOSELEY ET AL.[1]

Citation: Moseley JB, O'Malley K, Petersen NJ, Menke TJ, Brody BA, Kuykendall DH, Hollingsworth JC, Ashton CM, Wray NP. A controlled trial of arthroscopic surgery for osteoarthritis of the knee. N Engl J Med. 2002;347:81–8.

Research Question: Does arthroscopic knee surgery (washout/debridement) provide any benefit over a placebo/sham procedure?

Funding: Grant from the Department of Veteran Affairs

Year Study Began: 1995

Year Study Published: 2002

Study Location: Houston Veterans Affairs Medical Center

Who Was Studied: Age < 75 years with documented knee osteoarthritis (OA). These patients had persistent knee pain despite having completed at least 6 months of nonoperative treatment.

Who Was Excluded: Patients who have had previous knee arthroscopy in the preceding 2 years and those with advanced OA of the knee with a severity score of over 9 or severe clinical deformity. Patients with serious medical comorbidities were also excluded.

How Many Patients: 180

Study Overview: See Figure 21.1

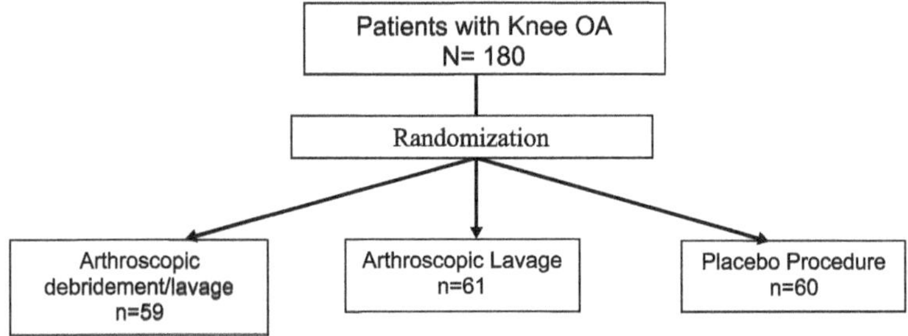

Figure 21.1. Summary of the trial design.

Study Intervention: 180 patients were split into 3 groups: (1) arthroscopic debridement/lavage group that included a standard setup under general anesthesia (GA), with diagnostic arthroscopy, a washout with 10 liters of normal saline, removal of any loose bodies, osteophytes, and debridement of the meniscus; (2) arthroscopic lavage group with a standard setup under GA, followed by a diagnostic arthroscopy and lavage including just a washout with 10 liters of normal saline; and (3) sham procedure performed under sedation using an opiate and short-acting benzodiazepine, with arthroscopy portal incisions only and no instrumentation placed into the knee; however, the knee was taken through a range of movements to simulate an arthroscopy. A standard postoperative protocol was followed for all patients, which included a stay overnight and then a gradual physiotherapy regime together with monitored analgesic intake.

Follow-Up:

- 2 weeks
- 6 weeks
- 3 months
- 6 months
- 12 months
- 18 months
- 24 months

Endpoints: The primary endpoint was assessing the mean Knee Specific Pain Scale (KSPS) score at 2 years after the surgery. Secondary outcomes were measured based on scoring systems for pain utilizing Arthritis Impact Measurement Scales[2] (AIMS2-P; arthritis-specific health status measure assessing physical function, pain, psychological status, social support, health perceptions, demographics, and treatment) and physical function with AIMS2-WB (5-item Walking–Bending subscale), the Physical Functioning Scale (PFS; objective measure of time taken to walk 30 m and to ascend/descend a flight of stairs as quickly as possible), and SF-36[3] (outcome measure tool utilized for self-reported measure of health and quality of life).

RESULTS (TABLE 21.1)

- *Demographics*: Average age 52.3 years, 92.8% male, and 60% Caucasian
- *Participation*: 44% declined
- *OA severity*: Mild 28.9%, moderate 46.1%, and severe 25%
- *Intervention comparisons*: At no point did either arthroscopic intervention (i.e., lavage or debridement) group outperform (i.e., statistically insignificant) the placebo group (sham) with respect to:
  - *Pain*: No significant difference in arthritis pain at 1 or 2 years (Figure 21.2)

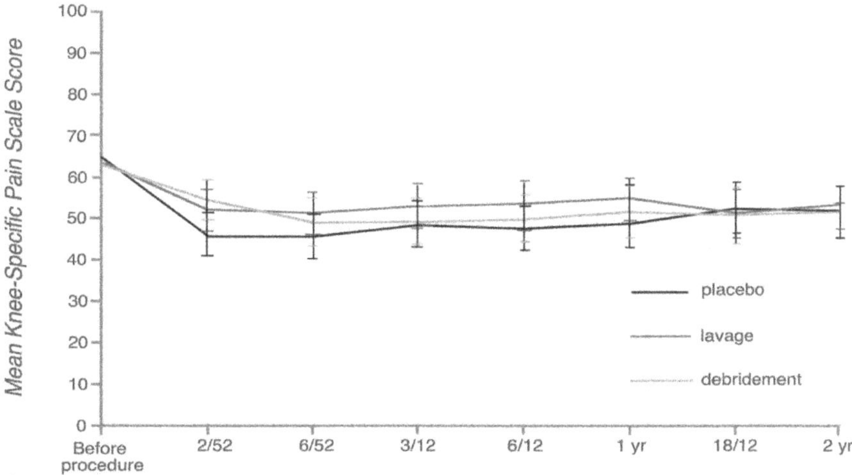

Figure 21.2. Mean (±95% CI) on the Knee-Specific Pain Scale. Assessments were made before the procedure and 2 weeks, 6 weeks, 3 months, 6 months, 12 months, 18 months, and 24 months after the procedure. Higher scores indicate poorer functioning.

- *Function:* Mean AIMS2-WB (Figure 21.3)

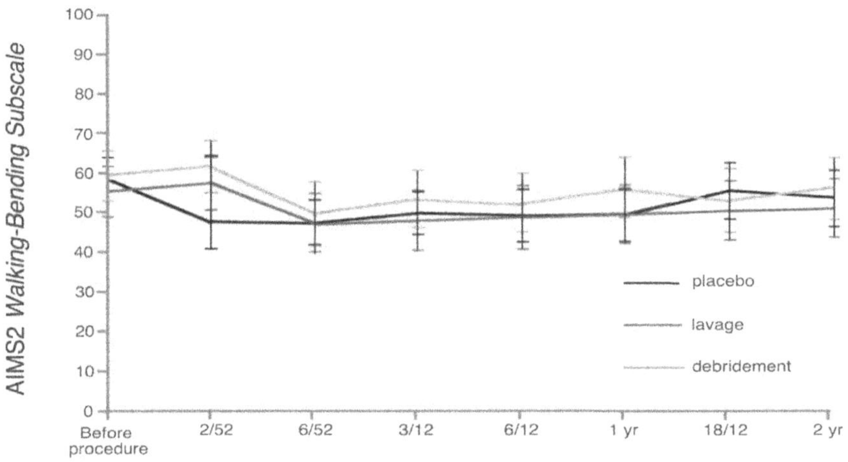

Figure 21.3. Mean (± 95% CI) on the Walking–Bending subscale of the AIMS2. Assessments were made before the procedure and 2 weeks, 6 weeks, 3 months, 6 months, 12 months, 18 months, and 24 months after the procedure. Higher scores indicate poorer functioning.

- *Mean PFS:* Scores were poorer in the debridement group vs. placebo group at 2 weeks (56.0 ± 21.8 vs. 48.3 ± 13.4; $p = 0.02$) and 1 year (52.5 ± 20.3 vs. 45.6 ± 10.2; $p = 0.04$) and showed a trend toward worse functioning at 2 years (52.6 ± 16.4 vs. 47.7 ± 12.0; $p = 0.11$)
- *Statistical analysis:* At almost all time points during follow-up, the CI excluded minimal clinically important differences

Table 21.1 Summary of Results

Follow-Up	Debridement	Lavage	Placebo	*p* Value[a]
		KSPS		
1 year	51.7 ± 22.4	54.8 ± 19.8	48.9 ± 21.9	0.14/0.51
2 years	51.4 ± 23.2	53.7 ± 23.7	51.6 ± 23.7	0.64/0.96
		AIMS2-WB		
1 year	56.4 ± 28.4	49.6 ± 29.1	49.4 ± 25.5	0.98/0.19
2 years	56.4 ± 29.4	51.1 ± 28.3	53.8 ± 27.5	0.61/0.64

[a] *p* value: debridement:placebo/lavage:placebo.

Criticisms and Limitations: This study consisted of a small sample size, single center, and single surgeon data set with most patients being Caucasian males. The study may not be representative of younger patients with early OA or those from an ethnic diversification. The KSPS is not a validated scoring tool for knee OA.

Other Relevant Studies and Information:

- Other studies[4–6] that have utilized validated outcome measures, including randomized controlled trials (RCTs) and meta-analyses, have concurred that arthroscopic debridement in knee OA does not offer much improvement to the patient when compared to nonoperative measures. Although these procedures can lead to a mild improvement, it does not last for too long. The risks of surgery should also be taken into account. Nonoperative measures deserve particular attention in improving patient outcomes and delaying the need for surgery.
- National Institute for Health and Care Excellence (NICE) guidance[7] for knee OA has incorporated this trial as part of its background literature search, suggesting arthroscopic knee surgery is not indicated for the treatment of OA in most circumstances.

Summary and Implications: This landmark RCT was one of the earliest to show no clinical or significant improvement between arthroscopic knee surgery and placebo surgery for knee OA. This trial has helped to establish guidelines toward the role of arthroscopy in OA and was used as evidence to formulate NICE guidelines[5] in the UK. On the other hand, this study has been deemed controversial due to its limitations and conclusions being generalized to all indications for knee arthroscopy. As such, the results of this trial are not representative for younger patients with isolated meniscal or chondral pathology and the treatment of mechanical symptoms (e.g., locking and instability) that may benefit from arthroscopic intervention.

CLINICAL CASE: A CASE OF OSTEOARTHRITIS OF THE KNEE

Case History

A 70-year-old patient presents with a chronic history of knee pain, stiffness, and reduction in his ability to carry out activities of daily living. She has tried conservative management options without success. Weight-bearing radiographs suggest mild to moderate OA. There are no mechanical symptoms mentioned. She is a retired lecturer with no significant past medical or social history. The patient is keen to get back to her usual premorbid activities. Based on this case history, how should this patient be managed according to this trial?

Suggested Answer

This patient clearly has symptoms of early OA of the knee. She has undergone nonoperative measures, but it is important to ascertain exactly what has been attempted. Based on conclusions from the literature, it would be prudent to continue to explore and exhaust all nonoperative interventions for as long as possible and to their maximum capacity prior to considering any surgical options. It is key to be aware that injection therapy with corticosteroids can cause a transient flare-up of OA and can take months to reach maximal effect. According to the study findings, arthroscopic knee surgery would not be beneficial in this case, as there is underlying OA as an irreversible pain trigger as well as an absence of mechanical symptoms. Applying the NICE guideline recommendations would include pain-relieving medication, physiotherapy, and weight reduction programs through a multidisciplinary approach. Conversely, arthroscopy may have a role in such cases with mechanical symptoms as demonstrated by clinical examination and radiological imaging. However, a balance of benefits and risks of surgery is crucial.

References

1. Moseley et al. A controlled trial of arthroscopic surgery for osteoarthritis of the knee. N Engl J Med. 2002;347:81–8.
2. Meenan et al. AIMS2: the content and properties of a revised and expanded Arthritis Impact Measurement Scales health status questionnaire. Arthritis Rheum. 1992;35:1–10.
3. Ware Jr et al. The MOS 36-Item Short-Form Health Survey (SF-36). I. Conceptual framework and item selection. Med Care. 1992;30:473–83.
4. Kirkley et al. A randomized trial of arthroscopic surgery for osteoarthritis of the knee. N Engl J Med. 2008;359(11):1097–107.
5. Thorlund et al. Arthroscopic surgery for degenerative knee: systematic review and meta-analysis of benefits and harms. Br J Sports Med. 2015;49:1229–35.
6. Brignardello-Petersen et al. Knee arthroscopy versus conservative management in patients with degenerative knee disease: a systematic review. BMJ Open. 2017;7: e016114.
7. National Institute for Health and Care Excellence. Arthroscopic knee washout, with or without debridement, for the treatment of osteoarthritis. August 22, 2007. https://www.nice.org.uk/guidance/ipg230/resources/arthroscopic-knee-washout-with-or-without-debridement-for-the-treatment-of-osteoarthritis-pdf-1899865329261253.

22

Surgical versus Nonoperative Treatment for Lumbar Spinal Stenosis Four-Year Results of the Spine Patient Outcome Research Trial

ABDUL NAZEER MOIDEEN AND ASHISH KHURANA

Nickname: SPORT (Spine Patient Outcomes Research Trial) trial

> Patients with spinal stenosis treated surgically showed significantly greater improvement in pain, function, satisfaction, and self-rated progress over four years compared to patients treated non-operatively.
>
> —Weinstein et al.[1]

Citation: Weinstein JN, Tosteson TD, Lurie JD, Tosteson A, Blood E, Herkowitz H, Cammisa F, Albert T, Boden SD, Hilibrand A, Goldberg H, Berven S, An H. Surgical versus nonoperative treatment for lumbar spinal stenosis four-year results of the Spine Patient Outcomes Research Trial. Spine. 2010;35(14):1329–38.

Research Question: Does surgery provide better outcomes for spinal stenosis in comparison to nonoperative care?

Funding: National Institute of Arthritis and Musculoskeletal and Skin Diseases (U01-AR45444), Office of Research on Women's Health, National Institutes of Health, National Institute of Occupational Safety and Health, and Centers for Disease Control and Prevention

Year Study Began: March 2000

Year Study Published: June 2010

Study Location: 13 US medical centers in 11 states

Who Was Studied: All patients with neurogenic claudication and/or radicular symptoms with confirmatory imaging showing lumbar spinal stenosis at 1 or more levels, who were judged to be surgical candidates, and who had ongoing symptoms for a minimum of 12 weeks.

Who Was Excluded: Age < 18 years, symptoms < 12 weeks, previous lumbar spine surgery, not a surgical candidate, cancer, current fracture, infection, and/or spinal deformity.

How Many Patients: 654

Study Overview: See Figure 22.1.

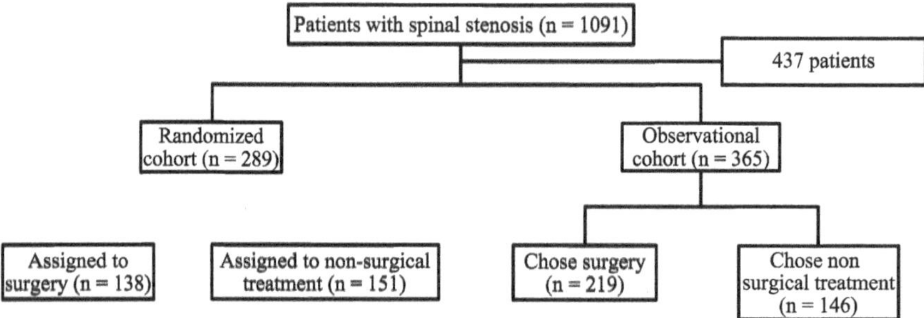

Figure 22.1. Summary of study design.

Study Intervention: Patients in the surgical group received a standard posterior decompressive laminectomy. Patients in the nonsurgical group received physiotherapy, education/counseling with home exercise, and nonsteroidal anti-inflammatory drugs (NSAIDs) if tolerated. Some patients received injections at the discretion of the treating surgeon. Patients willing to participate in the study were randomized, and those who were not willing were treated within the observational cohort. Patients in the surgical group who delayed or declined surgery and those in the nonoperative group who wanted surgery were crossed over.

Follow-Up: 4 years

Endpoints: Primary outcomes were the Oswestry Disability Index[2] (ODI; patient-completed questionnaire resulting in a percentage score of level of function [disability] in activities of daily living in those rehabilitating from low back pain) and SF-36[3] (outcome measure tool utilized for self-reported measure of health and quality of life) bodily pain (BP) and physical function (PF) scales measured at 6 weeks, 3 months, and annually up to 4 years. Secondary outcomes included patient self-reported improvement and satisfaction with current symptoms and care.

RESULTS (TABLE 22.1)

- *Randomized cohort (RC)*
  - 138 were assigned to surgery and 151 to nonoperative treatment.
  - Of those randomized to surgery, 68% received surgery by 4 years.
  - Of those randomized to nonoperative treatment, 49% received surgery by 4 years.
- *Observational cohort (OC)*
  - 219 patients initially chose surgery, and 146 patients initially chose nonoperative treatment.
  - Of those choosing surgery, 97% received surgery by 4 years.
  - Of those choosing nonoperative treatment, 26% received surgery by 4 years.
- *Combined:* In both cohorts combined, 419 patients received surgery, and 235 chose nonoperative treatment.
- *Intention to treat:* The intention-to-treat analysis of the RC showed no differences between surgery and nonoperative care.
- *As treated:* The "as treated" treatment effects significantly favored surgery in both cohorts.
- *Combined analysis*: Treatment effects were significant in favor of surgery for all primary and secondary outcome measures at each time point up to 4 years.

Table 22.1 Summary of Results[a]

	Surgery	**Nonoperative**	**Treatment Effect (95% CI)**	***p* Value**
At 1 year	64.7%	30.7%	33.9% (26.1–41.7)	< 0.001
At 4 years	60.6%	32.4%	28.2% (18.6–37.7)	< 0.001

[a] Proportion of patients who had a change of ≥ 15 on the ODI from baseline. Combined randomized and observational cohort based on the adjusted "as treated" analysis.

Criticisms and Limitations: There was considerable cross-over between the 2 treatment arms, which makes interpretation of results difficult. In addition, there was no clear protocol for nonoperative management, with only 44% of patients receiving physical therapy. Moreover, some patients in the RC reported receiving injections.

Other Relevant Studies and Information:

- Another randomized controlled trial (RCT) involving patients with long-standing moderate lumbar spinal stenosis showed that patients who underwent surgery had a consistent improvement in functional ability up to 6 years.[4]
- A well-designed prospective cohort study showed similar results to the SPORT study for patients who had surgery compared to nonoperative treatment over 4 years.[5]
- As a part of the SPORT trial, other RCTs were performed between surgical and nonoperative management for lumbar disc herniation and degenerative spondylolisthesis.
- For lumbar disc herniation, patients in both the operative and nonoperative groups improved substantially over a 2-year period. However, because of large numbers of patients who crossed over in both directions, conclusions about the superiority or equivalence of the treatments are not possible based on intention-to-treat analysis.[4]
- For degenerative spondylolisthesis and associated spinal stenosis, patients who are treated surgically maintain greater pain relief and improvement in function for 4 years when compared to nonoperative treatment.[5]

Summary and Implications: In this study, an "as treated" analysis combining the RC and OC of patients with spinal stenosis showed significantly greater improvement in pain, function, satisfaction, and self-rated progress over 4 years among patients treated surgically vs. nonoperatively. The 4-year mortality rate was similar in both treatment groups. However, the standard intention-to-treat analysis could not be interpreted due to high crossover, and thus these findings are not definitive.

CLINICAL CASE: SURGERY VERSUS CONSERVATIVE TREATMENT FOR SPINAL STENOSIS

Case History

A 68-year-old man presents to the clinic complaining of lower back pain radiating to both thighs that has been worse on walking for the past year. His symptoms are becoming worse, which is limiting his mobility to 150 yards before he must sit down due to pain. He has no severe comorbidities and no signs of peripheral vascular disease. Clinical examination revealed mild to moderate tenderness in the lumbar spine with no neurological deficit. Magnetic resonance imaging confirmed significant stenosis at L4/5. How should this patient be treated according to the SPORT trial?

Suggested Answer

The patient has severe spinal stenosis with significant symptoms. The results from the SPORT trial have demonstrated that patients with symptomatic spinal stenosis for at least 12 weeks who underwent posterior decompressive laminectomy had significant improvement in as early as 6 weeks. The positive surgical outcome appeared to reach maximal levels by 3–12 months and persisted over 4 years. Patients can be treated conservatively with physical therapy, NSAIDs, and possibly epidural injections; however, the improvement would likely be modest and temporary over time.

References

1. Weinstein et al. Surgical versus nonoperative treatment for lumbar spinal stenosis four-year results of the Spine Patient Outcomes Research Trial. Spine. 2010;35(14):1329–1338.
2. Fairbank et al. The Oswestry disability index. Spine. 2000;25(22):2940–53.
3. Ware Jr et al. The MOS 36-Item Short-Form Health Survey (SF-36). I. Conceptual framework and item selection. Med Care. 1992;30:473–83.
4. Slätis et al. Long-term results of surgery for lumbar spinal stenosis: a randomised controlled trial. Eur Spine J. 2011;20(7):1174–81.
5. Atlas et al. Surgical and nonsurgical management of lumbar spinal stenosis: four-year outcomes from the Maine lumbar spine study. Spine. 2000;25(5):556–62.
6. Weinstein et al. Surgical vs nonoperative treatment for lumbar disk herniation: the Spine Patient Outcomes Research Trial (SPORT): a randomized trial. JAMA. 2006;296(20):2441–50.
7. Weinstein et al. Surgical compared with nonoperative treatment for lumbar degenerative spondylolisthesis. four-year results in the Spine Patient Outcomes Research Trial (SPORT) randomized and observational cohorts. J Bone J Surg. 2009;91(6):1295–304.

23

Long-Term Survivorship of the Hip Following Operatively Treated Acetabular Fracture

ALEXANDER MARTIN AND HANI B. ABDUL-JABAR

> Open reduction and internal fixation of displaced acetabular fractures can successfully prevent the need for subsequent total hip arthroplasty within twenty years in 79% of patients.
>
> —TANNAST ET AL.[1]

Citation: Tannast M, Najibi S, Matta, JM. Two to twenty-year survivorship of the hip in 810 patients with operatively treated acetabular fractures. J Bone Joint Surg. Am. 2012;94(17):1559–67.

Research Question: What are the long-term outcomes following an operatively managed acetabular fracture, and what factors are predictive of conversion to total hip arthroplasty (THA) or hip arthrodesis?

Funding: Swiss National Science Foundation and Association for Orthopaedic Research

Year Study Began: Prospective data collection commenced 1980

Year Study Published: 2012

Study Location: Hip and Pelvis Institute, Santa Monica, California

Who Was Studied: A prospectively collected database recorded all adult patients presenting with an acetabular fracture. Only those who underwent operative management with a minimum of 2 years of follow-up (F/U) were included.

Who Was Excluded: Patients with an acetabular fracture that were treated nonoperatively, who required acute primary THA in the opinion of the treating surgeon, and with periprosthetic acetabular fractures were excluded.

How Many Patients: 816

Study Overview: See Figure 23.1.

Study Intervention: This was a prospective cohort study in which all patients managed with fixation of acetabular fracture were included. This was a single-surgeon series spanning over a 26-year period. The operative intervention was formal open reduction and internal fixation (ORIF) via an approach utilizing a standardized decision-making protocol based upon the original work by Letournel and Judet.[2] The approach utilized was selected at the discretion of the senior author and included Kocher-Langenback, ilioinguinal, and extended iliofemoral techniques. Plate and screw or screw-only fixation constructs were performed based upon preoperative planning and intraoperative findings.

Follow-Up: The mean F/U was 10.3 ± 6.9 years (range 2–28.6 years); 299 hips had F/U spanning over 10 years.

Endpoints: The primary outcome was conversion to total hip replacement (THR), providing a survivorship value of the hip following treatment. The THR rate was utilized as a surrogate marker of a successful outcome. Other postoperative outcomes included accuracy of reduction as graded by the treating surgeon both intraoperatively and on postoperative plain radiographs.

RESULTS

- Cumulative native hip survival of 816 acetabular fracture fixations, with conversion to THR or hip arthrodesis as endpoint, was 85% at 10 years and 79% at 20 years (Figure 23.2).
- 124 hips (15%) required conversion to THR, and 4 hips (0.5%) required conversion to arthrodesis.
- Mean time to failure (THR or arthrodesis) was 4.5 years. Notably, 50% of all conversions to THR occurred within the first 2 years postinjury.
- Fracture pattern only demonstrated a significant association with survivorship in associated both column (ABC) fractures, which fared better, and anterior wall fractures, which fared worse (87% and 34% survivorship respectively).

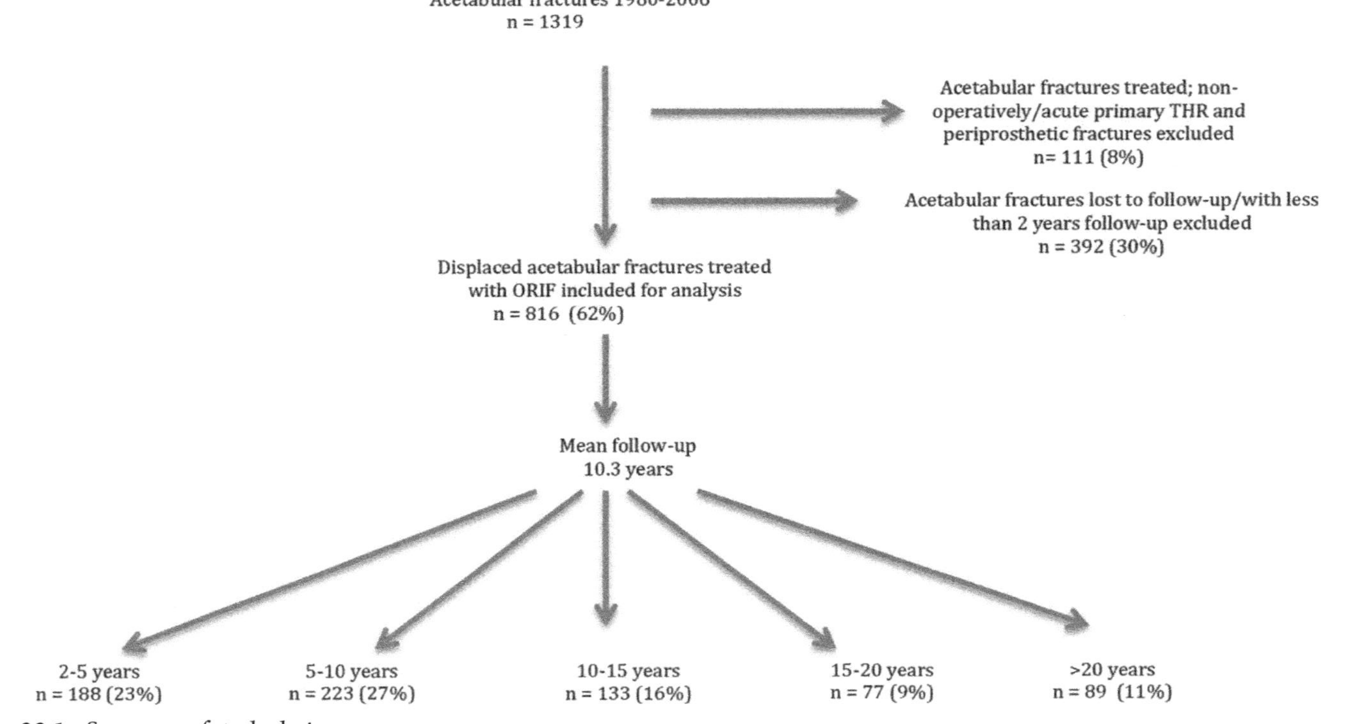

Figure 23.1. Summary of study design.

- Multivariate analysis identified 9 significant independent factors that were predictive of a poor outcome:
  - *6 factors predetermined at time of injury:*
    - Age > 40 years
    - Anterior hip dislocation
    - Femoral head cartilage lesion
    - Posterior wall involvement
    - Marginal impaction
    - Initial displacement > 20 mm
  - *3 factors related to surgical treatment:*
    - Nonanatomic reduction
    - Postoperative acetabular roof incongruence
    - Extended iliofemoral surgical approach
- The authors created an 8-factor nomogram (Figure 23.3) appropriate for clinical use to help predict the probability of early failure and requirement of conversion to THR by 2 years postoperatively following acetabular fracture fixation.

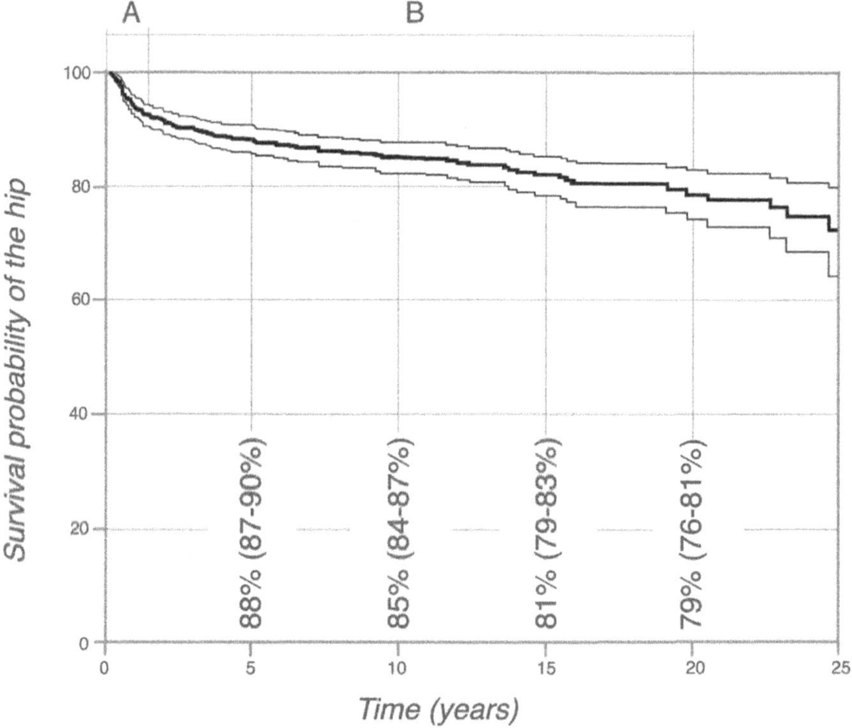

Figure 23.2. Survivorship curve (including 95% CI) for all acetabular fractures. Section A covers the first 1.5 years and represents an exponential decrease of the survivorship. Section B covers the time period from 1.5 to 20 years postoperatively and represents a linear decrease of the survivorship. The first 50% of hips that failed did so by 1.5 years postoperatively.

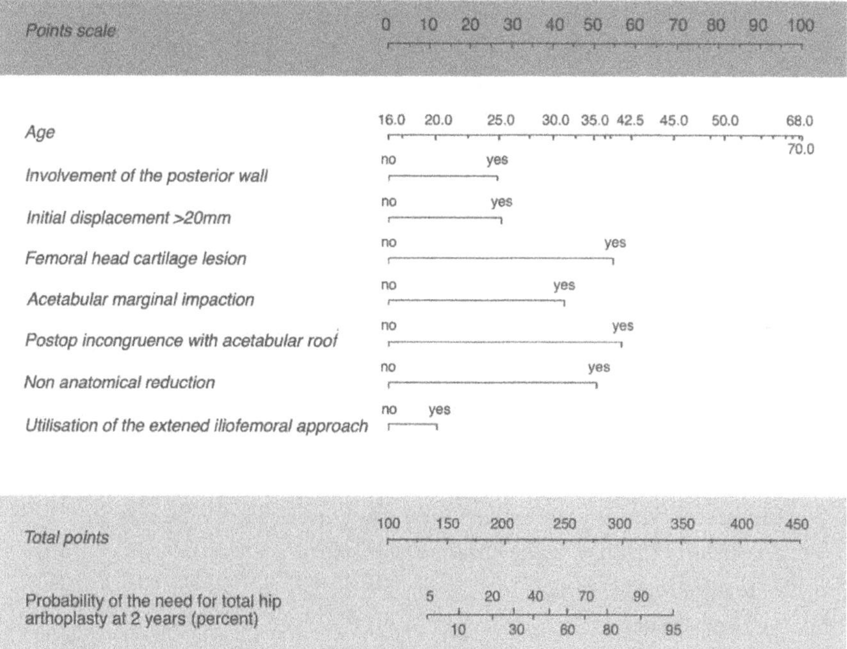

Figure 23.3. Nomogram to predict the need for early THA within 2 years following acetabular fracture fixation.

Criticisms and Limitations: This was a single-center and single-expert-surgeon series, which may not be generalizable to all hospitals. While the use of conversion to THR/fusion provides a straightforward, easily identifiable endpoint, this may overestimate the chances of a successful outcome. Without a formal radiographic or clinical F/U, patients who are in pain but are either unsuitable for or not offered THR will not be identified.

Other Relevant Studies and Information:

- Given the rarity and complexity of acetabular fractures, the literature with respect to long-term outcomes following fracture fixation has historically been almost exclusively limited to retrospective case series, often from a single institution or surgeon.
- Since publication of this seminal article, several articles assessing the long-term outcome following acetabular fracture management have been published.[3–5] None, however, have matched the large sample size of this study. The literature has also significantly expanded to assess outcomes of specific subtypes of acetabular fractures.[6,7]

- A comprehensive series of 161 surgically treated acetabular fractures from a single British surgeon utilized radiographic and clinical outcome scores in their series to demonstrate an “excellent” outcome in 47% and a “poor” outcome in 20%.[8] The publications also utilized multivariate analysis to identify poor prognostic indicators including increasing age, delay in time to surgery, quality of reduction, and certain fracture patterns. Regarding fracture pattern, the authors identified posterior column and T-shaped fractures as faring worst.
- One of the only meta-analyses assessing outcomes following operatively managed acetabular fractures provides an important overview of outcomes and treatment complications.[9] This study highlighted the paucity of high-quality data regarding acetabular fracture management, with just 5 prospective studies and 29 retrospective series suitable for inclusion. From a total of 3670 surgically managed acetabular fractures, this meta-analysis identified an 80% good or excellent outcome at 5 years and highlighted key prognostic factors:
  - Femoral head damage
  - Time to surgery
  - Quality of reduction
  - Type of fracture

Summary and Implications: This study represents the largest and longest series of operatively managed acetabular fractures. It highlights that with appropriate and skilled management, patients can expect a “survival” of their native hip joint in 79% at 20 years without progressing to THR. It also highlights the fact that 50% of all treatment failures occurred within the first 2 years postinjury. The nomogram can be used clinically to provide an estimation of the likelihood of early failure taking into account patient, injury, and surgical factors.

CLINICAL CASE: PREDICTING OUTCOME FOLLOWING A DISPLACED ACETABULAR FRACTURE

Case History

A 34-year-old male cyclist is knocked off his bicycle and lands directly onto his left hip. He is taken to his local hospital and managed according to Advanced Trauma Life Support guidelines. Following investigation, he is found to have sustained an isolated, closed, displaced acetabular fracture. His fracture is classified, according to Letournel and Judet,[2] as an ABC injury. He remained hemodynamically well and stable throughout his stay in the resus bay before being transferred to the ward. He was told to remain non–weight bearing. The patient has no significant past medical history and is a nonsmoker. How should this patient be treated, and what is the likely long-term outlook for his hip?

Suggested Answer

This is a young patient with a displaced acetabular fracture. He would benefit from ORIF aiming for perfect anatomic reduction of his joint surface. While this is a significant injury, the study by Tannast et al.[1] has demonstrated that at 20 years postinjury 79% of patients will not require conversion to THR. The same study highlighted that certain factors are predictive of a high chance of early treatment failure and conversion to THR. These include old age, posterior wall involvement, femoral head cartilage lesion, nonanatomic fracture reduction, and utilization of extensile surgical approaches. If any of these poor prognostic predictors are present, the patient should be counseled appropriately with respect to the severity of this injury.

References

1. Tannast et al. Two to twenty-year survivorship of the hip in 810 patients with operatively treated acetabular fractures. J Bone Joint Surg. Am. 2012;94(17):1559–67.
2. Letournel et al. Fractures of the Acetabulum. New York, NY: Springer; 1993.
3. Verbeek et al. Long-term patient reported outcomes following acetabular fracture fixation. Injury. 2018;49(6)11316.
4. Dunet et al. Acetabular fracture: long-term follow-up and factors associated with secondary implantation of total hip arthroplasty. Orthop Traumatol Surg Res. 2013;99(3):281–90.
5. Verbeek et al. Predictors for long-term hip survivorship following acetabular fracture surgery: importance of gap compared with step displacement. J Bone Joint Surg Am. 2018;100(11):922–9.
6. Firoozabadi et al. Risk factors for conversion to total hip replacement after acetabular fractures involving the posterior wall. J Orthop Trauma. 2018;32(12):607–11.
7. Borg et al. Quality of life after operative fixation of displaced acetabular fractures. J Orthop Trauma. 2012;26(8):445–50.
8. Briffa et al. Outcomes of acetabular fracture fixation with ten years' follow-up. J Bone Joint Surg Br. 2011;93(2):229–36.
9. Giannoudis et al. Operative treatment of displaced fractures of the acetabulum. A meta-analysis. J Bone Joint Surg Br. 2005;87(1):2–9.

24

Cemented or Uncemented Hemiarthroplasty for Displaced Intracapsular Fractures of the Hip

A Randomized Trial of 400 Patients

ASIM GHAFUR, ANDREW OSBORNE, AND IAN HOLLOWAY

> The results indicate that a contemporary cemented hemiarthroplasty gives better results than an uncemented hemiarthroplasty for patients with a displaced intracapsular fracture of the hip. When the condition of the patient permits, a cemented hemiarthroplasty should be used.
>
> —Parker et al.[1]

Citation: Parker MJ, Cawley S. Cemented or uncemented hemiarthroplasty for displaced intracapsular fractures of the hip: a randomized trial of 400 patients. Bone Joint J. 2020;102-B(1):11–16.

Research Question: Is it better to use a cemented or uncemented hemiarthroplasty (HA) to treat a displaced intracapsular neck of femur (NOF) fracture?

Funding: Not listed

Year Study Began: 2013

Year Study Published: 2020

Study Location: Peterborough, England

Who Was Studied: All patients with displaced intracapsular NOF fractures.

Who Was Excluded: Undisplaced intracapsular hip fracture, patients in another trial, younger patients, patients who declined to participate, patients who were unable to consent, equipment not available, pathological fracture, patients considered medically unfit for cemented arthroplasty, patients with arthritis of hip joint, and lead trialist not available.

How Many Patients: 400

Study Overview: See Figure 24.1.

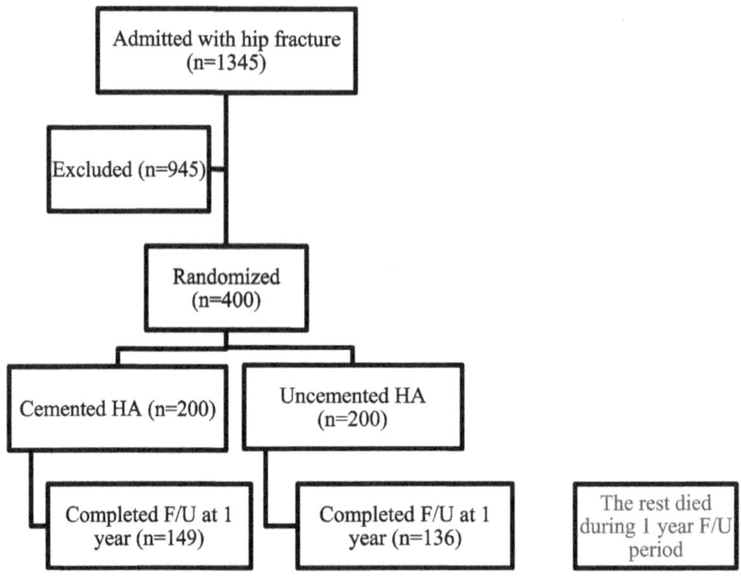

Figure 24.1. Summary of study design.

Study Intervention: A displaced intracapsular NOF fracture is one of the most common reasons for an elderly patient to be admitted to a hospital. These are treated by replacement HA usually. This study, conducted at a single center, randomized patients between a cemented unipolar double-tapered stem HA (Exeter Trauma Stem, Stryker Medical, Portgage, Michigan, USA, or CPT Zimmer/Biomet, Warsaw, Indiana, USA) or an uncemented fully hydroxyapatite-coated Furlong HA (JRI Orthopaedics, Sheffield, UK). The patients were followed up for 1 year. All the operations were performed through a Hardinge direct lateral approach with minimal-length skin incisions. After surgery all patients were mobilized with no restrictions on hip movements or weight bearing.

Follow-Up: This was divided into the following:

- 8 weeks after discharge in fracture clinic
- Telephone follow-up (F/U) at 3, 6, 9, and 12 months
- All assessments were undertaken by a research nurse blinded to the treatment

Endpoints: Primary outcomes were level of pain (scale 1–8 from modified Charnley score;[2] grades pain, mobility, and walking in relation to one hip, with lower scores indicating greater disability) after operation and effect on mobility (scale adapted from a hip fracture mobility score). Secondary outcomes were limb shortening, postoperative complications (e.g., pneumonia, deep vein thrombosis, pulmonary embolism, cerebrovascular accident, myocardial infarction, acute renal failure, pressure sores, delirium, and implant-related complications). Social dependence was assessed using a dependency score.

RESULTS

Demographic data is outlined in Table 24.1.

Table 24.1 PATIENT CHARACTERISTICS

	Cemented HA	**Uncemented HA**
Number (*n*)	200	200
Mean age (y; range)	84.2 (60–102)	85.3 (58–98)
Male (%)	67 (33.5%)	60 (30%)
From own home (%)	160 (80%)	169 (84.5%)
Mean mobility grade	4.0	4.1
Mean social dependency grade	3.4	3.5
Mean mental test score (/10)	6.6	6.4
Mean ASA score (/4)	3	3
Mean hemoglobin on admission	125	124

Cemented outperformed uncemented prosthesis with respect to the following (Table 24.2, Figure 24.2):

- There was an improved return of mobility in the cemented group.

- In the uncemented group there were 14 intraoperative femoral fractures as compared to 3 fractures in the cemented group.
- There was increased need for blood transfusion in the uncemented group.

Cemented HA did not outperform in regard to the following (Table 24.2, Figure 24.2):

- Mean duration of surgery and anesthesia was circa 5 minutes longer for cementing the prosthesis ($p \leq 0.001$).
- There were no statistically significant differences between the 2 cohorts in relation to general anesthesia, mean blood loss, residual pain, leg length discrepancy and loss of hip flexion, general postoperative complications (e.g., cardiorespiratory, venous thromboembolism) and implant-related complications (dislocation, secondary surgery), mean length of stay, and mortality (30, 120, and 365 days postoperatively).

Table 24.2 Perioperative Details and Mortality (Only Significant Factors)

	Cemented HA	**Uncemented HA**
Surgical time	4.7 minutes longer	
Anesthetic time	4.9 minutes longer	
Blood transfusion		Increased need twice as many times
Mean units of blood transfusion		Increased
Recovery of mobility	Rapid return of mobility	
Intraoperative fractures	3	14

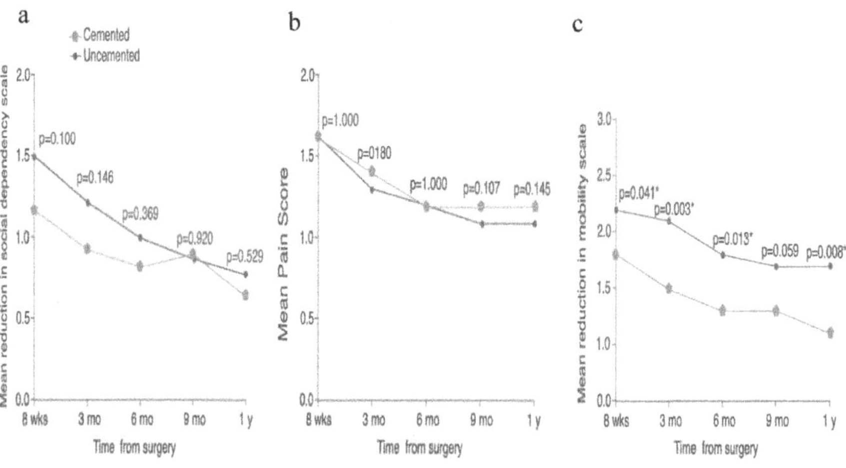

Figure 24.2. Plots observing for (a) mean reduction in social dependency, (b) mean pain, and (c) main reduction in mobility at set time intervals from surgery. *p* values calculated using unpaired *t*-test.

Criticisms and Limitations: The F/U period was only 1 year. It is possible that if the patients were followed up longer there may be clinical differences surfacing. The operations were all performed or supervised by the lead trialist (MJP) except for 8 operations. Although the number of total patients was 400, which satisfied the power study, there were only 200 patients in each group, which may not be representative on a wider scale.

Other Relevant Studies and Information:

- Cemented total hip replacement (THR) is similar if not superior to uncemented THR and provides better short-term clinical outcomes. There were better short-term clinical outcomes (mainly improvement in pain) after a cemented implant. There was no significant difference between the 2 groups in terms of implant survival as measured by the revision rate.[3]
- Survival of uncemented THA is inferior to that of cemented THA, and this may be because of the poorer performance of the uncemented cups. Although the uncemented stems performed better, there is an increased incidence of unrecognized intraoperative femoral fractures, which is the principal reason for early failure.[4]
- A meta-analysis on the topic concludes that there is better survival (if failure is defined as revision of 1 or both components) with cemented fixation in patients of all ages as compared to those that studied patients aged < 55 years.[5]
- National Institute for Health and Care Excellence guidelines recommend replacement arthroplasty in patients with a displaced intracapsular hip fracture and use of cemented implants (with a proven femoral stem design rather than Austin Moore or Thompson stems) through an anterolateral approach (in favor of a posterior approach).[6]
- In the most recent and largest randomized controlled trial[7] ($N = 1225$), among patients aged > 60 years, cemented HA resulted in a modestly but significantly improved quality of life and a lower risk of periprosthetic fracture than uncemented HA (0.5% vs. 2.1%; odds ratio [OR] = 4.37; 95% CI: 1.19–24.00). Mortality at 12 months was 23.9% in the cemented group and 27.8% in the uncemented group (OR = 0.80; 95% CI: 0.62–1.05). The incidences of other complications were similar in both groups.

Summary and Implications: This study found that after a displaced intracapsular NOF fracture patients who underwent cemented HA achieved better recovery in terms of mobility. The study found that there was neither a significant difference in the pain score nor an increase in postoperative complications or mortality with the use of cement. This study suggests that when HA is used for a hip fracture, it should be cemented in place.

CLINICAL CASE: OUTCOME OF UNCEMENTED HIP HEMIARTHROPLASTY IN A SERIOUSLY ILL PATIENT

Case History

An 85-year-old male was admitted after a mechanical fall and sustained a right-sided intracapsular hip fracture. He had a similar fracture on the other side around a decade ago, which was treated with a cemented Thompson prosthesis at the time. He recovered well after that surgery. On admission he was found to have severe cardiorespiratory comorbidities (including chronic obstructive pulmonary disorder and heart failure) and was a high-risk anesthetic patient with American Society of Anesthesiologists (ASA) class 3. It was agreed that he would benefit from a quicker operation. Would one opt for a cemented or an uncemented prosthesis according to this study, and what are their contraindications?

Suggested Answer

Cemented hip hemiarthroplasties have fewer intraoperative complications, such as iatrogenic fractures, which are more of a problem especially with a background of likely osteoporosis. This patient is at higher risk for bone cement implantation syndrome due to ASA classification, old age, being male, severe cardiorespiratory disease, and osteoporosis. According to the research, a cemented prosthesis would be considered gold standard even if it takes longer (without affecting mortality rate), but there is also an argument for resorting to implanting an uncemented stem as long as the risk of intraoperative fractures is accounted for. Intraoperative fractures can in turn take much longer to manage than working with cement, so the presence of an attending/consultant is mandatory. Furthermore, uncemented prostheses may also lead to more postoperative blood transfusions and slower return to mobility.

References

1. Parker et al. Cemented versus uncemented hemiarthroplasty for intracapsular hip fractures: a randomised controlled trial in 400 patients. Bone Joint J. 2020;102-B(1):11–16.
2. Charnley. The long-term results of low-friction arthroplasty of the hip performed as a primary intervention. J Bone Joint Surg Br. 1972;54-B(1):61–6.

3. Marques et al. The choice between hip prosthetic bearing surfaces in total hip replacement: a protocol for a systematic review and network meta-analysis. Syst Rev. 2016;5:19.
4. Hailer et al. Uncemented and cemented primary total hip arthroplasty in the Swedish Hip Arthroplasty Register. Evaluation of 170,413 operations. Acta Orthop. 2010;81(1):34–41.
5. Morshed et al. Comparison of cemented and uncemented fixation in total hip replacement. A meta-analysis. Acta Orthop. 2007;78:3315–26.
6. National Institute for Health and Care Excellence. Hip fracture management. Clinical guideline (CG124). Published June 22, 2011. Updated May 10, 2017. Available at https://www.nice.org.uk/guidance/cg124/chapter/recommendations
7. Fernandez et al. WHiTE 5 Investigators. Cemented or uncemented hemiarthroplasty for intracapsular hip fracture. N Engl J Med. 2022;386(6):521–30.

25

Vertebroplasty versus Sham Procedure for Management of Painful Osteoporotic Vertebral Fractures

SHIREEN IBISH AND CHRIS BROWN

> We found no beneficial effect of vertebroplasty as compared with a sham procedure in patients with painful osteoporotic vertebral fractures, at 1 week or at 1, 3, or 6 months after treatment.
>
> —Buchbinder et al.[1]

Citation: Buchbinder R, Osborne RH, Ebeling PR, Wark JD, Mitchell P, Wriedt C, Graves S, Staples MP, Murphy B. A randomized trial of vertebroplasty for painful osteoporotic vertebral fractures. N Engl J Med. 2009;361(6): 557–68.

Research Question: Is vertebroplasty a safe and efficient approach for managing pain and improving physical functioning from painful osteoporotic vertebral fractures in the initial short-term period?

Funding: National Health and Medical Research Council of Australia, Arthritis Australia, Cabrini Education and Research Institute, Cook Australia, National Health and Medical Research Council Practitioner Fellowship, National Health and Medical Research Council Population Health Career Development Award

Year Study Began: 2004

Year Study Published: 2009

Study Location: 4 hospitals in Australia

Who Was Studied: Adults with back pain of no more than 12 months' duration and magnetic resonance imaging (MRI)-proven 1 or 2 recent vertebral fractures, defined as vertebral collapse of grade 1 or higher according to the grading system of Genant et al.[2] and edema, a fracture line, or both within the vertebral body.

Who Was Excluded: Presence of > 2 recent vertebral fractures, spinal cancer, neurologic complications, osteoporotic vertebral collapse of > 90%, fracture through or destruction of the posterior wall, bony fragments that are either retropulsed or impinging on the spinal cord, medical conditions that would make the patient ineligible for emergency decompressive surgery if needed, previous vertebroplasty, inability to give informed consent, and a likelihood of noncompliance with follow-up (F/U). All analyses were on an intention-to-treat principle.

How Many Patients: 78

Study Overview: See Figure 25.1.

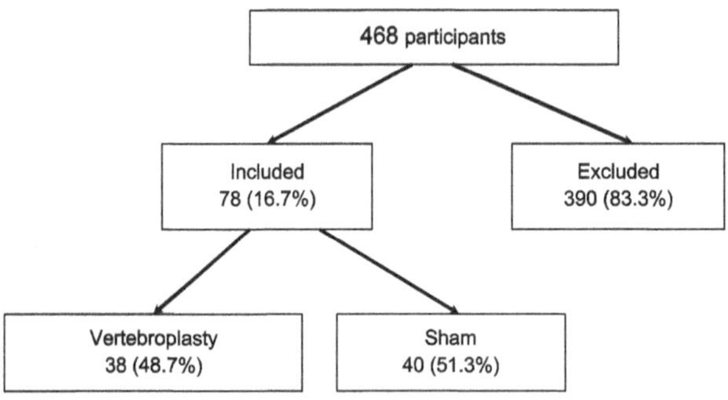

Figure 25.1. Summary of study design.

Study Intervention: Both groups were managed by interventional radiologists as seen in Table 25.1.

Table 25.1 Management Options for Each Cohort

Vertebroplasty/Intervention Group	**Sham Group**
1. Left pedicle identified using metallic marker 2. Skin infiltrated using 25-gauge needle 3. Periosteum of posterior lamina infiltrated using 23-gauge 4. Skin incision made and 13-gauge needle inserted posterolaterally to pedicle 5. Needle gently taped to guide through pedicle into anterior two-thirds of the vertebral body 6. Anteroposterior and lateral radiographs confirmed position of needle before proceeding 7. ~3 ml of polymethylmethacrylate (PMMA) slowly injected into the vertebral body and confirmed with fluoroscopy 8. Injection stopped when either enough resistance was met, cement reached posterior quarter of vertebral body, or there was cement leakage 9. Intravenous cephalothin injected immediately after cementing	Steps 1–3 as for Intervention group 4. Skin incision made and 13-gauge needle inserted then let rest on lamina 5. PMMA prepared (to release smell) and vertebral body gently tapped to simulate vertebroplasty

Follow-Up: 6 months

Endpoints: Primary outcome was score for overall pain (0–10), with 1.5 points signifying minimal clinical relevance. Secondary outcomes were quality of life (QOL) measures using the following scores:

- Quality of Life Questionnaire of the European Foundation for Osteoporosis (QUALEFFO):[3] Range from 0 to 100, with higher scores indicating worse QOL
- Assessment of Quality of Life (AQoL) questionnaire:[4] Range from −0.04 to 1.0, with 1 indicating perfect health and 0.06 representing the minimal clinically important difference
- European Quality of Life–5 Dimensions (EQ-5D) scale:[5] Range from 0 to 1, with 1 indicating perfect health and 0.074 representing the minimal clinically important difference
- Pain score[6] at rest and at night
- Modified 23-item version of the Roland-Morris Disability Questionnaire (RDQ)[7]: Range from 0 to 23, with higher scores indicating worse physical functioning and 2 to 3 points representing the minimal clinically important difference

RESULTS (TABLE 25.2)

- *Baseline characteristics:* Age, sex, duration of back pain, corticosteroid use, pain, and QOL score were largely similar between both cohorts.
- *F/U*: At 6 months, 35 (92.1%) participants from the vertebroplasty group and 36 (90%) from the placebo group returned completed questionnaires (91% return).
- *Patient-reported outcome measures:* Participants from both groups experienced similar improvements in their overall perceived pain (including night pain), physical functioning, and QOL.
- *Outcomes:* No significant difference in the primary or secondary outcomes was observed between both groups at 6 months, irrespective of duration of symptoms, sex, treatment center, and presence or absence of previous vertebral fracture.
- *Complications:* 1 participant in the vertebroplasty group did not receive prophylactic antibiotics and developed adjacent osteomyelitis; 7 participants reported vertebral fractures within 6 months after study intervention.

Table 25.2 Summary of Key Findings

Outcome	**Vertebroplasty Baseline**	**6 Months**	**Sham Baseline**	**6 Months**	**Adjusted Between-Group Mean Difference (95% CI)**
Overall pain	7.4 ± 2.1	2.4 ± 3.3	7.1 ± 2.3	2.1 ± 3.3	0.1 (−1.2–1.4)
Pain at rest	4.5 ± 2.3	2.0 ± 3.2	4.8 ± 2.8	0.9 ± 3.1	0.3 (−0.9–1.5)
Pain at night	4.8 ± 3.0	1.5 ± 3.6	3.6 ± 3.2	1.6 ± 3.6	−0.2 (−1.6–1.1)
QUALEFFO total score	56.9 ± 13.4	6.4 ± 13.4	59.6 ± 17.1	6.1 ± 13.4	0.6 (−5.1–6.2)
AQoL score	0.33 ± 0.25	0.0 ± 0.3	0.27 ± 0.26	0.1 ± 0.3	0.1 (−0.1–0.2)
RDQ score	17.3 ± 2.8	4.1 ± 5.8	17.3 ± 2.9	3.7 ± 5.8	0.0 (−3.0–2.9)

Criticisms and Limitations: The limitations of the study include a selection bias with 30% of eligible participants declining to partake in the study, potentially limiting the generalizability of the findings. In addition, the study was relatively small with just 78 participants with a F/U duration of 6 months only.

Other Relevant Studies and Information:

- Kallmes et al.[8] conducted a randomized controlled trial (RCT) with 131 participants, concluding no difference in outcome measures between participants treated with vertebroplasty compared with a sham procedure.

- Firanescu et al.[9] conducted the VERTOS IV double-blinded RCT of 180 participants comparing percutaneous vertebroplasty to sham procedure for acute osteoporotic vertebral fractures with a 12-month F/U. They concluded that there was no significant difference between both groups.
- Buchbinder et al.[10] published a Cochrane database literature review on the use of vertebroplasty for osteoporotic vertebral fractures and concluded that there is no role for vertebroplasty for the treatment of acute and subacute vertebral fractures.
- National Institute for Health and Care Excellence[11] guidelines published in 2013, subsequently reviewed in 2016, concluded that the use of vertebroplasty should be used only in people:
  - "who have severe ongoing pain after recent, unhealed vertebral fracture despite optimal pain management" and
  - "in whom the pain has been confirmed to be at the level of the fracture by physical examination and imaging"

Summary and Implications: There was no beneficial effect of vertebroplasty compared to sham procedure in painful osteoporotic vertebral fractures, either at 1 week or at 1, 3, or 6 months after treatment. Guidelines recommend that vertebroplasty should be reserved for patients with pain clearly linked to the site of the vertebral fracture who remain in significant discomfort despite optimal pain management.

CLINICAL CASE: THE ROLE OF SURGERY IN PAINFUL OSTEOPOROTIC VERTEBRAL FRACTURES

Case History

A 74-year-old male was brought in by ambulance to the Emergency Department following a first-time nocturnal seizure, witnessed by his wife. His past medical history included hypertension and neck pain from a known C6–C7 protrusion. He was investigated in the department for a possible aortic dissection following complaint of radiating chest pain. A computed axial tomography scan ruled out aortic dissection but confirmed a T5 wedge fracture. Blood results showed no abnormalities of note. On discharge home the patient was provided with regular oral analgesia to manage his back pain. The patient was followed up a week later and due to ongoing back pain was referred to the spine team for further management. Should the spine team proceed with a vertebroplasty procedure to manage this patient's symptoms based on the findings of this study?

Suggested Answer

Buchbinder et al.[1] showed that vertebroplasty did not show superior benefit when compared to a sham procedure at 6 months. A vertebroplasty is not an effective approach to manage the above patient's symptoms at this stage of his treatment. Clinicians should be aware of the high levels of pain experienced by patients following vertebral fractures and the importance of ensuring that patients are provided with regular and titrated analgesia to reach a balance between therapeutic effect and manageable side-effect profile. This case study fits the description of patients studied by Buchbinder et al.[1] and would therefore be suitable for management with analgesia in the acute phase of treatment. This was the option chosen when reviewed in the spine outpatient clinic. On subsequent F/U, he showed improvement in symptoms and returned back to work, and an MRI of his spine 8 weeks following his injury showed reduction in both marrow edema and prevertebral soft tissue edema.

References

1. Buchbinder et al. A randomized trial of vertebroplasty for painful osteoporotic vertebral fractures. N Engl J Med. 2009;361:557–68.
2. Genant et al. Vertebral fracture assessment using a semiquantitative technique. J Bone Miner Res. 1993;8:1137–48.
3. Lips et al. Quality of life in patients with vertebral fractures: validation of the Quality of Life Questionnaire of the European Foundation for Osteoporosis (QUALEFFO). Osteoporos Int. 1999;10:150–60.
4. Hawthorne et al. Population norms and meaningful differences for the Assessment of Quality of Life (AQoL) measure. Aust N Z J Public Health. 2005;29:136–42.
5. Walters et al. Comparison of the minimally important difference for two health state utility measures: EQ-5D and SF-6D. Qual Life Res. 2005;14:1523–32.
6. Buchbinder et al. Efficacy and safety of vertebroplasty for treatment of painful osteoporotic spinal fractures: a randomised controlled trial. BMC Musculoskelet Disord. 2008;9:156.
7. Trout et al. Evaluation of vertebroplasty with a validated outcome measure: the Roland-Morris Disability Questionnaire. AJNR Am J Neuroradiol. 2005;26:2652–7.
8. Kallmes et al. A randomized trial of vertebroplasty for osteoporotic spinal fractures. N Engl J Med. 2009;361:569–79.
9. Firanescu et al. Vertebroplasty versus sham procedure for painful acute osteoporotic compression fractures (VERTOS IV): randomised sham controlled clinical trial. BMJ. 2018;361:k1551.

10. Buchbinder et al. Percutaneous vertebroplasty for osteoporotic vertebral compression fracture. Cochrane Database Syst Rev. 2018;4.
11. National Institute for Health and Care Excellence. Percutaneous vertebroplasty and percutaneous balloon kyphoplasty for treating osteoporotic vertebral compression fractures. April 24, 2013. www.nice.org.uk/guidance/ta279/resources/percutaneous-vertebroplasty-and-percutaneous-balloon-kyphoplasty-for-treating-osteoporotic-vertebral-compression-fractures-pdf-82600620856261

26

Graft Selection in Anterior Cruciate Ligament Reconstructions

Hamstring versus Patellar Tendon Autograft

THOMAS C. EDWARDS AND HENRY EDMUND BOURKE

> Both HT and PT autograft ACL reconstructions have excellent 10-year results. Radiographic osteoarthritis in PT-reconstructed knees is greater at 10 years. Kneeling pain is greater in PT-reconstructed knees. Ten-year survivorship and subjective function is no different between graft types.
>
> —PINCZEWSKI ET AL.[1]

Citation: Pinczewski LA, Lyman J, Salmon LJ, Russell VJ, Roe J, Linklater J. A 10-year comparison of anterior cruciate ligament reconstructions with hamstring tendon and patellar tendon autograft: a controlled, prospective trial. Am J Sports Med. 2007;35(4):564–74.

Research Question: Which graft is superior in primary arthroscopic anterior cruciate ligament (ACL) reconstructions: hamstring tendon (HT) or patella tendon (PT) autograft?

Funding: Smith and Nephew

Year Study Began: 1993

Year Study Published: 2007

Study Location: Sydney, Australia

Who Was Studied: Patients were aged 13–52 years with ACL tears who wished to return to sports requiring pivoting/side-stepping or those with recurrent instability following conservative treatment with physiotherapy.

Who Was Excluded: Patients who had associated ligament injuries, evidence of chondral damage or degenerative joint disease/abnormal radiographs, contralateral knee pathology, previous meniscectomy, or excision of greater than one-third of meniscus at the time of surgery and those seeking compensation for their injury were excluded.

How Many Patients: 180

Study Overview: See Figure 26.1.

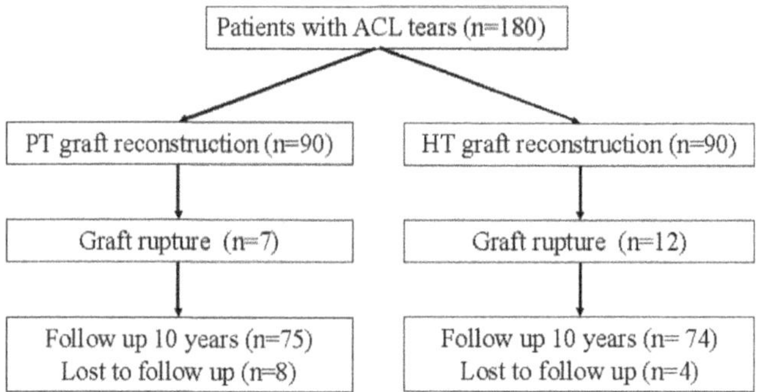

Figure 26.1. Overview of study design.

Study Intervention: In this prospective and nonrandomized study, patients with primary ACL injuries were recruited to undergo arthroscopic ACL reconstruction using either PT or HT autograft. All operations were performed by the senior author. HT grafts were 4-strand from the gracilis and semitendinosus tendons. PT grafts were from the ipsilateral middle third portion. Fixation was with RCI screws (Smith and Nephew, London, UK) proximally and distally in both groups. All patients underwent the same postoperative rehabilitation program.

Follow-Up: Annually at 2, 5, 7, and 10 years postoperatively

Endpoints: ACL graft rupture, contralateral ACL rupture, complications, harvest site symptoms, kneeling pain, subjective functional assessment using the International Knee Documentation Committee[2] (IKDC; the patient-reported questionnaire examines 3 categories: symptoms, athletic activity, and knee function) score and Lysholm knee score (a questionnaire designed to assess the degree of knee instability at both impairment and limitation levels, with a high score correlating to a low degree of instability),[3] ligament laxity as measured by instrumented testing, Lachman test and pivot-shift test, and radiographic evidence of osteoarthritis (OA) as measured using the IKDC radiographic grading system (knee examination portion of the IKDC form includes a radiographic grading system to grade degenerative changes).[2,4]

RESULTS (TABLE 26.1)

- *Graft survival (Figure 26.2):* There was no significant difference observed between both groups with graft rupture rates of 7.8% in the PT group vs. 13.3% in the HT group ($p = 0.24$).
- *Knee function:* 97% reported normal (or nearly normal) knee function at 10-year follow-up (F/U) on the IKDC subjective functional assessment score in both groups with no significant difference detected.
- *Knee stability:* No differences in instrumented ligament laxity ($p = 0.53$), pivot-shift testing ($p = 0.48$), or Lachman test ($p = 0.78$) between both groups were observed at 10-year F/U.
- *Postoperative symptoms:* The PT group reported a significantly higher incidence of graft harvest site symptoms (i.e., tenderness, irritation, numbness) at 10-year F/U ($p = 0.001$), with 34.7% reporting mild, moderate, or severe symptoms compared with 5.4% in the HT group.
- *Kneeling pain:* The PT group reported a higher incidence of kneeling pain at 10 years: 59% vs. 27% in the HT group ($p < 0.01$).
- *Postoperative complications:* No significant differences between the groups were observed.
- *OA sequelae:* Radiographic assessment showed a significantly higher incidence of OA in the PT group with 39% of patients having grade B or C changes (i.e., joint space narrowing that is barely detectable and up to 50% respectively) on the IKDC grading system at 10-year F/U compared to 18% in the HT group ($p = 0.04$).

Table 26.1 Summary of Key Findings

Outcome at 10-Year F/U	PT Group	HT Group	*p* Value
Graft rupture	7/90 (7.8%)	12/90 (13.3%)	0.24
Contralateral ACL	20/90 (22.2%)	9/90 (10%)	0.02
Kneeling pain	59%	27%	< 0.01
Harvest site symptoms	34.7%	5.4%	0.001
Knee function score (grade A or B)	97%	97%	N/A
Radiographic OA (grade B or C)	39%	18%	0.04

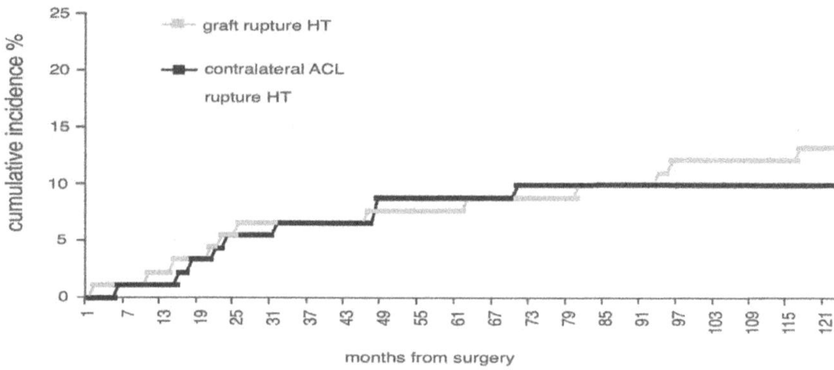

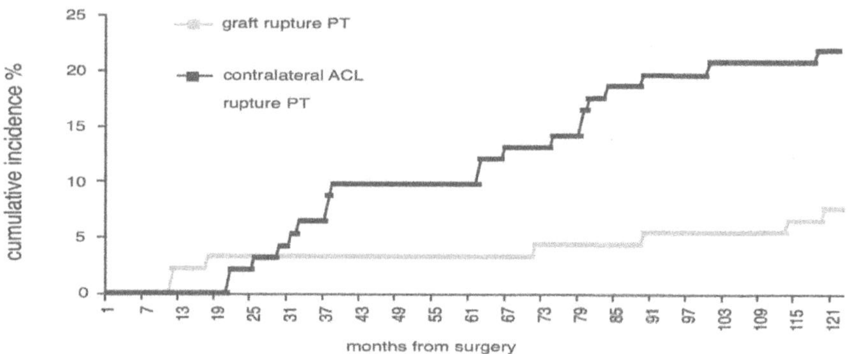

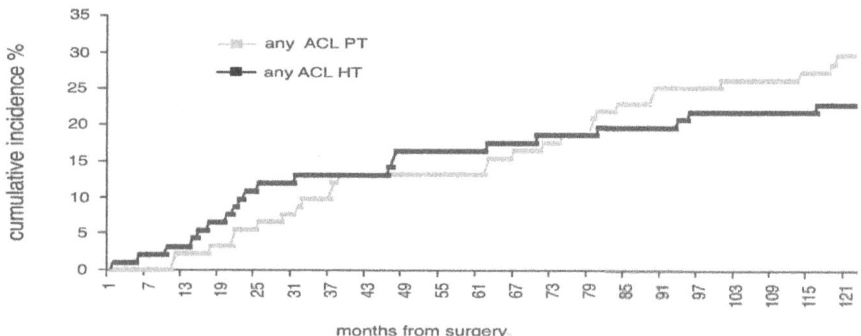

Figure 26.2. Incidence of ACL graft and contralateral ACL rupture in the HT group and the PT group with combined incidence of ACL graft or contralateral ACL injury in the HT and PT groups.

Criticisms and Limitations: The main limitation was absence of randomization with no attempt at blinding the patients or examiners, which may have introduced selection bias. No sample size calculation was made, so the lack of statistical significance demonstrated in graft rupture rates could be the result of a type II error due to the study being underpowered. No attempt was made to stratify the sample populations according to variables including age, body mass index (BMI), or usual level of activity. The HT group was recruited after the PT group, which took place at the beginning of the senior surgeon's learning curve with performing the HT technique, whereas the PT patients were recruited after the senior surgeon had amassed significant experience in the operative technique. Postoperative radiographs were interpreted by a single rater with no documentation of reliability testing.

Other Relevant Studies and Information:

- Several studies support these findings, reporting equivalent graft longevity[5] and, similarly, a higher incidence of harvest site morbidity and kneeling pain associated with PT grafts.[6–8]
- A randomized study of 220 patients with 5-year F/U compared PT, HT, and double-bundle ACL reconstruction. Similar to this study, a higher incidence of kneeling pain in the PT group was observed. However, a significantly higher chance of traumatic reinjury in the HT group was also observed.[9]
- 1 recent randomized study with a 14-year F/U reported a similar risk of developing knee OA between PT and HT grafts. The authors report a 3-fold increase in the risk of OA in ACL-injured knees compared to healthy knees.[10]
- According to British Orthopaedic Association,[11] graft choice should be decided based on individual patient characteristics and surgeon experience. However, allografts are not recommended for primary reconstructions in younger patients (< 35 years old), while synthetic ligaments are not recommended for routine primary reconstruction. Differences in clinical outcomes between grafts have been reviewed by the British Association for Surgery of the Knee.[12]

Summary and Implications: This study demonstrates that both PT and HT grafts perform well with respect to longevity and knee function at 10-year F/U. The HT graft had a lower incidence of harvest site symptoms and kneeling pain as well as a lower incidence of early radiographic OA. It is worth noting that even though there was no significant difference in graft rupture between both cohorts ($p = 0.24$), the graft rupture rate was almost halved when comparing the PT group with the HT group (7.8% vs. 13.3% respectively). The authors suggest that for the majority of cases a HT graft would be preferred, due to the lower risk of harvest site morbidity, kneeling pain, and potential reduction in radiographic OA at 10-year F/U. However, since this was not a randomized trial it is possible that confounding factors influenced the results, and thus firm conclusions cannot be drawn.

CLINICAL CASE: PT VERSUS HT GRAFTING IN ACL RECONSTRUCTION

Case History

A 38-year-old gardener is seen in the outpatient department after twisting his knee while skiing 2 weeks ago. His knee swelled up immediately and has subsequently been feeling unstable. He is fit and well and is a semiprofessional footballer. On examination he has a mild effusion, range of motion of 0–110 degrees of flexion, and a grade 2 Lachman test with no firm endpoint. His magnetic resonance imaging scan shows a complete tear of his ACL with no other injuries. He wants to know his options for treatment and likely prognosis. How should this patient be managed based on the findings of this study? If surgically, which graft should be chosen for his ACL reconstruction and why?

Suggested Answer

Because this patient is keen on returning to football, the authors would recommend surgical management to restore knee stability and allow him to perform pivoting or side-stepping activities. The results of this study showed low rates of graft rupture and excellent functional outcomes using both grafts. Given his job as a gardener, he may spend a considerable amount of time kneeling, and so the lower chance of kneeling pain and harvest site morbidity with an HT graft may make this the more favorable option in this case. With surgery, he has a high (97%) chance of restoration of normal knee function; however, his injury does carry an elevated risk of developing future OA (potentially a 3-fold increase[7]) and a 13.3% chance of subsequent graft rupture. However, when choosing a graft, it is important to discuss these findings with the patient and make an operative plan that considers individual patient needs, including activity levels and type of employment.

References

1. Pinczewski et al. A 10-year comparison of anterior cruciate ligament reconstructions with hamstring tendon and patellar tendon autograft: a controlled, prospective trial. Am J Sports Med. 2007;35(4):564–74.

2. Irrgang et al. Development and validation of the international knee documentation committee subjective knee form. Am J Sports Med. 2001;29(5):600–13.
3. Tegner et al. Rating systems in the evaluation of knee ligament injuries. Clin Orthop. 1985;198:43–9.
4. Hefti et al. Evaluation of knee ligament injuries with the IKDC form. Knee Surg Sports Traumatol Arthrosc. 1993;1(3–4):226–34.
5. Beard et al. Hamstrings vs. patella tendon for anterior cruciate ligament reconstruction: a randomised controlled trial. Knee. 2001;8(1):45–50.
6. Samuelsson et al. Treatment of anterior cruciate ligament injuries with special reference to graft type and surgical technique: an assessment of randomized controlled trials. Arthroscopy. 2009;25(10):1139–74.
7. Biau et al. Bone-patellar tendon-bone autografts versus hamstring autografts for reconstruction of anterior cruciate ligament: meta-analysis. BMJ. 2006;332(7548): 995–1001.
8. Aglietti et al. Anterior cruciate ligament reconstruction: bone-patellar tendon-bone compared with double semitendinosus and gracilis tendon grafts. A prospective, randomized clinical trial. J Bone Joint Surg Am. 2004;86(10):2143–55.
9. Mohtadi et al. A randomized clinical trial comparing patellar tendon, hamstring tendon, and double-bundle ACL reconstructions: patient-reported and clinical outcomes at 5-year follow-up. J Bone Joint Surg Am. 2019;101(11):949–60.
10. Barenius et al. Increased risk of osteoarthritis after anterior cruciate ligament reconstruction: a 14-year follow-up study of a randomized controlled trial. Am J Sports Med. 2014;42(5):1049–57.
11. British Orthopaedic Association. BOAST—Best practice for management of anterior cruciate ligament (ACL) injuries. September 2020. https://www.boa.ac.uk/resources/best-practice-management-for-acl-injuries-pdf.html
12. British Orthopaedic Association. BOA, BASK, BOSTAA elective care standards: best practice for management of anterior cruciate ligament (ACL) injuries. September 2020. https://www.boa.ac.uk/static/88a4c3e3-df3e-4e51-a92e7d2f86d7d82a/Best-Practice-Book-for-management-of-Anterior-Cruciate-Ligament-injuries.pdf

27

A Randomized, Controlled Trial of Total Knee Replacement

BRANAVAN RUDRAN AND LUKE D. JONES

> This randomized, controlled trial showed that total knee replacement followed by nonsurgical treatment is more efficacious than nonsurgical treatment alone in providing pain relief and improving function and quality of life after 12 months in patients with knee osteoarthritis who are eligible for unilateral total knee replacement.
>
> —Skou et al.[1]

Citation: Skou ST, Roos EM, Laursen MB, Rathleff MS, Arendt-Nielsen L, Simonsen O, Rasmussen S. A randomized, controlled trial of total knee replacement. N Engl J Med. 2015;373(17):1597–606.

Research Question: In patients with established knee osteoarthritis (OA), does total knee replacement (TKR) + nonoperative treatment result in better outcomes at 12 months compared to nonoperative strategies alone?

Funding: Obel Family Foundation, Danish Rheumatism Association, Health Science Foundation of the North Denmark region, Foot Science International, Spar Nord Foundation, Bevica Foundation, Association of Danish Physiotherapists Research Fund, Medical Specialist Heinrich Kopp's Grant, and Danish Medical Association Research Fund

Year Study Began: 2011

Year Study Published: 2015

Study Location: Aalborg University Hospital, Denmark

Who Was Studied: Patients with radiographically confirmed knee OA as defined by a Kellgren and Lawrence (KL)[2] score ≥ 2, who were determined to be eligible for a TKR by an experienced orthopaedic surgeon.

Who Was Excluded: Patients with a previous TKR of the ipsilateral knee, simultaneous bilateral TKRs, and knee pain during the previous week rated > 60 mm on a visual analog scale (VAS).

How Many Patients: 100

Study Overview: See Figure 27.1.

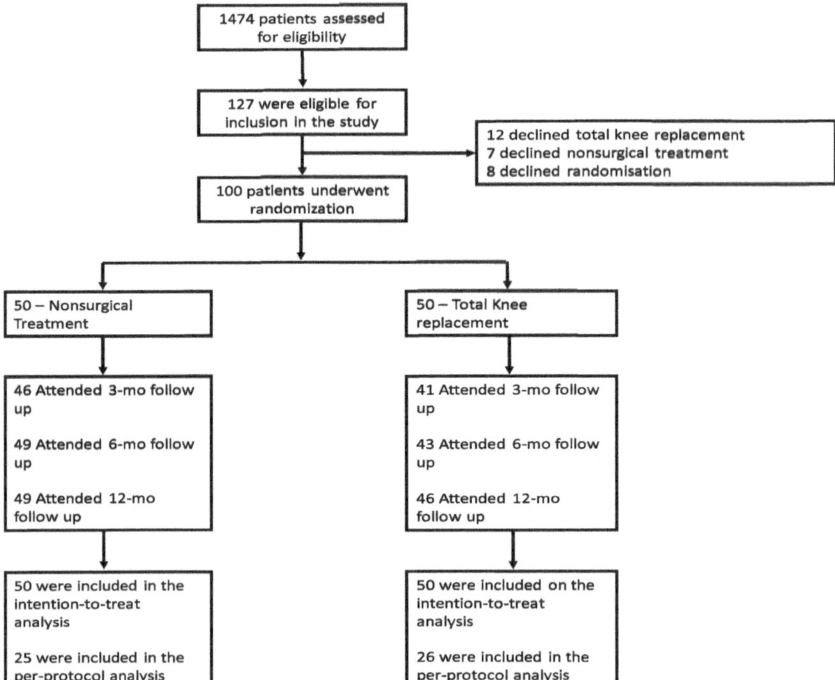

Figure 27.1. A flow diagram to illustrate the study enrollment, randomization, treatment, and F/U.

Study Intervention: One hundred patients with moderate to severe knee OA and eligible for unilateral TKR were enrolled in this randomized controlled trial (RCT). Half of the patients were equally assigned to either the treatment or the control group. The treatment group underwent TKR followed by 12 weeks of nonsurgical treatment. The control group received only 12 weeks of nonsurgical treatment that was delivered by physiotherapists and dietitians and consisted of exercise, education, dietary advice, use of insoles, and pain medication.

Follow-Up: Single blinded follow-up (F/U) assessments were performed at 3, 6, and 12 months following the initiation of nonsurgical treatment.

Endpoints: Primary outcome measure was a change of mean score from baseline to 12 months between both groups in 4 Knee injury and Osteoarthritis Outcome Score[3] ($KOOS_4$; knee-specific tool that was developed to assess the patients' opinions about their short- and long-term consequences of knee injury) subscales:

- Pain
- Symptoms
- Activities of daily living (ADLs)
- Quality of life (QOL)

Secondary outcomes consisted of the following:

- Change from baseline to 12 months in $KOOS_4$ subscales including a fifth component covering function in sport and recreation
- Time for the timed up-and-go test
- EuroQol group 5-Dimension Self-Report questionnaire (EQ-5D; standardized measure of health-related QOL to provide a simple, generic questionnaire for use in clinical and economic appraisal or population health status surveys)[4]
- Weight in kilograms
- Type, dose, and quantity of painkillers taken over the previous week

RESULTS

- *Baseline:* There were no significant differences between groups in the reported characteristics.
- *Outcomes:* Mean improvement from baseline to 12 months for $KOOS_4$ score was twice as much in the TKR group (Table 27.1, Figure 27.2). The TKR group had significantly greater improvements in the scores on all 5 KOOS subscales, EQ-5D scores, timed up-and-go test, and time on 20-m walk tests vs. the nonsurgical treatment group.
- *Serious adverse events:* These were 4 times greater in the TKR group ($p = 0.005$).

Table 27.1 Summary of Key Results—Outcomes at 12 Months

Outcome	Total Number of Assessments[a]		Mean Improvement in Outcome from Baseline to 12 Months (95% CI)		Between-Group Difference in Mean Improvement (95% CI)	
	Nonsurgical	TKR	Nonsurgical	TKR	Crude	Adjusted[b]
Primary Outcome						
$KOOS_4$	179	193	16.0 (10.1–21.9)	32.5 (26.6–38.3)	16.5 (10.2–22.7)	15.8 (10.0–21.5)
Secondary Outcomes						
KOOS subscale score						
Pain	180	194	17.2 (10.4–24.1)	34.8 (28.1–41.5)	17.6 (10.1–25.1)	17.1 (10.4–23.8)
Symptoms	179	194	11.4 (4.4–18.4)	26.4 (21.5–31.4)	15.0 (8.3–21.7)	12.7 (6.6–18.8)
ADLs	180	193	17.6 (11.4–23.9)	30.0 (22.7–37.2)	12.3 (5.5–19.2)	12.9 (6.8–19.1)
QOL	180	194	17.8 (11.2–24.4)	38.2 (30.6–45.8)	20.4 (12.8–27.9)	20.2 (13.2–27.1)
Sports and recreation	177	193	19.3 (10.8–27.7)	34.5 (27.9–41.0)	15.2 (6.7–23.7)	15.6 (7.3–23.9)
Time on up-and-go test (s)	163	185	−1.2 (−1.8 to −0.6)	−2.4 (−3.1 to −1.6)	1.2 (0.4–1.9)	0.9 (0.2–1.6)
Time on 20-m walk tests (s)	163	185	−1.0 (−1.5 to −0.4)	−2.9 (−3.8 to −1.9)	1.9 (0.9–2.8)	1.5 (0.7–2.4)
EQ-5D scores						
Descriptive index	178	194	0.115 (0.063–0.166)	0.206 (0.141–0.270)	0.091 (0.026–0.155)	0.078 (0.023–0.132)
VAS	180	193	10.2 (4.6–15.7)	15.0 (8.6–21.5)	4.9 (2.2–12.0)	4.4 (1.8–10.6)
Weight (kg)[c]	134	160	−2.6 (−3.9 to −1.4)	0.1 (−1.5–1.7)	2.8 (1.4–4.1)	2.8 (1.4–4.1)

[a] There were 200 possible assessments for each study group (50 each at baseline and at 3, 6, and 12 months).

[b] The results were adjusted for time of assessment (baseline and 3, 6, and 12 months), clinic (Frederikshavn or Farsoe), baseline values, and the interaction between time of assessment and study group

[c] Data are presented only for patients with a body mass index ≥ 25 at baseline (43 patients in the nonsurgical treatment group and 39 patients in the TKR group).

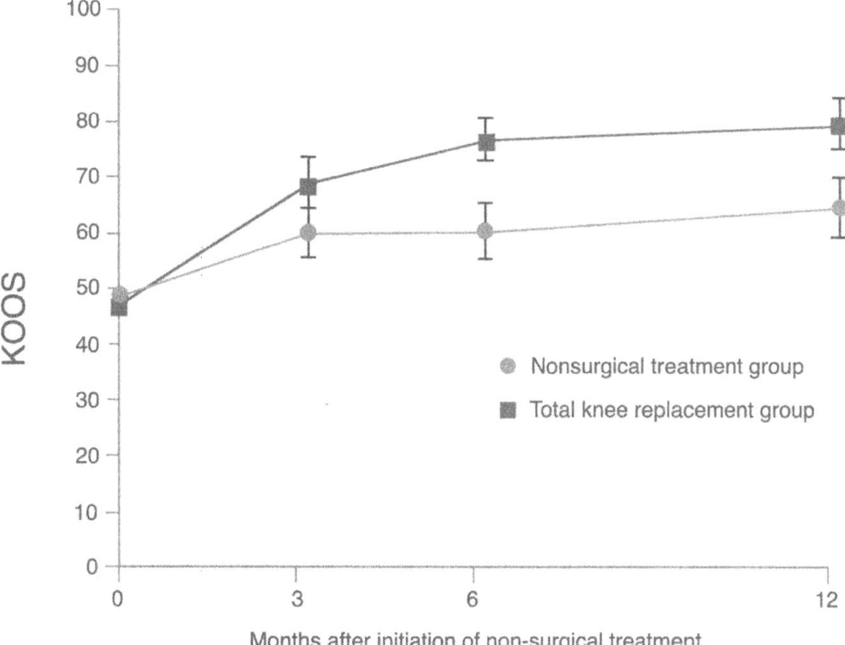

Figure 27.2. Graph showing the mean score on 4 $KOOS_4$ subscales, covering pain, symptoms, ADLs, and QOL, for groups randomly assigned to undergo TKR followed by 12 weeks of nonsurgical treatment (i.e., TKR group) or to receive only the 12 weeks of nonsurgical treatment (i.e., nonsurgical treatment group), which consists of exercise, education, dietary advice, use of insoles, and pain medication. The $KOOS_4$ ranges from 0 (worst) to 100 (best). Bars indicate 95% CI.

Criticisms and Limitations: Of those allocated to nonoperative management, 25% had a TKR during the study, which would have dampened the apparent efficacy and safety of surgical treatment. The ethnicity of the patients was not mentioned. Patients in the control group did not undergo a sham operation, which may have biased their qualitative assessments of symptom improvement. Patients with severe knee pain were excluded, limiting generalizability. F/U was only 12 months, limiting conclusions of the long-term efficacy of nonoperative management strategies. Finally, this trial only included experienced surgeons, which may have biased the results in favor of surgical treatment.

Other Relevant Studies and Information:

- There are no other high-quality RCTs that have investigated surgical vs. nonsurgical intervention for knee OA.[5]

- American Academy of Orthopaedic Surgeons guidelines[6,7] for managing knee OA:
  - They strongly recommend management with strengthening and engaging in physical activity consistent with international guidelines. They also moderately recommend weight loss to alleviate symptoms of knee OA.
  - Surgical management with early-stage supervised mobilization improves function and reduces pain after TKR.
  - They support the findings by Skou et al.[1] that supervised exercise programs, diet control, and surgical intervention can improve function and alleviate pain.
- Evidence-based guidelines to guide indications and timing of TKR are not known[8] and are currently being developed by the American Academy of Rheumatology.[9] There are consensus statements from professional bodies from Osteoarthritis Research International (OARSI)[10] and the European Alliance of Associations for Rheumatology (EULAR).[11] The National Institute for Health and Care Excellence[12] supports indications for knee replacement including prolonged and established functional limitation and severe pain that have a substantial impact on QOL and are refractory to nonsurgical treatments.

Summary and Implications: This RCT comparing surgical vs. nonsurgical intervention for moderate to severe knee OA with radiological signs found that treatment with TKR followed by nonsurgical treatment for 3 months performed significantly better than nonsurgical treatment alone in terms of functional outcomes and pain. Both groups in the study improved from baseline in terms of $KOOS_4$ subscales.

CASE STUDY: KNEE PAIN: A 78-YEAR-OLD MAN WITH RIGHT KNEE PAIN

Case History

A 78-year-old gentleman presents to the clinic with global right knee pain. He reports pain at rest and at night and struggles to walk for more than 10 minutes. He is unable to do his shopping or do the housework because of his knee. He walks with a stick. He has well-controlled hypertension. Medications include losartan and codydramol. Examination reveals normal hip range of motion (ROM), 10-degree varus knee deformity, crepitus and effusion, a fixed flexion deformity of 10 degrees, and reduction in ROM compared to his normal contralateral side. The radiograph shows KL grade 4 tricompartmental knee OA. How should this patient be managed according to this study?

Suggested Answer

This gentleman is demonstrating a significant decline in his QOL most likely due to the disabling extent of right knee OA. He walks with a walking aid and is unable to participate in activities. The plain film radiograph confirms severe knee OA. Skou et al.[1] suggest that this patient would benefit from a TKR followed by a supervised exercise regime, diet control, and pain relief for at least 3 months to improve his mobility and pain. If the patient refuses operative management, he should be offered a full nonoperative management strategy but should be counseled that although he can expect to improve, he should expect inferior clinical outcomes to that of joint replacement. After all, surgery should always be considered as the final resort and the patient must be appropriately consented for both the benefits and risks of the procedure including pain, bleeding, infection, fracture, loosening, revision surgery, blood clots, neurovascular ± soft tissue injuries, scarring, instability, anesthetic risks, foot drop, complex regional pain syndrome, numbness, and dislocation. Numbness, redness, and swelling may persist for up to 2 years postoperatively. The patient is expected to take responsibility for the aftercare and must partake in the rehabilitation program as there is a dissatisfaction rate of circa 15%–20%.

References

1. Skou et al. A randomized, controlled trial of total knee replacement. N Engl J Med. 2015. 373(17):1597–606.
2. Kellgren et al. Radiological assessment of osteo-arthrosis. Ann Rheum Dis. 1957;16(4):494–502.
3. Roos et al. The Knee injury and Osteoarthritis Outcome Score (KOOS): from joint injury to osteoarthritis. Health Qual Life Outcomes. 2003;1:64.
4. Rabin et al. EQ-5D: a measure of health status from the EuroQol Group. Ann Med. 2001;33(5):337–43.
5. Lim et al. Randomised trial support for orthopaedic surgical procedures. PLoS One. 2014;9(6):e96745.
6. Brown. AAOS clinical practice guideline: treatment of osteoarthritis of the knee: evidence-based guideline, 2nd edition. J Am Acad Orthop Surg. 2013;21(9):577–9.
7. Weber et al. AAOS clinical practice guideline: surgical management of osteoarthritis of the knee: evidence-based guideline. J Am Acad Orthop Surg. 2016;24(8):e94–6.
8. Gossec et al. OARSI-OMERACT Task Force Total Articular Replacement as Outcome Measure in OA. OARSI/OMERACT initiative to define states of severity and indication for joint replacement in hip and knee osteoarthritis. An OMERACT 10 Special Interest Group. J Rheumatol. 2011;38(8):1765–9.

9. American College of Rheumatology. 2023 American College of Rheumatology (ACR) and American Association of Hip and Knee Surgeons (AAHKS) guideline: indications for total hip and knee replacement. https://www.rheumatology.org/Portals/0/Files/Total-Joint-Arthroplasty-Project-Plan.pdf
10. Zhang et al. OARSI recommendations for the management of hip and knee osteoarthritis, part II: OARSI evidence-based, expert consensus guidelines. Osteoarthr Cartil. 2008;16(2):137–62.
11. Jordan et al. EULAR recommendations 2003: an evidence based approach to the management of knee osteoarthritis: Report of a Task Force of the Standing Committee for International Clinical Studies Including Therapeutic Trials (ESCISIT) Ann Rheum Dis. 2003;62:1145–55.
12. National Institute for Health and Care Excellence. Osteoarthritis: care and management (CG177). December 2020. https://www.nice.org.uk/guidance/cg177/chapter/1-Recommendations#referral-for-consideration-of-joint-surgery-2

28

Surgery versus Physical Therapy for a Meniscal Tear and Osteoarthritis

KHALID AL-DADAH AND SHERIF EL-TAWIL

Study Nickname: METEOR trial

> Given that improvements in functional status and pain at 6 months did not differ significantly between patients assigned to arthroscopic partial meniscectomy and those assigned to physical therapy alone—these data provide considerable reassurance regarding an initial non-operative strategy.
>
> —KATZ ET AL.[1]

Citation: Katz JN, Brophy RH, Chaisson CE, de Chaves L, Cole BJ, Dahm DL, Donnell-Fink LA, Guermazi A, Haas AK, Jones MH, Levy BA, Mandl LA, Martin SD, Marx RG, Miniaci A, Matava MJ, Palmisano J, Reinke EK, Richardson BE, Rome BN, Safran-Norton CE, Skoniecki DJ, Solomon DH, Smith MV, Spindler KP, Stuart MJ, Wright J, Wright RW, Losina E. Surgery versus physical therapy for a meniscal tear and osteoarthritis. N Engl J Med. 2013;368(18):1675–84.

Research Question: Should patients aged > 45 years with a symptomatic meniscal tear and mild to moderate knee osteoarthritis (OA) be treated with arthroscopic partial meniscectomy or physiotherapy alone?

Funding: National Institute of Arthritis and Musculoskeletal and Skin Diseases, Maryland, USA

Year Study Began: 2008

Year Study Published: 2013

Study Location: 7 US tertiary referral centers

Who Was Studied: Patients aged > 45 years with symptomatic meniscal tears and evidence of mild to moderate OA on imaging (plain radiography or magnetic resonance imaging [MRI]).

Who Was Excluded: Patients with a locked knee as clear indication for surgery, progressed OA (Kellgren-Lawrence[2] [KL] grade 4), inflammatory arthritis, contraindications to surgery or physiotherapy, prior surgery on the same knee, or viscosupplementation injection in past 4 weeks.

How Many Patients: 351

Study Overview: See Figure 28.1.

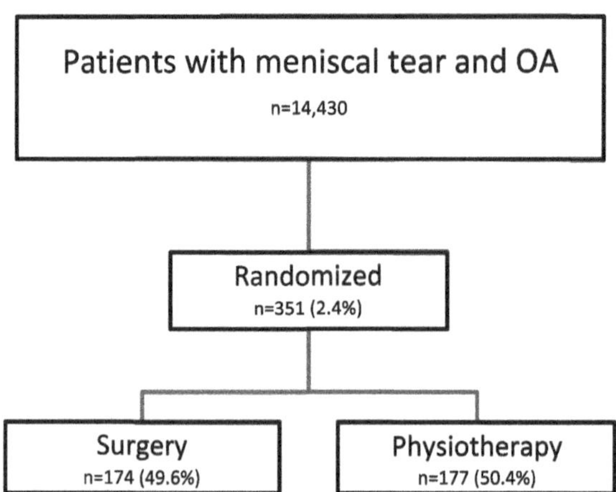

Figure 28.1. Summary of study design.

Study Intervention: In this study 351 patients aged > 45 years were randomized into 2 groups. Group 1 had arthroscopic partial meniscectomy (APM) and postoperative physiotherapy. Group 2 had a standardized physiotherapy (PT) regime alone with no surgical intervention; however, there was the opportunity to cross over to surgery if the patient and surgeon thought it was clinically appropriate.

Group 1—Surgery: Fellowship-trained surgeons, who perform ≥ 50 arthroscopic meniscectomies a year, followed the study protocol. The damaged meniscus was trimmed to a stable rim. Any loose bone or cartilage was debrided without penetration to subchondral bone. Patients could then weight-bear as tolerated without a brace. Then they were referred to a physiotherapist to undergo the same standardized physiotherapy regimen as group 2.

Group 2—Physiotherapy: A protocol was devised by experienced physiotherapists. This addressed inflammation, range of motion, muscle conditioning, and proprioception. Patients attended physiotherapy sessions once or twice weekly and performed exercises at home, with patients progressing at their own pace, for a total of about 6 weeks. Standard analgesia and intra-articular glucocorticoid injections were allowed in both groups throughout their management.

Follow-Up: Baseline and at 3, 6, and 12 months

Endpoints: Primary outcome was difference between the study groups' scores on the physical function scale of the Western Ontario and McMaster Universities Osteoarthritis Index[3] (WOMAC; self-administered questionnaire consisting of 24 items divided into 3 subscales of pain, stiffness, and physical function affected by hip/knee OA) at 6 months. Secondary outcomes included WOMAC scores at 3 and 12 months, pain scores on the Knee injury and Osteoarthritis Outcome Score[4] (KOOS; self-administered knee-specific tool extended from the WOMAC OA index that was developed to assess patients' opinions about their short- and long-term consequences of knee injury), and score on the physical activity scale of the SF-36[5] (self-reported measure of health and quality of life) at each time point. A binary outcome of treatment success or failure was based on whether or not patients improved by 8 points on the WOMAC physical function score.

RESULTS (TABLE 28.1)

- *Clinical scores (Figure 28.2)*
  - *WOMAC*: Surgical group score improved from baseline to 6 months by 13%, but this was insignificant. However, at 6 months, treatment success (as defined above) was 67% in the surgical group vs. 44% in the physiotherapy group ($p = 0.001$).
  - *KOOS*: Surgical group score improved by 14%, but this was insignificant.
  - *SF-36:* Scores were similar for both groups.

- *Cross-over:* At 6 months, 51 patients in the physiotherapy group (30%) went on to have arthroscopic surgery; 9 patients in the surgical group (6%) did not end up having surgery as they either withdrew, went on to have a TKR, or died.
- *TKR conversion:* 5 patients (3%) in the surgical group went on to have TKR compared to 3 patients (2%) in the physiotherapy group.
- *Follow-up (F/U):* In the surgical group, 18 did not complete the study at 12 months, while 13 did not complete it from the physiotherapy-alone group. There was a mixture of reasons, including patient withdrawal, progression to TKR, lost to F/U, and death. Attendance to physiotherapy appointments was 90%–93% for both groups.
- *Steroid injections:* 21 patients (12%) in the physiotherapy group received intra-articular glucocorticoid injections vs. 9 patients (6%) in the surgical group.
- *Adverse events:* No significant between-group adverse events were observed.
- *Mortality:* 1 death (0.6%) occurred in each group (pulmonary embolism in the surgical group and sudden death in physiotherapy group).

Table 28.1 Score Outcomes between Both Groups

Outcome Mean (95% CI)	**Arthroscopic Partial Meniscectomy (*n* = 161)**	**Physiotherapy (*n* = 169)**	**Between-Group Difference in Improvement from Baseline**
		6 Months	
WOMAC	14.7 (12.0–17.5)	19.0 (16.3–21.7)	2.4 (−1.8–6.5)
KOOS	21.1 (18.3–23.9)	25.2 (22.4–28.0)	2.9 (−1.2–7.0)
SF-36	69.2 (65.2–73.2)	66.1 (62.1–70.1)	1.1 (−4.4–6.6)
Crossover within 6 months, no./total (%)	8/40 (20)	51/82 (62)	
Data missing, *no. (%)*	13 (8)	13 (8)	
		12 Months	
WOMAC	13.7 (11.2–16.2)	14.5 (12.0 –16.9)	0.7 (−3.5–4.9)
KOOS	19.1 (16.4–21.9)	19.3 (16.6–22.0)	−0.4 (−4.8–4.0)
SF-36	69.0 (64.6–73.4)	71.4 (67.0–75.7)	−3.0 (−8.8–2.7)

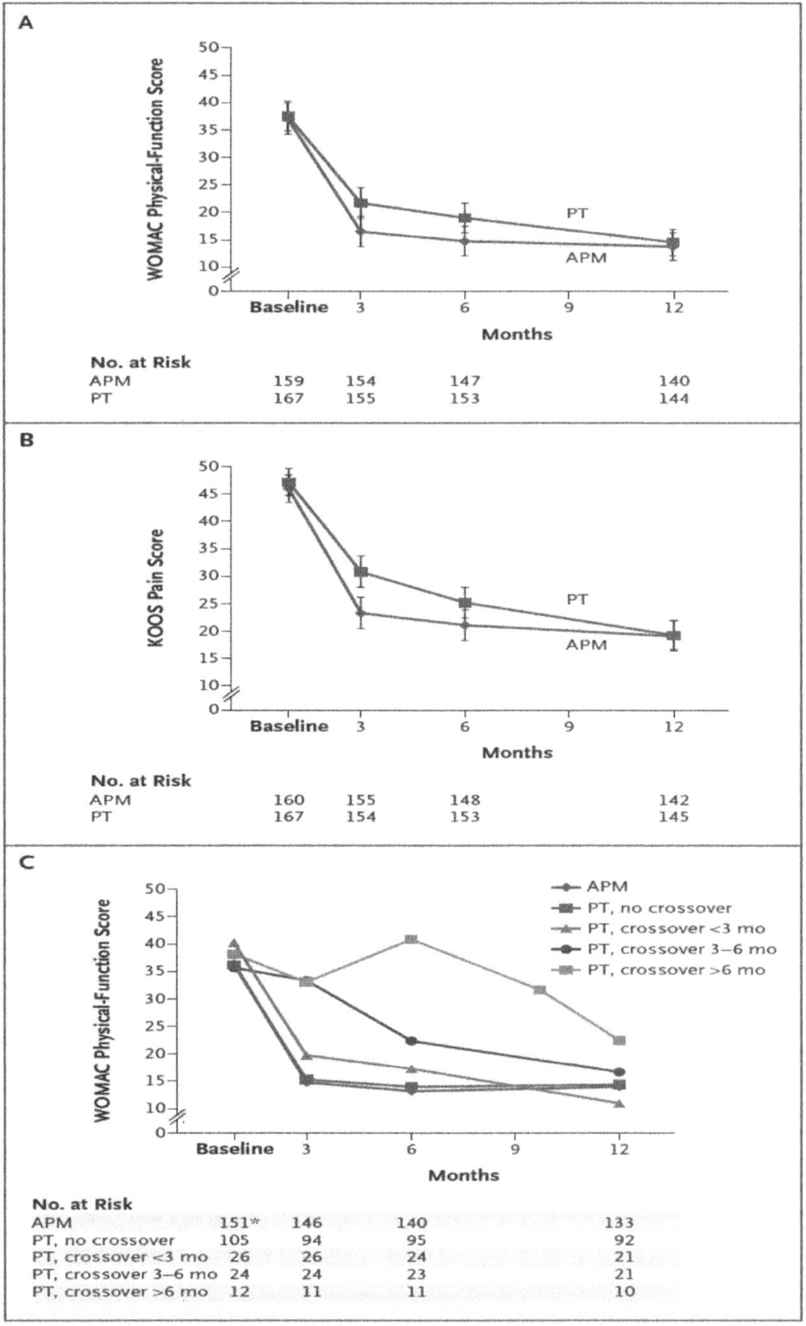

Figure 28.2. Scores on the WOMAC physical function scale and KOOS pain scale over the 12-month F/U. (A) shows the scores on the physical-function scale of the WOMAC. (B) shows the scores on the pain scale of the KOOS; scores on both scales range from 0-100, with higher scores indicating more severe symptoms. Bars indicate 95% CI. (C) shows WOMAC physical-function scores in the APM group and in the PT group according to crossover status. * indicates that 9 patients assigned to APM did not undergo surgery.

Criticisms and Limitations: Only 26% of eligible patients were enrolled, as the patient or surgeon had a strong preference for one treatment or the other, making it vulnerable to selection bias. The study was not blinded, as a sham comparison group was not feasible. The trial was conducted at an academic tertiary referral center; therefore, care must be taken when generalizing the findings in the community or district general hospital settings.

Other Relevant Studies and Information:

- The more recent ESCAPE trial is a similar multicenter randomized controlled trial taking place across 9 hospitals in The Netherlands; 321 patients aged > 45 years were randomized to arthroscopic meniscectomy and physiotherapy. Subjects had symptomatic, nonobstructive meniscal tears (no locking) and mild to moderate OA. Self-reported knee functional scores were obtained over a 2-year period. There was no significant difference between the operative group and physiotherapy group.[6]
- A systematic review and meta-analysis looked at 9 eligible trials comparing arthroscopic partial meniscectomy and physiotherapy in patients who were of middle or older age, with or without signs of OA. At 6 months, there was a marginal functional benefit in the operative group; however, outcomes were equal at the 12- and 24-month postoperative mark between both groups.[7]
- Most high-impact trials are in favor of trialing a period of physiotherapy in the first instance, before proceeding with surgery.[8]
- The British Association for Surgery of the Knee[9,10] has prepared a meniscal tear management guideline flow chart outlining indications for conservative vs. operative options. Likewise, the European Society for Sports Traumatology, Knee Surgery and Arthroscopy (ESSKA),[11] Australian Knee Society,[11] and American Physical Therapy Association[13] have also published their guidelines. The American Academy of Orthopaedic Surgeons[14] went as far as to deem the recommendation regarding arthroscopic partial meniscectomy (in knee OA) from a consensus to inconclusive. Furthermore, the National Institute for Health and Care Excellence has no guidelines published on this.

Summary and Implications: In this trial of patients with mild to moderate OA and meniscal tears, there was no clear benefit of early surgical intervention compared to physiotherapy. At 6 months, there was a trend toward benefit with surgical treatment; however, after 12 months of F/U this trend became equivocal. Based on this and other studies, among patients with symptomatic, nonobstructive (i.e., no locking) meniscal tears, it is appropriate to begin treatment with a period of physiotherapy, reserving surgery for cases in which symptoms persist despite exhausting conservative management options.

CLINICAL CASE: SURGERY VERSUS PHYSICAL THERAPY FOR A MENISCAL TEAR AND OA

Case History

A 52-year-old gentleman comes to the clinic presenting with medial joint line tenderness of the right knee. It occurred while he was gardening around 6 weeks ago. As he knelt down to pull weeds from the ground, he felt a pop and pain in his knee with a slow effusion over the next few days. The pain has settled with simple analgesia over the recent weeks; however, he has pain in the posteromedial aspect on deep squatting and kneeling and in bed when his leg rolls over. He is otherwise fit, well, and active, and works as an IT consultant. Based on the METEOR trial, what is the most appropriate management for this patient?

Suggested Answer

This is a very common scenario seen in the clinic. Clearly there is a history of an exacerbating onset, and the temptation is to elect a surgical option to rectify the acute problem. The METEOR trial provides a sensible treatment pathway for this scenario. It is advisable to obtain imaging in the form of a plain radiograph in the first instance to assess for a traumatic bone injury or degenerative changes. Depending on the patient's symptoms, an MRI may characterize the offending pathology further. As long as there are no obstructive symptoms, such as a locked knee, the evidence suggests that it is appropriate to begin with a standardized physiotherapy regimen. It ought to be emphasized that the patient must also take responsibility by performing exercises at home regularly, and not only in the presence of physiotherapists. A review can be made at 6 months, allowing sufficient time to rehabilitate the knee, especially if this patient has had a recent improvement in the severity of symptoms. If in the F/U visit the patient has persisting symptoms affecting his activities of daily living, or worsening of symptoms sooner, a discussion can be had with the patient regarding arthroscopic partial meniscectomy. It is then up to the patient to decide if the severity of his symptoms outweighs the risks of surgery following a formal consenting process.

References

1. Katz et al. Surgery versus physical therapy for a meniscal tear and osteoarthritis. N Engl J Med. 2013;368(18):1675–84.
2. Kellgren et al. Radiological assessment of osteo-arthrosis. Ann Rheum Dis. 1957;16(4):494–502.
3. Bellamy et al. Validation study of WOMAC: a health status instrument for measuring clinically important patient relevant outcomes to antirheumatic drug therapy in patients with osteo-arthritis of the hip or knee. J Rheumatol. 1988;15:1833–40.
4. Roos et al. The Knee injury and Osteoarthritis Outcome Score (KOOS): from joint injury to osteoarthritis. Health Qual Life Outcomes. 2003;1:64.
5. Ware Jr et al. The MOS 36-Item Short-Form Health Survey (SF-36). I. Conceptual framework and item selection. Med Care. 1992;30:473–83.
6. Van de Graaf et al. Effect of early surgery vs physical therapy on knee function among patients with nonobstructive meniscal tears. The ESCAPE randomized clinical trial. JAMA. 2019;320(13):1328–37.
7. Thorlund et al. Arthroscopic surgery for degenerative knee: systematic review and meta-analysis of benefits and harms. Br J Sports Med. 2015;49:1229–35.
8. Khan et al. Arthroscopic surgery for degenerative tears of the meniscus: a systematic review and meta-analysis. CMAJ. 2014;186(14):1057–64.
9. Abram et al. BASK Meniscal Working Group. Arthroscopic meniscal surgery: a national society treatment guideline and consensus statement. Bone Joint J. 2019;101-B(6):652–9.
10. British Association for Surgery of the Knee (BASK). BASK meniscal surgery guideline 2018. https://baskonline.com/professional/wp-content/uploads/sites/5/2018/07/BASK-Meniscal-Surgery-Guideline-2018.pdf
11. Kopf et al. Management of traumatic meniscus tears: the 2019 ESSKA meniscus consensus. Knee Surg Sports Traumatol Arthrosc. 2020;28(4):1177–94.
12. Australian Knee Society. Australian Orthopaedic Association. Position statement from the Australian Knee Society on Arthroscopic Surgery of the Knee, including reference to the presence of osteoarthritis or degenerative joint disease. 2019. https://www.kneesociety.org.au/resources/Position-Statement-from-the-Australian-Knee-Society-on-Arthroscopic-Surgery-of-the-Knee-Final-2019.pdf
13. Logerstedt et al. Knee pain and mobility impairments: meniscal and articular cartilage lesions revision 2018. J Orthop Sports Phys Ther. 2018;48(2):A1–50.
14. Jevsevar DS. Treatment of osteoarthritis of the knee: evidence-based guideline, 2nd edition. J Am Acad Orthop Surg. 2013;21(9):571–6.

29

Compression Plating versus Intramedullary Nailing for Humeral Shaft Fractures Requiring Operative Fixation

CATRIN MORGAN, KEWAL SINGH, AND ALEXANDER MAGNUSSEN

> Open reduction and internal fixation with dynamic compression plating remains the best treatment for unstable fractures of the shaft of the humerus. Fixation by intramedullary nailing may be indicated for specific situations, but is technically more demanding and has a higher rate of complications.
>
> —McCormack et al.[1]

Citation: McCormack RG, Brien D, Buckley RE, McKee MD, Powell J, Schemitsch EH. Fixation of fractures of the shaft of the humerus by dynamic compression plate or intramedullary nail: a prospective, randomised trial. J Bone Joint Surg Br. 2000;82(3):336–9.

Research Question: In acute and unstable humeral shaft fractures, which method of fixation provides the most optimal functional outcome with the least complications?

Funding: No funding declared

Year Study Began: 1994

Year Study Published: 2000

Study Location: Canada

Who Was Studied: Skeletally mature patients of all ages who sustained fractures to the humeral shaft that required surgical stabilization.

Who Was Excluded: Any patient with an injury > 3 weeks old, previous humerus fractures, pre-existing humerus pathology, pathological fractures, or grade III (Gustilo Anderson classification) open fractures, and those who would not be able to cooperate with functional assessment.

How Many Patients: 44

Study Overview: See Figure 29.1.

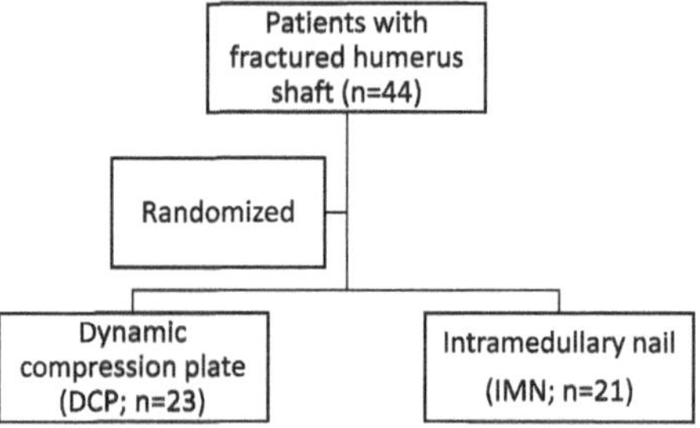

Figure 29.1. Study overview.

Study Intervention: All patients were operated on by specialist surgeons across the 3 centers. Those randomized to plate fixation had a dynamic compression plate (DCP) applied through either a posterior or an anterolateral approach. The length of the plate and need for bone grafting were dependent on the fracture pattern and not part of the final analysis. The second group received an intramedullary nail (IMN) using the Russell-Taylor Locked Nail (Smith and Nephew, Memphis, Tennessee, USA). Initially all nails were inserted antegrade, but after an interim analysis as well as publication of new literature reporting shoulder problems, retrograde insertion was performed wherever possible.

Follow-Up: Mean of 14.3 months (range 6–33)

Endpoints: The primary outcomes consisted of function using the American Shoulder and Elbow Surgeons' (ASES) score[2] (based on a mixed-outcome reporting measure, applicable for use in all patients with shoulder pathology regardless of their specific diagnosis) and pain using a visual analog scale (VAS).

Secondary outcomes consisted of incidence of complications and need for further surgery.

RESULTS (TABLES 29.1 AND 29.2)

- *Complications*: 16 complications and 8 secondary operations were documented. Complications (81%) and the need for further surgery (87.5%) were significantly more common in the IMN group ($p < 0.02$).
- *Nonunion:* Only 1 case of nonunion in the DCP group required further surgery, whereas the rest ($n = 2$) had good outcomes with conservative treatment.
- *Revisions/reoperations:* In the IMN group, the late fracture and nonunions ($n = 3$) required revision to DCP. Cases leading to impingement and infection ($n = 4$) required removal of the nail. The adhesive capsulitis case ($n = 1$) required manipulation under anesthesia but still did not regain full function.
- *Pain and function:* Insignificant differences were found for both at final follow-up (F/U) between groups.

Table 29.1 Details of Complications in Both Groups

Complication	DCP	IMN
Iatrogenic palsy of radial nerve	0	3 (23%)
Late fracture	0	1 (8%)
Nonunion	1 (33%)	2 (15%)
Intraoperative comminution	1 (33%)	2 (15%)
Infection	0	1 (8%)
Severe impingement	0	3 (23%)
Adhesive capsulitis (shoulder)	0	1 (8%)
Minimal loss of fixation	1 (33%)	0
Total	**3**	**13**

Table 29.2 Details of Secondary Surgery Required in Both Groups

Indication	DCP	IMN
Nonunion	1 (100%)	2 (28.5%)
Infection	0	1 (14.3%)
Nerve palsy	0	1 (14.3%)
Failure of fixation	0	1 (14.3%)
Impingement	0	2 (28.5%)
Total	**1**	7

Criticisms and Limitations: The study consisted of a small number ($n = 44$) of patients and had a change in study protocol during the trial (antegrade insertion of nail changed to retrograde), which could have influenced the outcomes. Recruitment halted when an increased incidence of complications and need for further surgery were identified in the IMN group. This study used curved nails, whereas contemporary practice, especially in the UK, leans more toward using a straight nail to avoid violating the rotator cuff at the watershed vascular zone. This also diminishes the risk of iatrogenic rotator cuff injury.

Other Relevant Studies and Information:

- This study was included in a Cochrane systematic review[3] along with another 4 small trials totaling 260 patients. Findings were similar in that IMN was associated with a significantly increased risk of shoulder impingement as well as need for further surgery. Additionally, there was no significant difference found in blood loss, operating time, nerve injury, ASES score, or return to preinjury occupation.
- A meta-analysis published in 2006 including 2 additional studies ($n = 155$) also reached a similar conclusion.[4]
- The HUMMER (HUMeral Shaft Fractures: MEasuring Recovery after Operative versus Non-operative Treatment) study, a multicenter prospective cohort, compared primary osteosynthesis and nonoperative management for AO type 12A and 12B humeral shaft fractures. This study included 390 patients and found that primary osteosynthesis was superior to nonoperative treatment with an earlier functional recovery, better shoulder and elbow range of motion, and reduced risk of nonunion.[5]
- A prospective randomized study compared locking IMN and locking plates in the treatment of 2-part proximal humeral surgical neck fractures.[6] This study included 51 patients with a minimum 3-year F/U. The results demonstrated no difference in ASES scores between both groups. In contrast to McCormack et al.,[1] the complication rate was lower in the locking IMN group; however, locking plate fixation had better 1-year outcomes.

Summary and Implications: In this study involving patients with acute and unstable humeral shaft fractures, open reduction and internal fixation with DCP was associated with similar functional outcomes as fixation by IMN. Still, this study and the wider literature have suggested significantly higher complication rates (including shoulder impingement), revision rates, and a technically more challenging procedure with IMN. Based on the evidence, DCP should be the primary consideration for surgical fixation of humeral shaft fractures.

CLINICAL CASE: HIGH ENERGY SHAFT OF HUMERUS FRACTURE IN MANUAL LABORER

Case History

A 32-year-old right-hand-dominant male builder presents after having fallen 3 meters off of scaffolding. He is otherwise fit and healthy. He drinks alcohol socially and is an ex-smoker for 2 years. The patient is also sporty. He has sustained an isolated, closed fracture to the diaphysis of his right humerus. There is no neurovascular deficit. Plain radiographs show a long oblique fracture pattern with a large butterfly segment at the level of the spiral groove. There is significant displacement and a rotational deformity. Based on the results of this study, how should this patient be treated?

Suggested Answer

The study conducted by McCormack et al.[1] demonstrated no difference in functional outcome between DCP and IMN in humeral shaft fractures; however, it did report a significantly higher complication and revision rate with IMN. The patient is a young and active patient with an unstable fracture. Therefore, this injury requires surgical fixation. This patient should be treated with DCP fixation. However, his functional outcome will likely not differ between plating and nailing. DCP fixation has lower complication rates, and the patient is less likely to require metalwork removal in the future. Moreover, this approach avoids violating an otherwise healthy rotator cuff and has a lower risk of shoulder impingement compared to IMN.

References

1. McCormack et al. Fixation of fractures of the shaft of the humerus by dynamic compression plate or intramedullary nail: a prospective, randomised trial. J Bone Joint Surg Br. 2000;82(3):336–9.
2. Angst et al. Measures of adult shoulder function: Disabilities of the Arm, Shoulder, and Hand Questionnaire (DASH) and its short version (QuickDASH), Shoulder Pain and Disability Index (SPADI), American Shoulder and Elbow Surgeons (ASES) Society standardized shoulder assessment form, Constant (Murley) Score (CS), Simple Shoulder Test (SST), Oxford Shoulder Score (OSS), Shoulder Disability Questionnaire (SDQ), and Western Ontario Shoulder Instability Index (WOSI). Arthritis Care Res (Hoboken). 2011 Nov;63(Suppl 11):S174–88.

3. Kurup et al. Dynamic compression plating versus locked intramedullary nailing for humeral shaft fractures in adults. Cochrane Database Syst Rev. 2011 Jun 15;(6):CD005959.
4. Bhandari et al. Compression plating versus intramedullary nailing of humeral shaft fractures—a meta-analysis. Acta Orthop. 2006;77(2):279–84.
5. Den Hartog et al. Functional and clinical outcome after operative versus nonoperative treatment of a humeral shaft fracture (HUMMER): results of a multicenter prospective cohort study. Eur J Trauma Emerg Surg. 2022;48(4):3265–77.
6. Zhu et al. Locking intramedullary nails and locking plates in the treatment of two-part proximal humeral surgical neck fractures: a prospective randomized trial with a minimum of three years of follow-up. J Bone Joint Surg Am. 2011;93(2):159–68.

30

Autologous Chondrocyte Implantation Compared with Microfracture in Isolated Symptomatic Chondral Defect of the Knee

AMIN ABUKAR AND KESAVAN SRI-RAM

> Both methods (autologous chondrocyte implantation and microfracture) had acceptable short-term clinical results. There was no significant difference in macroscopic or histological results between the two treatment groups and no association between the histological findings and the clinical outcome at the two-year time-point.
>
> —KNUTSEN ET AL.[1]

Citation: Knutsen G, Engebretsen L, Ludvigsen TC, Drogset JO, Grontvedt T, Solheim E, Strand T, Roberts S, Isaksen V, Johansen O. Autologous chondrocyte implantation compared with microfracture in the knee: a randomized trial. J Bone Joint Surg Am. 2004;86-A(3):455–64.

Research Question: Should patients with an isolated symptomatic chondral defect of the knee be managed with autologous chondrocyte implantation (ACI) or microfracture (MF)?

Funding: Norwegian Ministry of Health

Year Study Began: January 1999

Year Study Published: March 2004

Study Location: 4 university hospitals in Norway

Who Was Studied: Adult patients (aged 18–45 years) with a single symptomatic cartilage defect (Outerbridge grade 3 or 4, measuring between 2 and 10 cm^2 postdebridement; osteochondral lesions < 10 mm in depth) in a stable knee (i.e., no fixed-flexion deformity).

Who Was Excluded: Patients with a history of substance (i.e., drug/alcohol) abuse during last 3 years, body mass index > 30 kg/m^2, presence of patellofemoral instability, or malalignment with > 5 degrees valgus or varus deformity. Patients with serious illness, arthroscopically verified general osteoarthritis (OA) but without a specified severity, gout, Bechterew syndrome (ankylosing spondylitis), or chondrocalcinosis.

How Many Patients: 80 patients

Study Overview: See Figure 30.1.

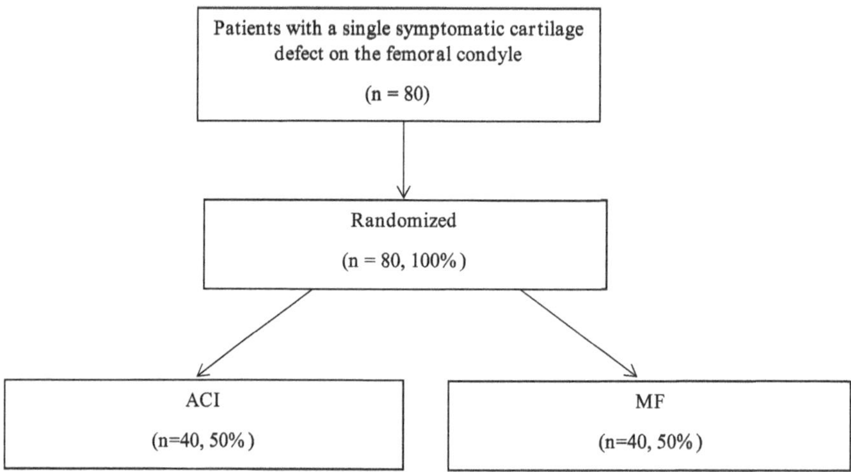

Figure 30.1. Summary of study design.

Study Intervention: Patients in the MF group underwent single-stage arthroscopy with microfracture following randomization. However, patients in the ACI group had a 2-stage intervention. The ACI group had cartilage cell samples harvested during the initial arthroscopy after randomization prior to returning approximately 4 weeks later for cell implantation through an arthrotomy. Both groups were subsequently treated with the same rehabilitation program.

Follow-Up: 2 years

Endpoints: The outcomes included a head-to-head comparison between the treatment groups involving clinical scores (Lysholm,[2] SF-36,[3] pain visual analog scale [VAS],[4] and Tegner[5]) and histological (macroscopic assessment at arthroscopy and microscopic assessment of the repair cartilage biopsy) parameters.

RESULTS (TABLE 30.1)

- *Lysholm score (LS):* This improved significantly *within* both groups and without significant difference *between* both groups (Figure 30.2).
- *VAS*: Pain was significantly improved *within* both groups without significant difference *between* both groups (Figure 30.2).
- *MF group*: There was significantly better improvement in the SF-36 physical component vs. the ACI group. However, with regard to the SF-36 mental health subscale score, there was no difference *between* the groups (Figure 30.2).
- *Age:* In both groups younger patients (aged < 30 years) had significantly better clinical outcomes than older patients.
- *Activity level*: More active patients (Tegner score > 4) had significantly better clinical results (i.e., LS, VAS, and SF-36 scores) than less active patients.
- *Size of defect:* Patients in the MF group with a lesion < 4 cm^2 had significantly better clinical results (i.e., LS, VAS, and SF-36 scores) than those with a larger defect. In the ACI group, no association between defect size and clinical outcome was detected.
- *Histology:* Macroscopically, there were no differences between both groups. Microscopically, there was no significant difference between the groups in regard to the frequency with which hyaline and fibrocartilage repair tissues were found. No association was found between the histological quality of the cartilage biopsy and clinical outcomes (i.e., LS, SF-36, and VAS scores).
- *Complications:* There were 2 failures at 6 and 12 months in the ACI group and 1 failure at 15 months in the MF group. In both groups no serious complications such as deep infection or thromboembolic events were recorded.

Table 30.1 SUMMARY OF KEY FINDINGS

Outcome	**Significant Improvement Compared with Baseline**		**Significant Difference between the Groups**
	Microfracture	**Autologous Cartilage Implantation**	
Lysholm score	Yes ($p < 0.0001$)	Yes ($p = 0.003$)	NS
Visual analog score	Yes ($p < 0.0001$)	Yes ($p < 0.0001$)	NS
SF-36 physical[1] component			Yes ($p = 0.004$)[a]
Macroscopic evaluation			NS
Microscopic evaluation			NS

[a] The MF group had a significantly better improvement in the SF-36 physical component compared with ACI.
NS, not significant.

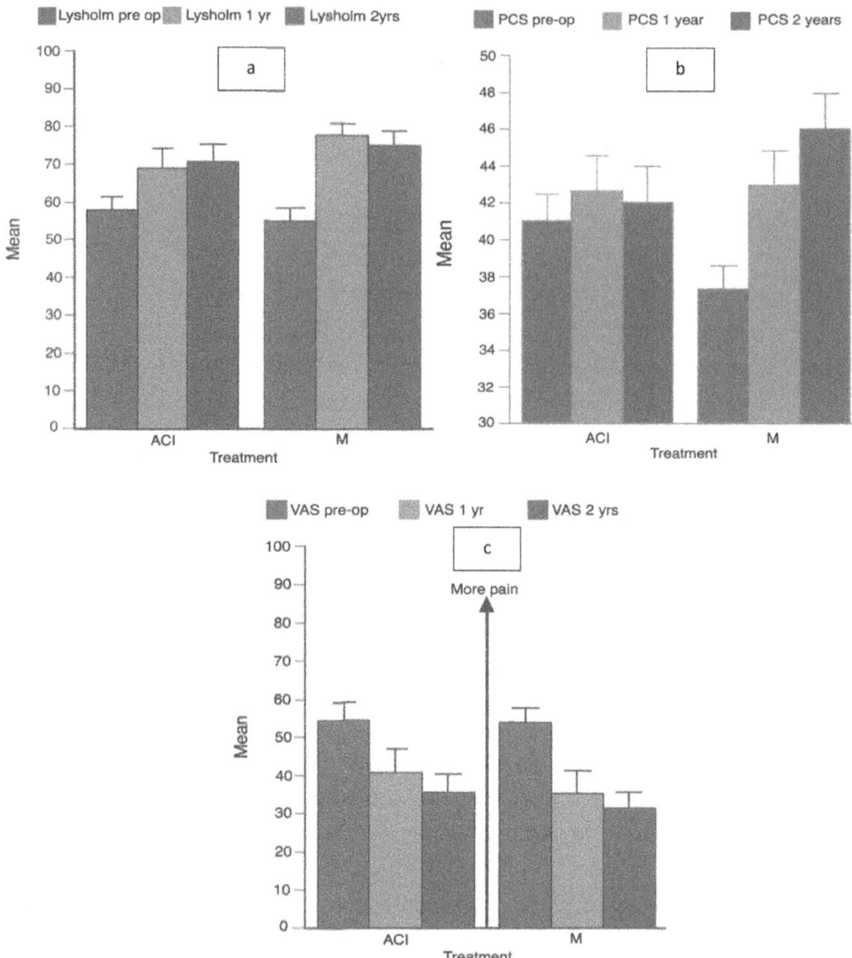

Figure 30.2. Histograms demonstrating preoperative vs. 1- and 2-year postoperative scores for (a) mean Lysholm scores, where score at 2 years was significantly improved compared to both groups at baseline ($p < 0.003$) but without any significant difference *between* groups detected ($p = 0.092$); (b) mean SF-36 physical component scores (PCS), where improvement was significantly better in the MF group ($p = 0.004$); (c) mean pain scores from VAS, where pain at 2 years was significantly improved compared with the baseline value in both groups ($p < 0.0001$) but without any significant difference *between* the groups detected ($p = 0.292$).

Criticisms and Limitations: It was not possible to blind the surgeon or the patient in this study due to the 2-stage nature of the ACI. The study results cannot be generalized to all patients presenting with cartilage problems, as the authors assessed cartilage defects only on weight-bearing medial and lateral femoral condyles; hence, patellofemoral joint cartilage defects were not included. Also, the authors reported that they did not detect a significant difference between either MF or ACI with regard to histological findings. However, it was acknowledged that the present study was not sufficiently powered to detect a difference between the 2 interventions.

Other Relevant Studies and Information:

- The authors from the original study published the results of their long-term F/U. Surviving patients (who did not have a failure) had significant improvements in their clinical scores compared with their own baseline at long-term F/U (14–15 years). There was no significant difference between the groups; 57% in the ACI group and 48% in the MF group had evidence of early OA, highlighting concerns about the efficacy of interventions in delaying OA and preventing further surgery.[6]
- A number of studies comparing MF with ACI have come to similar conclusions as the study conducted by Knutsen et al.,[1] although in some studies an evolved version of the ACI technique (second and third generations) were utilized, which revealed similar or somewhat better clinical results than MF.[7–12] Moreover, Aae et al. conducted cost-effective analysis using published trials and observed that MF was associated with lower costs and lower cost per point increase in patient-reported outcome measures.[13]
- The American Academy of Orthopaedic Surgeons[14] was unable to recommend for or against a specific cartilage repair technique in symptomatic skeletally immature/mature patients with unsalvageable osteochondritis dissecans lesions. The Cochrane group[15] was also unable to draw any conclusions due to insufficient evidence. The National Institute for Health and Care Excellence (NICE)[16,17] summarizes the available evidence only supporting the use of ACI (using chondrosphere) in patients without previous repair to articular cartilage defects, minimal osteoarthritic damage to the knee, and osteochondritis dissecans lesions > 2 cm^2. Yet it is as effective in the short term as MF, which is the most commonly used surgical option. The International Cartilage Repair Society[18] supported the NICE guidelines but added that ACI ought to be conducted in a tertiary referral center and proposing exhaustive guidelines on the design and conduct of associated clinical studies in knee articular cartilage repair.[19] Insurance companies have written extensive policies on their indications for supporting ACI treatment.[20,21]

Summary and Implications: In patients with a single symptomatic cartilage defect, autologous use of either ACI or MF provided significant clinical improvements in the short term (i.e., 2 years). There was no significant difference between the groups in regard to Lysholm and VAS scores; however, at the 2-year mark those in the MF group had a significantly better SF-36 physical component than the ACI group. Additionally, within the MF group, patients with smaller cartilage lesions (< 4 cm^2) had significantly better clinical results. The results, however, cannot be generalized to all patients presenting with cartilage defects as the study was limited to patients with lesions located only on the weight-bearing portions of the medial and lateral femoral condyles.

CLINICAL CASE: ACI VERSUS MF IN THE KNEE

Case History

A 28-year-old man with no significant past medical history presented with knee pain and swelling. His clinical examination was unremarkable except for a mild effusion and medial joint line tenderness. The affected knee was initially assessed with a plain radiograph, which was within normal limits; he was then sent for magnetic resonance imaging (MRI). The MRI study revealed a chondral defect on the medial femoral condyle. This chondral defect was further evaluated at arthroscopy, where he was noted to have an isolated Outerbridge grade 3 defect on his medial femoral condyle. The chondral defect measured 1.5 × 1.0 cm in size after debridement to healthy cartilage. Which definitive treatment option will you advise according to this study?

Suggested Answer

The recommendation leans toward MF. The study by Knutsen et al.[1] showed that in the MF group chondral defect sizes < 4 cm^2 had significantly better results clinically (i.e., Lysholm, VAS, and SF-36 physical component scores) compared to those with a larger defect. In contrast, this association between chondral defect size and clinical outcome was not observed in the ACI group. As noted by the authors, MF is a relatively simple and single-stage procedure, whereas ACI is more technically demanding, requiring 2 separate surgical procedures. For the patient this means less surgery with MF and hence rehabilitation is easier. This may account for the MF group having a significantly better improvement in the SF-36 physical component compared with ACI.

References

1. Knutsen et al. Autologous chondrocyte implantation compared with microfracture in the knee: a randomized trial. J Bone Joint Surg Am. 2004;86-A(3):455–64.
2. Smith et al. Modification and validation of the Lysholm Knee Scale to assess articular cartilage damage. Osteoarthr Cartil. 2009;17:53–8.
3. Ware Jr et al. The MOS 36-Item Short-Form Health Survey (SF-36): I. Conceptual framework and item selection. Med Care. 1992 (30):473–83.
4. Scott et al. Graphic representation of pain. Pain. 1976;2:175–84.
5. Briggs et al. Lysholm score and Tegner activity level in individuals with normal knees. Am J Sports Med. 2009;37:898–901.
6. Knutsen et al. A randomized multicenter trial comparing autologous chondrocyte implantation with microfracture. J Bone Joint Surg Am. 2016;98-A(16):1332–9.
7. Vanlauwe et al. Five-year outcome of characterized chondrocyte implantation versus microfracture for symptomatic cartilage defects of the knee. Am J Sports Med. 2011;39(12):2566–74.
8. Lim et al. Current treatments of isolated articular cartilage lesions of the knee achieve similar outcomes. Clin Orthop Relat Res. 2012;470(8):2261–7.
9. Petri et al. CaReS (MACT) versus microfracture in treating symptomatic patellofemoral cartilage defects: a retrospective matched-pair analysis. J Orthop Sci. 2013;18(1):38–44.
10. Van Assche et al. Physical activity levels after characterized chondrocyte implantation versus microfracture in the knee and the relationship to objective functional outcome with 2-year follow-up. Am J Sports Med. 2009;37(1_Suppl):42–9.
11. Kon et al. Arthroscopic second-generation autologous chondrocyte implantation compared with microfracture for chondral lesions of the knee. Am J Sports Med. 2009;37(1):33–41.
12. Basad et al. Matrix-induced autologous chondrocyte implantation versus microfracture in the treatment of cartilage defects of the knee: a 2-year randomised study. Knee Surg Sports Traumatol Arthrosc. 2010;18(4):519–27.
13. Aae et al. Microfracture is more cost-effective than autologous chondrocyte implantation: a review of level 1 and level 2 studies with 5 year follow-up. Knee Surg Sports Traumatol Arthrosc. 2018;26:1044–52.
14. Chambers et al. American Academy of Orthopaedic Surgeons clinical practice guideline on: the diagnosis and treatment of osteochondritis dissecans. J Bone Joint Surg Am. 2012;94(14):1322–4.
15. Gracitelli et al. Surgical interventions (microfracture, drilling, mosaicplasty, and allograft transplantation) for treating isolated cartilage defects of the knee in adults. Cochrane Database Syst Rev. 2016;(9):CD010675.
16. National Institute for Health and Care Excellence. Interventional Procedures Programme. Interventional procedure overview of mosaicplasty for symptomatic articular cartilage defects of the knee. IP 283/2 (IPG607). 2018. https://www.nice.org.uk/guidance/ipg607/evidence/overview-final-pdf-4778837965
17. National Institute for Health and Care Excellence. Autologous chondrocyte implantation using chondrosphere for treating symptomatic articular cartilage defects of the knee (TA508). March 2018. https://www.nice.org.uk/guidance/ta508/resour

ces/autologous-chondrocyte-implantation-using-chondrosphere-for-treating-symptomatic-articular-cartilage-defects-of-the-knee-pdf-82606726260421

18. International Cartilage Regeneration and Joint Preservation Society. NICE (National Institute for Clinical Excellence) guidance on ACI. October 2017. https://cartilage.org/news/nice-national-institute-for-clinical-excellence-issued-guidance-on-aci
19. Mithoefer et al. Guidelines for the design and conduct of clinical studies in knee articular cartilage repair: International Cartilage Repair Society recommendations based on current scientific evidence and standards of clinical care. Cartilage. 2011;2(2):100–21.
20. Aetna. Autologous chondrocyte implantation. February 2021. http://www.aetna.com/cpb/medical/data/200_299/0247.html
21. UnitedHealthcare® Commercial Medical Policy. Articular cartilage defect repairs. Policy Number: 2021T0030U. July 2021. https://www.uhcprovider.com/content/dam/provider/docs/public/policies/comm-medical-drug/articular-cartilage-defect-repairs.pdf

31

Comparison of Adverse Outcomes after Total Knee versus Unicompartmental Knee Replacements

RAVI POPAT, SUBHAJIT GHOSH, AND DINESH NATHWANI

> In decisions about which procedure to offer, the higher revision/reoperation rate of [unicompartmental knee replacement] than of [total knee replacement] should be balanced against a lower occurrence of complications, readmission, and mortality, together with known benefits for [unicompartmental knee replacement] in terms of postoperative function.
>
> —LIDDLE ET AL.[1]

Citation: Liddle A, Judge A, Pandit H, Murray D. Adverse outcomes after total and unicompartmental knee replacement in 101,330 matched patients: a study of data from the National Joint Registry for England and Wales. Lancet. 2014;384(9952):1437–45.

Research Question: Is there a significant difference in the rate of adverse outcomes in a matched cohort of patients receiving a total knee replacement (TKR) vs. unicompartmental/unicondylar knee replacement (UKR)?

Funding: Royal College of Surgeons of England and Arthritis Research UK

Year Study Began: 2012 (data collection began April 2003)

Year Study Published: 2015

Study Location: Nuffield Department of Orthopedics, Rheumatology and Musculoskeletal Science, University of Oxford, Oxford

Who Was Studied: 25 334 UKRs were matched to 75 996 TKRs on the basis of propensity score.

Who Was Excluded: Patellofemoral replacements, complex primary TKR, primary operations with augmentation and stems.

How Many Patients: 101 330

Study Overview: See Figure 31.1.

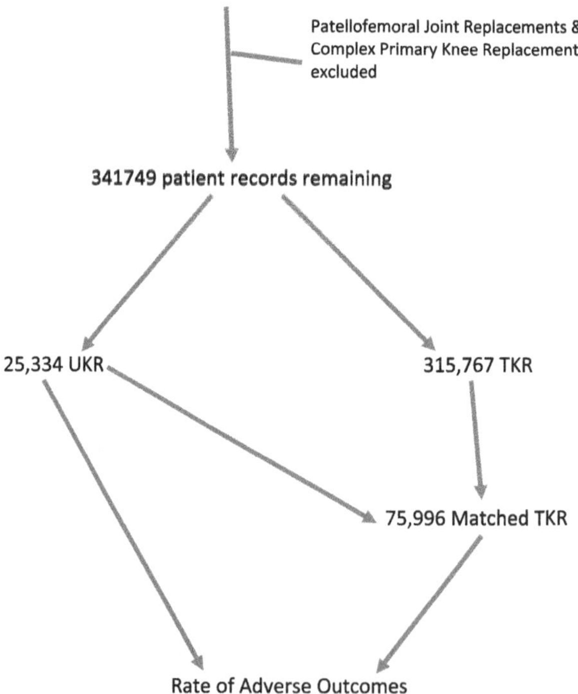

Figure 31.1. Study overview.

Study Intervention: A total of 101 330 patient records were analyzed from the original 552 015 records. Outcomes from the National Joint Registry for

England and Wales, Hospital Episode Statistics (HES), and the Office for National Statistics were reviewed. Propensity score matching was used to generate a matched cohort on a 1:3 ratio producing 75 996 TKRs for comparison to reduce bias due to confounding variables. Matched confounders included:

- Age
- Sex
- Ethnic origin
- Implant fixation
- American Society of Anesthesiologists score
- Type of mechanical or chemical thromboprophylaxis
- Surgical caseload done by the surgeon in charge in the year of surgery
- The grade of the primary surgeon (consultant or trainee)

Follow-Up: Implant survival reported at 8 years

Endpoints: Analyses were performed to compare the outcomes of TKR and UKR using 6 measures:

- Rates of revision
- Revision/reoperation
- Readmission
- Length of stay (LOS)
- Complications of surgery
- Mortality

RESULTS

Analysis of the matched cohorts demonstrated the following:

- *Reoperation rate (Table 31.1):*
    - In the first 3 months, the revision/reoperation rate was significantly higher for TKR than for UKR.
    - Between 3 months and 8 years, the risk of revision/reoperation was significantly higher for UKR than TKR (subhazard ratio [SHR] 1.38; 95% CI: 1.31–1.44).
    - Although aseptic loosening was the most common reason for revision after either operation, significantly more TKRs than UKRs were revised for infection and stiffness. Yet, unexplained pain, aseptic loosening, malalignment, wear, and periprosthetic fracture for revision were significantly more common in UKR than TKR.

  - Most revisions of TKRs involved augments or constrained implants; revisions of UKRs typically involved conversions to TKR.
- *Mortality rate (Figure 31.1)*: There was a significantly higher mortality rate for TKR at all time points—cumulative mortality at 30 days was 0.24% for TKR vs. 0.06% for UKR. Absolute difference in death rate increased to 1.1% at 4 years.
- *Implant survival (Figure 31.2):* This was greater for TKR than UKR at 8 years (SHR 2.12; 95% CI: 1.99–2.26).
- *Mean LOS*: There was a 1.38-day significantly shorter stay for UKR than TKR.
- *Readmission:* Within the first year readmission was significantly less likely with UKR.
- *Complications:* Intraoperative complications, blood transfusion, venous thromboembolism, stroke, and myocardial infarction were significantly less likely for UKR than TKR.

Table 31.1 Revision, Reoperation, and Mortality Results for TKR and UKR Using Propensity-Score-Matched Cohorts (Hazard Ratios < 1 Favor UKR)

	Survival of TKR (%; 95% CI)	**Survival of UKR (%; 95% CI)**	**Hazard/Subhazard Ratio (95% CI)**
		Revision	
4 years	96.4% (96.2–96.5)	92.7% (92.3–93.1)	1.97 (1.84–2.12)
8 years	94.6% (94.2–94.9)	87.0% (86.2–87.9)	2.12 (1.99–2.26)
		Revision/Reoperation	
Overall	87.2% (86.7–87.8)	80.4% (79.4–81.4)	1.38 (1.31–1.44)
		Mortality	
30 days	99.76% (99.71–99.81)	99.94% (99.88–99.97)	0.23 (0.11–0.50)
90 days	99.53% (99.45–99.59)	99.78% (99.68–99.85)	0.47 (0.31–0.69)
1 year	99.22% (99.15–99.28)	99.47% (99.37–99.55)	0.69 (0.58–0.83)
4 years	95.66% (95.46–95.84)	96.71% (96.41–96.98)	0.75 (0.68–0.82)
8 years	88.52% (87.85–89.16)	89.10% (88.06–90.06)	0.85 (0.79–0.92)

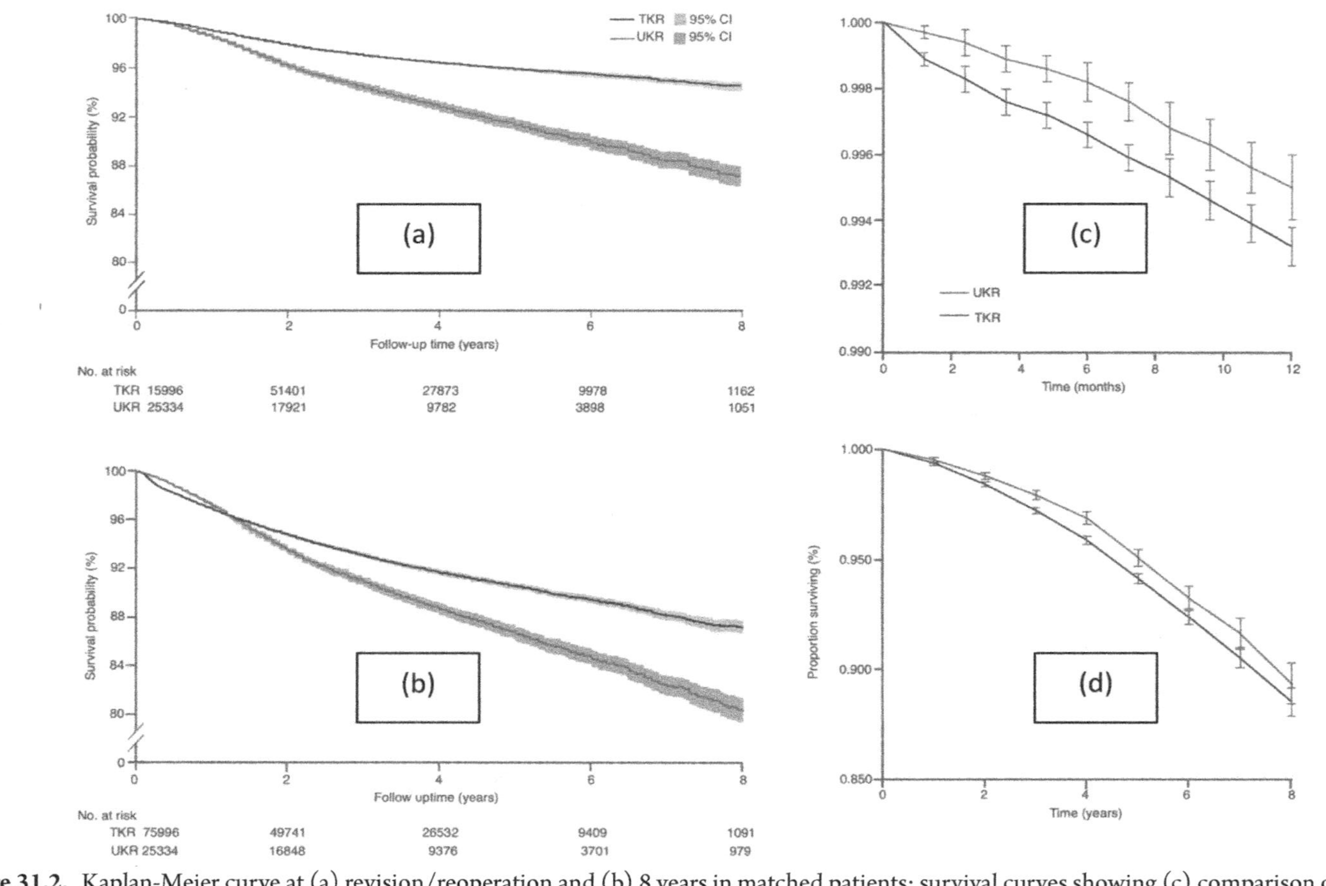

Figure 31.2. Kaplan-Meier curve at (a) revision/reoperation and (b) 8 years in matched patients; survival curves showing (c) comparison of mortality at 1 year and (d) at 8 years. Error bars show 95% CI.

Criticisms and Limitations: This is an observational study, where propensity scoring is used to match cohorts; however, all observational studies will have a degree of confounding and the results therefore cannot prove causality.

Other Relevant Studies and Information:

- The Total or Partial Knee Arthroplasty Trial (TOPKAT) trial[2] aimed to assess the clinical and cost effectiveness of TKR vs. partial knee replacement (PKR) in patients with medial compartment osteoarthritis (OA). This was a multicenter, pragmatic randomized controlled trial performed at 27 UK hospitals with 528 patients and 5-year data. There was no significant difference in Oxford Knee Scores (OKSs) or number of reoperations and revisions; however, patients receiving TKR had more complications ($p = 0.036$). A within-trial cost-effectiveness analysis was performed indicating that PKR is more cost effective (0.240 additional quality-adjusted life years, 95% CI: 0.046–0.434) and less expensive than TKR (–£910, 95% CI: −1503 to −317) during the 5 years of follow-up (F/U).
- Harbourne et al.[3] observed that 75% of UKA vs. 59% of TKA patients returned to desired activity at 12 months postoperatively. Preoperative predictors evaluated were age, sex, body mass index (BMI), education, comorbidities, pain expectations, OKS, University of California Los Angeles Activity Score, and EQ-5D. TKA patients ($n = 575$) were older with a greater BMI than patients undergoing UKA ($n = 420$). TKA patients had a greater risk of nonreturn to desired activity than patients undergoing UKA. Predictors of nonreturn to desired activity following UKA were worse OKSs, higher BMI, and worse expectations. Predictors of nonreturn to desired activity following TKA were worse EQ-5D and OKSs. UKA patients were more likely to return to desired activity than TKA patients.
- National Institute for Health and Care Excellence (NICE) guidelines[4] have recognized that UKR has important benefits including improved patient-reported outcome measures (PROMs), reduced LOS, higher cost effectiveness, and reduced risk for deep venous thrombosis, minor revisions, and reoperations after 5 years.

Summary and Implications: This large, propensity-score-matched cohort study suggests better implant survival and a lower reoperation rate for TKR when compared to UKR at 8 years. UKR was associated with lower mortality rates, complication rates, LOS, and readmission rates than TKR at all measured time points. This was not a randomized trial, but it is possible that residual confounding factors influenced the results. NICE guidelines highlight the benefits of UKR vs. TKR, including improved PROM, lower rates of some complications, and greater cost effectiveness. The pros and cons of each procedure should be considered when determining the appropriate surgical option for each patient.

CLINICAL CASE: UKR VERSUS TKR IN MEDIAL COMPARTMENT OA

Case History

A 73-year-old gentleman with a past medical history of diabetes mellitus and ischemic heart disease presents to an elective knee clinic complaining of chronic right medial knee pain that has gradually deteriorated over the last 12 months. His activities of daily living are limited and he can walk 100 meters before pain on the medial aspect of his knee forces him to stop. The knee pain also disturbs his sleep frequently. On examination, this patient has a correctible 10-degree varus deformity and a range of motion between 0 and 120 degrees of flexion, and the collateral and cruciate ligaments appear to be intact. Plain radiograph illustrates more medial compartment degenerative signs, as seen in Figure 31.3. This gentleman has exhausted all nonoperative treatment options and is keen on exploring surgical intervention. Based on this study, how should this patient be counseled and managed?

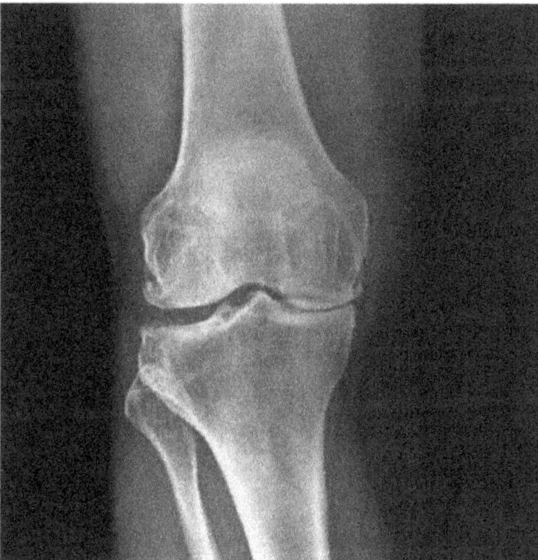

Figure 31.3. Weight-bearing anteroposterior radiograph demonstrating medial compartment OA.

Suggested Answer

This gentleman is a candidate for UKR or TKR. When deciding which procedure to offer, the higher revision/reoperation rate of UKR when compared against TKR should be balanced against a lower occurrence of complications, readmission, and mortality associated with UKR. Data from the TOPKAT study also demonstrates a higher complication rate with TKR; however, the reoperation rate and revision rate (with 5-year F/U) are similar between both options. Informing patients of the evidence can enable them to make a decision in their best interest.

References

1. Liddle et al. Adverse outcomes after total and unicompartmental knee replacement in 101,330 matched patients: a study of data from the National Joint Registry for England and Wales. Lancet. 2014;384(9952):1437–45.
2. Beard et al. The clinical and cost-effectiveness of total versus partial knee replacement in patients with medial compartment osteoarthritis (TOPKAT): 5-year outcomes of a randomised controlled trial. Lancet. 2019;394(10200):746–56.
3. Harbourne et al. Predictors of return to desired activity 12 months following unicompartmental and total knee arthroplasty. Acta Orthop. 2019;90(1):74–80.
4. National Institute for Health and Care Excellence (NICE). Joint replacement (primary): hip, knee and shoulder. Evidence review for total knee replacement (NG157). March 2020. www.nice.org.uk/guidance/ng157/evidence/k-total-knee-replacement-pdf-315756469334

32

Total or Partial Knee Replacement for Treating Medial Compartment Osteoarthritis

THOMAS W. HAMILTON AND ABTIN ALVAND

Study Nickname: TOPKAT

> Both TKR and PKR are effective, offer similar clinical outcomes, and result in a similar incidence of re-operations and complications. Based on our clinical findings, and results regarding the lower costs and better cost-effectiveness with PKR during the 5-year study period, we suggest that PKR should be considered the first choice for patients with late-stage isolated medial compartment osteoarthritis.
>
> —Beard et al.[1]

Citation: Beard DJ, Davies LJ, Cook JA, MacLennan G, Price A, Kent S, Hudson J, Carr A, Leal J, Campbell H, Fitzpatrick R, Arden N, Murray D, Campbell MK; TOPKAT Study Group. The clinical and cost-effectiveness of total versus partial knee replacement in patients with medial compartment osteoarthritis (TOPKAT): 5-year outcomes of a randomised controlled trial. Lancet. 2019;394:746–56.

Research Question: Should patients with late-stage medial compartment osteoarthritis (OA) be managed with total knee replacement (TKR) or partial knee replacement (PKR)?

Funding: National Institute for Health Research Health Technology Assessment Programme, UK

Year Study Began: 2010

Year Study Published: 2019

Study Location: UK (27 sites, 68 surgeons)

Who Was Studied: Patients with medial compartment knee OA with exposed bone on both the femur and tibia, functionally intact anterior cruciate ligament (where superficial damage or splitting were acceptable), full-thickness and good-quality lateral cartilage, and correctable intra-articular varus deformity (suggestive of an adequate medial collateral ligament) and who were medically fit (i.e., American Society of Anesthesiologists grade 1 or 2).

Who Was Excluded: History of rheumatoid arthritis (or other inflammatory disorders), significant damage to the patellofemoral joint (especially on the lateral facet), simultaneous bilateral TKRs, and symptomatic foot, hip, or spinal pathology. Those with prior knee septic arthritis, knee surgery (other than diagnostic arthroscopy or medial meniscectomy), and inclusion in the study with the contralateral knee.

How Many Patients: 528

Study Overview: See Figure 32.1.

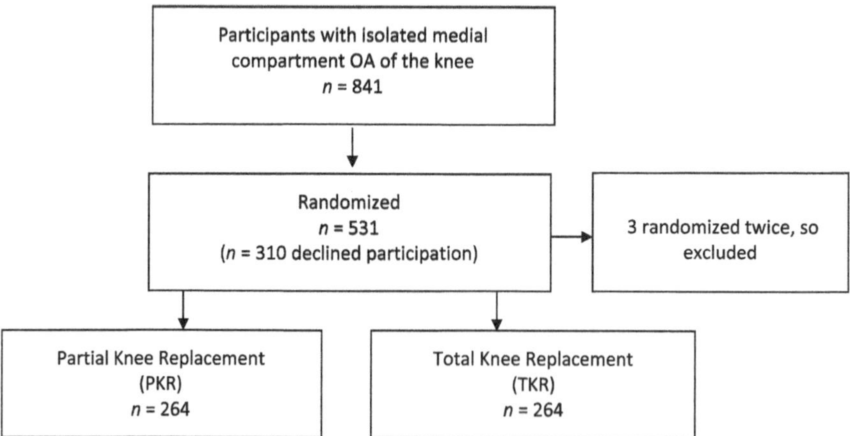

Figure 32.1. Overview of the study design for the TOPKAT trial.

Study Intervention: TOPKAT was a multicenter (27 sites, 68 surgeons), pragmatic, and randomized controlled trial (RCT) conducted within the UK National Health Service to compare TKR against PKR for the treatment of isolated medial compartment OA of the knee. Surgeons either performed *both* TKR and PKR (equipoise surgeon) or worked as a pair of surgeons at a delivery unit performing *either* TKR *or* PKR (expertise surgeon). Surgeons were required to have had appropriate training, to have practiced their technique for at least 1 year, and to have performed this operation at least 10 times in the previous year. Surgeons, patients, and follow-up (F/U) assessors were not masked to treatment allocation. Patients were randomized 1:1 to receive either TKR or PKR. A minimization algorithm that incorporated sex, age band (< 50, 50–70, or > 70 years), baseline Oxford Knee Score[2] (OKS; patient-reported outcome measure questioning level of function, activities of daily living [ADLs], and how they have been affected by knee pain with a maximum score of 48) band (≤ 14 or less, 15–21, or ≥ 22), and delivery unit (equipoise surgeon or pair of expertise surgeons) was used to balance baseline characteristics.

Follow-Up: Up to 5 years after randomization

Endpoints: Primary outcome was OKS. Secondary outcomes were the following scores: EuroQol EQ-5D-3L, High Activity Arthroplasty Score, University of California Los Angeles Activity Score, American Knee Society Score, Lund Satisfaction Score, complications, reoperation and revision, and health economic cost-effectiveness analysis.

RESULTS (TABLE 32.1)

At 5-year follow-up:

- *Functional outcomes:* Both groups had improved outcomes as compared to their preoperative status, but there was no difference in functional outcomes *between* both groups (Figure 32.2).
- *Health related quality of life (QOL):* This was assessed by the EuroQol EQ-5D-3L visual analog scale and was significantly better in those receiving PKR, but this was not judged to be clinically meaningful.
- *Patient satisfaction*: There was no difference between groups (82% PKR vs. 77% TKR; relative risk [RR] 1.06, 95% CI: 0.99–1.13; $p = 0.097$).
- *Complications:* More complications were recorded in participants receiving TKR than PKR (27% vs. 20% respectively; RR 0.72, 95% CI: 0.53–0.98; $p = 0.04$), unexplained pain (3.7% PKR vs. 3.0% TKR), and knee stiffness (0% PKR vs. 3.7% TKR).
- *Reoperations:* The rate was similar *between* groups (6% PKR vs. 8% TKA; RR 0.75; 95% CI: 0.37–1.53; $p = 0.432$).

- *Revisions:* The rate was similar *between* groups with 4% PKR (2 participants for unexplained pain, 3 participants for bearing dislocation) vs. 4% TKA (5 participants for unexplained pain).
- *Health economic cost-effectiveness analysis:* PKR was more effective (0.240 additional quality-adjusted life years, 95% CI: 0.046–0.434) and less expensive than TKR (–£910, 95% CI: –1503 to –317) during the F/U. The probability that PKR was the most cost-effective option was more than 99.9% for all reasonable threshold values.

Table 32.1 SUMMARY OF KEY FINDINGS

Outcome	PKR Mean (SD)	TKR Mean (SD)	Effect Size (95% CI)	*p* Value
Oxford Knee Score	38.0 (10.1)	37.0 (10.6)	1.04 (–0.42–2.50)	0.16
EuroQol EQ-5D-3L (score)	0.744 (0.29)	0.717 (0.32)	0.0018 (–0.033–0.069)	0.48
EuroQol EQ-5D-3L (visual analog scale)	75.4 (16.5)	71.7 (19.7)	4.02 (1.36–6.67)	**0.004**
High Activity Arthroplasty Score	7.9 (3.5)	7.6 (3.4)	0.22 (–0.24–0.67)	0.33
University of California Los Angeles Activity Score	5.0 (1.9)	4.9 (2.0)	0.17 (–0.09–0.43)	0.19
American Knee Society Score (objective)	85.8 (16.6)	86.6 (16.4)	–0.89 (–5.18–3.41)	0.68
American Knee Society Score (functional)	82.6 (18.5)	81.7 (19.0)	0.37 (–3.81–4.55)	0.86

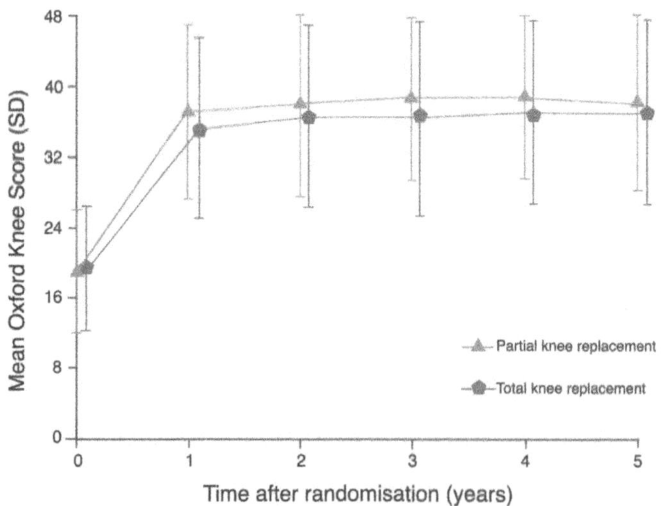

Figure 32.2. Oxford Knee Scores after randomization.

Criticisms and Limitations: The TOPKAT is the largest RCT to date comparing PKR and TKR. The limitations of this study include the absence of masking, as this was not felt to be feasible. Additionally, there was some data missing for healthcare resource and EQ-5D (12% across all time periods).

Other Relevant Studies and Information:

- A number of smaller RCTs comparing PKR against TKR have reported similar results as TOPKAT, finding no difference in clinical outcomes between both options.[3–6]
- Health economic analysis using large data sets of routinely collected data have reported that PKR can be expected to generate better health outcomes and lower lifetime costs than TKR.[7,8]
- National Institute for Health & Care Excellence guidelines recommend that surgeons "offer a choice of partial or total knee replacement to people with isolated medial compartmental osteoarthritis. Discuss the potential benefits and risks of each option with the person."[9]

Summary and Implications: The TOPKAT trial reported that at 5 years there was no difference in functional outcomes, health-related QOL, or patient satisfaction between participants receiving PKR and those receiving TKR. While no difference in reoperation or revision rates were noted between both groups, TKR was associated with an increase in complications, particularly knee stiffness. Health economic cost-effectiveness analysis found that PKR was more effective and less expensive compared to TKR during the 5 years of F/U, and that PKR represented the most cost-effective treatment option in more than 99.9% of reasonable threshold values. Based on better cost effectiveness with PKR, TOPKAT suggested that PKR should be considered as the first choice for patients with late-stage isolated medial compartment knee OA.

CASE STUDY: CHOOSING BETWEEN PKR VERSUS TKR

Case History

A 60-year-old patient presents to the clinic with a 2-year history of activity-related right knee pain. He has no significant medical or surgical history and is within a healthy weight range. His mild varus alignment of the right lower limb is correctable. There is mild fixed flexion deformity, but he can flex his knee to 120 degrees. He is tender to palpation along the medial joint line. Otherwise the knee is stable in both coronal and sagittal planes. There is no clinical evidence of patellofemoral joint irritability or spine or hip pathology. Imaging demonstrates bone-on-bone medial compartment arthritis with a radiographically normal lateral compartment and patellofemoral joint. Despite nonoperative treatment, the patient continues to have pain that limits his ADLs and he is keen to pursue surgical treatment. Based on the results of the TOPKAT study, how should this patient be treated?

Suggested Answer

The patient presents with isolated medial compartment OA that is refractory to nonoperative treatment. Both PKR and TKR can be offered in this scenario, and the potential benefits and risks of each option should be discussed. The TOPKAT reported that at 5 years there was no difference in functional outcomes, health-related QOL, or patient satisfaction between participants receiving PKR and those receiving TKR. While there was no difference in reoperation or revision rates between both groups, TKR was associated with an increase in complications, particularly knee stiffness. Health economic cost-effectiveness analysis found that PKR was more effective and less expensive compared to TKR. Based on better cost effectiveness with PKR, the results of TOPKAT suggest that PKR should be considered as the first choice for patients in this scenario.

References

1. Beard et al. The clinical and cost-effectiveness of total versus partial knee replacement in patients with medial compartment osteoarthritis (TOPKAT): 5-year outcomes of a randomised controlled trial. Lancet. 2019;394:746–56.
2. Dawson et al. Questionnaire on the perceptions of patients about total knee replacement. J Bone Joint Surg Br. 1998;80(1):63–9.
3. Costa et al. Unicompartmental and total knee arthroplasty in the same patient. J Knee Surg. 2011;24(4):273–8.
4. Newman et al. Unicompartmental or total knee replacement: the 15-year results of a prospective randomised controlled trial. J Bone Joint Surg Br. 2009;91(1):52–7.
5. Murray et al. A randomised controlled trial of the clinical effectiveness and cost-effectiveness of different knee prostheses: the Knee Arthroplasty Trial (KAT). Health Technol Assess. 2014;18(19):1–viii.
6. Sun et al. Mobile bearing UKA compared to fixed bearing TKA: a randomized prospective study. Knee. 2012;19(2):103–6.
7. Burn et al. Cost-effectiveness of unicompartmental compared with total knee replacement: a population-based study using data from the National Joint Registry for England and Wales. BMJ Open. 2018;8(4):e020977.

8. Burn et al. Choosing between unicompartmental and total knee replacement: what can economic evaluations tell us? A systematic review. Pharmacoecon Open. 2017;1(4): 241–53.
9. National Institute for Health & Care Excellence. Joint replacement (primary): hip, knee and shoulder (NG157). June 2020. https://www.nice.org.uk/guidance/ng157/resources/joint-replacement-primary-hip-knee-and-shoulder-pdf-66141845322181.

33

Randomized Trial of Reamed and Unreamed Intramedullary Nailing of Tibial Shaft Fractures

IRIS H. Y. KWOK AND PETER BATES

Study Nickname: SPRINT (Study to Prospectively evaluate Reamed Intramedullary Nails in patients with Tibial fractures) trial

> The present study demonstrates a possible benefit for reamed intramedullary nailing in patients with closed fractures. We found no difference between approaches in patients with open fractures. Delaying reoperation for nonunion for at least six months may substantially decrease the need for reoperation.
>
> —BHANDARI ET AL.[1]

Citation: SPRINT Investigators, Bhandari M, Guyatt G, Tornetta P 3rd, Schemitsch EH, Swiontkowski M, Sanders D, Walter SD. Randomized trial of reamed and unreamed intramedullary nailing of tibial shaft fractures. J Bone Joint Surg Am. 2008;90(12):2567–78.

Research Question: Is there a difference in reoperation rates and complications between reamed and unreamed intramedullary nailing (IMN) in the treatment of tibial shaft fractures?

Funding: Canadian Institutes of Health Research, National Institutes of Health,

Orthopaedic Research and Education Foundation, Orthopaedic Trauma Association, Hamilton Health Sciences research grant, Zimmer, and Canada Research Chair in Musculoskeletal Trauma at McMaster University

Year Study Began: July 2000

Year Study Published: 2008

Study Location: 29 centers in Canada

Who Was Studied: Skeletally mature patients who had sustained a closed or open tibial shaft fracture that was amenable to operative fixation with IMN.

Who Was Excluded: Pathological fractures, fractures not amenable to IMN, patients who were likely to have problems with follow-up (F/U).

How Many Patients: 1226

Study Overview: See Figure 33.1.

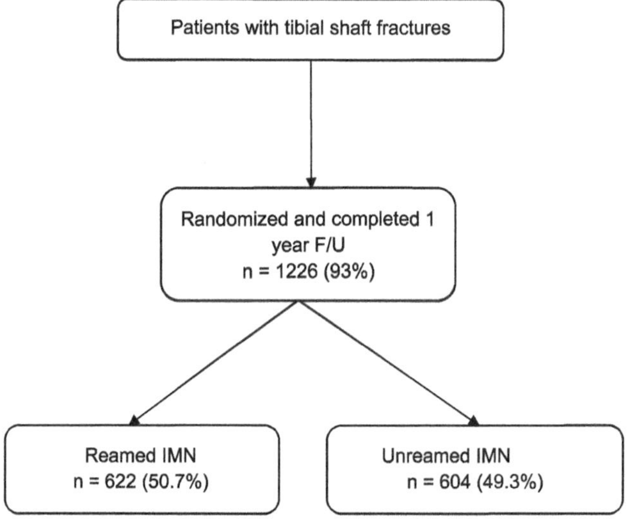

Figure 33.1. Summary of SPRINT trial design.

Study Intervention: Standardization of pre- and postoperative care for both closed and open fractures was carried out. Reoperations for nonunion < 6 months were disallowed. For both groups, surgeons were required to insert both proximal and distal locking screws (at least 1 screw each). The groups were divided into the following:

- *Reamed group:* Intramedullary reaming using power reamers was performed over a guidewire. Nail diameter choice was based on the first detection of "cortical chatter". Reaming continued until 1–1.5 mm larger than the first detection of cortical chatter.
- *Unreamed group:* An intramedullary nail was inserted across the fracture site, with an upper diameter limit of 10 mm, and a nail measuring at least 2 mm less than the diameter measured at the isthmus of the tibia on anteroposterior and lateral radiographs.

Follow-Up: 1 year

Endpoints: Primary composite outcome consisted of reoperation > 6 months including bone grafting, implant exchange, removal of metalwork (for breakage or loosening), dynamization in patients with a fracture gap of < 1 cm and drainage of hematomas, and fasciotomy for compartment syndrome and reoperation for infection at any time point.

RESULTS (TABLE 33.1)

- *Adherence:* 96% of patients adhered to the perioperative and technical aspects of the study protocol.
- *Reoperation and/or autodynamization within 1 year:* 105 (16.9%) reamed and 114 (18.9%) unreamed nailings experienced a primary outcome event (relative risk [RR] 0.90; 95% CI: 0.71–1.15; $p = 0.40$), which was insignificant.
- *Closed fractures:* 113 patients (13.7%; 95% CI: 12–16) underwent a reoperation within the first year. There was a higher number of reoperations in the unreamed group (68/410, 17%) vs. the reamed group (45/416, 11%; $p = 0.03$) with RR (0.67; 95% CI: 0.47–0.96; $p = 0.03$), mainly due to a difference in the rates of autodynamization (i.e., failure of the screw-bone construct [e.g., spontaneous screw breakage leading to fracture dynamization prior to healing]).
- *Open fractures*: 106 patients (26.5%; 95% CI: 22–31) underwent a reoperation or autodynamization within the first year. There was no

significant difference in reoperation rates between the unreamed group (46/194, 24%) vs. the reamed group (60/206, 29%; $p = 0.16$).

- *All patients:* There was no significant difference in primary composite outcome (reoperation and/or autodynamization within 1 year) in the unreamed (114/611, 18.9%) and reamed (105/637, 17%) nailing groups ($p = 0.4$).

Table 33.1 Key Results

Primary Outcome	Reamed Group	Unreamed Group	*p* Value
Closed fractures	11%	17%	0.03
Open fractures	29%	24%	0.16
All patients	17%	19%	0.4

- *Reoperations:* Reoperations to promote fracture healing were performed in 106 patients, with 48 (45%; 23 reamed and 25 unreamed; $p = 0.97$) reoperated on in < 6 months.
- *Nonunion:* Among all patients, 57 (4.6%) required implant exchange or bone grafting because of nonunion.
- *Adverse events:* 18 patients died, 9 had deep venous thromboses (DVTs), 7 has pulmonary embolisms (PEs), and 1 had sepsis. There were significantly more deaths in the reamed vs. the unreamed nailing group (14 vs. 4; $p = 0.03$). However, blinded adjudicators classified all deaths as unrelated to the IMN procedure itself.

Criticisms and Limitations: Participating surgeons had relatively more experience with the reamed nailing approach (shown in a survey of study investigators). There was no way to blind surgeons as 87% of surgeons believed that a reamed procedure was superior. This may have led to a differential threshold for reoperation. The primary composite endpoint used means where certain outcomes (e.g., autodynamization) are overrepresented, which may not necessarily reflect its actual importance to patients. The trial therefore provides little evidence of the superiority of reamed vs. unreamed IMN in terms of the more patient-important components.

Other Relevant Studies and Information:

- Systematic review and meta-analysis of 9 randomized controlled trials (RCTs) showed that reamed IMN of lower-extremity long-bone fractures significantly reduced the rates of nonunion and implant failure in comparison to unreamed nailing; 1 nonunion could be prevented for every 14 patients treated with reamed IMN (number needed to treat = 14).[2]

- Systematic review of 7 comparative studies showed an increased nonunion rate and screw breakage rate in the unreamed group in tibial shaft fractures.[3]
- Systematic review of 8 studies showed a reduced risk of reoperation with reamed IMN in open tibial fractures. The use of both reamed and unreamed nails reduced the risk of reoperation when compared to external fixators.[4]
- The Cochrane group[5] concluded that there was "moderate"-quality evidence demonstrating no clear difference in the rate of major reoperations and complications between reamed and unreamed techniques. However, reamed nailing has a lower incidence of implant failure. "Low"-quality evidence also suggests that reamed nailing may reduce the incidence of major reoperations related to nonunion in closed fractures only.

Summary and Implications: This study of 1226 patients with tibial shaft fractures showed a decrease in reoperation rate in reamed vs. unreamed IMN in patients with closed tibial shaft fractures. This is largely due to differences in the rate of autodynamization. There was an insignificant increase in the reoperation rate associated with reamed IMN in patients with open fractures. The overall reoperation rate in this study was 4.6%. There were significantly more deaths in the reamed compared to the unreamed group; however, the deaths were unrelated to the IMN procedure itself.

CLINICAL CASE: REAMED VERSUS UNREAMED IMN IN CLOSED TIBIAL SHAFT FRACTURE

Case History

A 26-year-old male was brought into the Emergency Department following an isolated closed right 2-part spiral midshaft tibial fracture during a football tackle. He is otherwise fit and healthy with no other past medical history, and he is a nonsmoker. The lower limb is neurovascularly intact on examination. This was confirmed by the presence of peripheral pulses, handheld Doppler, and saturation levels on the pulse oximetry. The orthopaedic surgeon performing his surgery decides to treat the fracture by IMN. According to the

SPRINT trial, should the surgeon choose to ream the tibia intraoperatively prior to nail insertion or not? What is the rationale? Does the current evidence support this?

Suggested Answer

The choice between reamed or unreamed IMN of tibial fractures remains controversial. In this patient, the surgeon should opt to ream the tibia prior to nail insertion. Reaming allows the use of larger nails, which affords greater stability across the fracture site. Proponents of unreamed nailing would argue that the endosteal blood supply is preserved and may improve fracture healing. The SPRINT study[1] from 2008 has shown that in closed tibial fractures, reamed nailing has a lower reoperation rate. This is also supported by a systematic review in 2001 conducted by Bhandari et al.[2] Nonunion and implant failure rates have also been shown to be lower in other systematic reviews.[3,4] Although reamed nailing has a higher theoretical risk of DVT/PE due to increased fat emboli entering the bloodstream, this has not been demonstrated in RCTs. This patient is otherwise fit and healthy with no risk factors for thromboembolism apart from his long-bone fracture; therefore, it would be reasonable to perform reamed IMN.

References

1. Study to Prospectively Evaluate Reamed Intramedullary Nails in Patients with Tibial Fractures Investigators et al. Randomized trial of reamed and unreamed intramedullary nailing of tibial shaft fractures. J Bone Joint Surg Am. 2008;90(12):2567–78.
2. Bhandari et al. Reamed versus nonreamed intramedullary nailing of lower extremity long bone fractures: a systematic overview and meta-analysis. J Orthop Trauma. 2000;14:2–9.
3. Forster et al. Should the tibia be reamed when nailing? Injury. 2005;36:439–44.
4. Bhandari et al. Treatment of open fractures of the shaft of the tibia. J Bone Joint Surg Br. 2001;83:62–8.
5. Duan et al. Intramedullary nailing for tibial shaft fractures in adults. Cochrane Database Syst Rev. 2012 Jan 18;1:CD008241.

34

Timing of Surgical Decompression after Onset of Cauda Equina Syndrome

Does It Matter?

WARRAN WIGNADASAN AND DUSHAN THAVARAJAH

> There was a significant advantage to treating patients within 48 hours versus more than 48 hours after the onset of cauda equina syndrome. A significant improvement in sensory and motor deficits as well as urinary and rectal function occurred in patients who underwent decompression within 48 hours versus after 48 hours.
>
> —Ahn et al.[1]

Research Question: What is the relationship between timing of surgical decompression from onset of cauda equina syndrome (CES) and clinical outcomes, and are there any preoperative variables correlated with outcomes?

Year Study Began: Meta-analysis initiated in 1999

Year Study Published: 2000

Study Location: Meta-analysis from Johns Hopkins University School of Medicine

Who Was Studied: A literature search was conducted for CES produced by lumbar disc herniation from January 1966 to May 1999; 104 articles were obtained, but only 42 articles met the inclusion criteria.

Who Was Excluded: Articles that described CES being caused by a pathology other than lumbar disc herniation as well as any animal studies on CES were excluded from the meta-analysis.

How Many Patients: 322

Study Overview: See Figure 34.1.

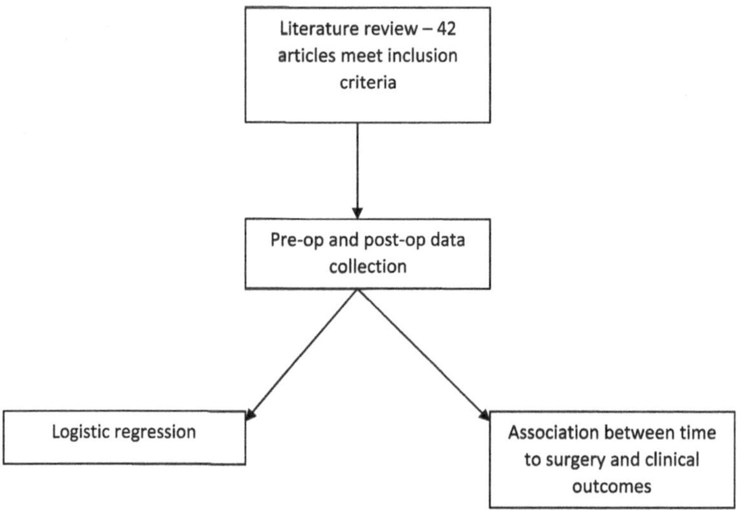

Figure 34.1. Summary of study design.

Study Intervention: Pre- and postoperative variables (shown in Table 34.1) were defined by the authors, with each patient needing to provide at least 1 of each to be included in the study. Data from 322 patients from the 42 articles that met the inclusion criteria were obtained. The logistic regression of postoperative outcomes on the preoperative variables was analyzed to assess for an association. Evaluation of time to surgery from the onset of CES was performed thereafter; 5 time intervals were defined between onset of CES and surgical decompression:

- < 24 hours
- 24–48 hours
- 2–10 days
- 11 days–1 month
- > 1 month

In this study the authors stipulated that a resolution of preoperative deficits represented a full resolution rather than a partial resolution, which subsequently was characterized as a failure to resolve.

Table 34.1 Pre- and Postoperative Variables Analyzed within the Meta-Analysis

Preoperative Variables	**Postoperative Variables**
Age	Resolution of:
Gender	• Pain
History of:	• Sensory deficit
• Previous spine surgery	• Motor deficit
• Chronic lower back pain	• Urinary incontinence
• Trauma with onset of CES	• Sexual dysfunction
Duration of chronic low back pain prior to CES	• Rectal dysfunction
Sudden onset of CES	
Presence of sciatica with CES	
Length of time to surgery from onset of CES	
Preoperative:	
• Weakness in lower extremities	
• Sensory deficit	
• Loss of reflexes	
• Rectal dysfunction	

Follow-Up: Months to years

Endpoints: Associations between (1) predefined postoperative and preoperative variables as seen in Table 34.1 and (2) timing to decompression from the onset of CES and clinical outcomes.

RESULTS (TABLE 34.2)

- *< 24 hours:* There was no significant difference in patient outcomes who underwent surgical decompression within < 24 hours vs. at between 24 and 48 hours.
- *> 48 hours*: There was no significant difference in outcomes in patients among all 3 groups (2–10 days, 11 days–1 month, and > 1 month) who underwent surgical decompression at > 48 hours.
- *< 24 vs. > 48 hours*: There were significant differences in clinical outcomes between the < 24-hour vs. > 48-hour groups as well as the 24–48-hour vs. > 48-hour groups, with better outcomes occurring in the < 24-hour and 24–48-hour groups. Therefore, combining

these findings, there was a significant difference in clinical outcomes between patients undergoing decompression within < 48 hours vs. at > 48 hours, with those being decompressed < 48 hours having better outcomes.

- *48-hour mark:* Patients who received decompression at > 48 hours vs. within < 48 hours were:
  - 2.5× more likely to continue experiencing urinary deficit
  - 3.5× more likely to continue having sensory deficits
  - 9.1× more likely to continue suffering from rectal dysfunction and motor deficits
- Associations when the postoperative variables were regressed on 13 preoperative variables:
  - Worse prognosis for urinary incontinence in patients with preoperative chronic back pain or rectal dysfunction
  - Worse prognosis for rectal dysfunction with chronic back pain
  - Worse prognosis for sexual function rectification with increasing age
  - Worse prognosis for sensory deficit with preoperative rectal dysfunction

Table 34.2 Decompression after 48 Hours versus before 48 Hours

	Surgery Performed within < 48 Hours (vs. at > 48 Hours)			
	OR	***p* Value**	**95% CI**	***N***
Resolution of pain	0.51	0.338	0.13–2.00	66
Resolution of sensory deficit	3.45	0.005	1.45–8.33	98
Resolution of motor deficit	9.09	0.001	2.56–33.33	73
Resolution of urinary deficit	2.5	0.01	1.19–5.26	189
Resolution of sexual dysfunction	3.85	0.09	0.79–2.06	51
Resolution of rectal dysfunction	9.09	0.003	2.13–33.3	47

OR, probability of a positive outcome with a positive risk factor; *p* value for calculated OR; 95% CI for OR; number of patients used in analysis.

Criticisms and Limitations: A limitation was the range of follow-up (F/U) duration. As these times vary from months to years, patients who were recorded as having a partial recovery of symptoms may have gone on to have a full resolution of deficits after their final F/U. Furthermore, the surgical decompressions performed in the various studies differed, and these different procedures could have produced different clinical outcomes, although the authors felt that the vital component of the procedures was decompression of the neural elements.

Other Relevant Studies and Information:

- The timing of surgery from the onset of CES symptoms is a vital factor that influences clinical outcomes, with further studies supporting the role of early surgical intervention.[2–5]
- Kohles et al.[4] critically assessed the meta-analysis and determined that while there is an advantage to surgically decompress within < 48 hours of symptoms, there is further benefit in operating within < 24 hours. This study concludes that there is a "flawed methodology and misinterpretation of results" in the review by Ahn et al.[1]
- Further studies have shown that surgical decompression within < 24 hours of onset of CES symptoms increased the likelihood of recovery of bladder function in incomplete CES.[5,6]
- Gleave et al. believe that "the die is cast at the time of prolapse" and that there is no evidence to favor emergency surgery benefiting recovery in patients with CES and urinary retention (i.e., CES-R).[7]
- The British Association of Spine Surgeons standards of care for CES recommend surgery as soon as possible, stating that there are "no safe time thresholds." CES is believed to be a continuous compressive process, with longer duration of compression of the nerve roots leading to worse prognosis.[8]

Summary and Implications: This meta-analysis suggests that the surgical decompression of neural components due to lumbar disc herniation within < 48 hours of the onset of CES symptoms is associated with a significant advantage compared to decompression at > 48 hours. Major guidelines recommend surgical decompression as soon as possible following onset of symptoms.

CLINICAL CASE: CES IN THE EMERGENCY DEPARTMENT

Case History

A 49-year-old man presents to the Emergency Department with acute lower back pain after lifting a heavy object 30 hours previously while at work. There is no significant past medical history. He complains of pain radiating down both legs with 3 episodes of urinary incontinence, starting 24 hours ago. On examination he has reduced power and sensation bilaterally and normal lower limb reflexes. He has reduced perianal sensation and a reduced anal tone. A postvoid bladder scan shows 5 ml. Magnetic resonance imaging (MRI) scan of the lumbar spine done within an hour of presentation shows complete compression of the cauda equina at L4/L5. How should this patient be managed on the basis of this study?

Suggested Answer

The meta-analysis by Ahn et al.[1] shows that the clinical outcomes of surgical decompression within < 48 hours of CES symptoms are significantly better compared to those decompressed at > 48 hours. This patient has confirmed compression of the cauda equina and has a 24-hour history of urinary symptoms. This patient should therefore be kept nil by mouth, be immediately discussed with the spinal team on call, be considered for emergent MRI, and be listed for an urgent lumbar decompression. He should be worked up for an operation immediately, with up-to-date blood tests and an anesthetic review. The procedure should take place as soon as possible, and operating theaters ought to be informed about the equipment required. The on-call radiographers should be informed too because an image intensifier is required for fluoroscopic-guided detection of the correct lumbar level.

References

1. Ahn et al. Cauda equina syndrome secondary to lumbar disc herniation. A meta-analysis of surgical outcomes. Spine. 2000;25:151522.
2. Chau et al. Timing of surgical intervention in cauda equina syndrome: a systematic critical review. World Neurosurg. 2014;81:640–50.
3. DeLong et al. Timing of surgery in cauda equina syndrome with urinary retention: meta-analysis of observational studies. J Neurosurg Spine. 2008;8:305–20.
4. Kohles et al. Time-dependent surgical outcomes following cauda equina syndrome diagnosis. Spine. 2004;29:1281–7.
5. Todd NV. Cauda equina syndrome: the timing of surgery probably does influence outcome. Br J Neurosurg. 2005;19:301–6.
6. Srikandarajah et al. Does early surgical decompression in cauda equina improve bladder outcome? Spine. 2015;40:580–3.
7. Gleave et al. Prognosis for recovery of bladder function following lumbar central disc prolapse. Brit J Neurosurg. 1990;4:205–10.
8. Germon et al. British Association of Spine Surgeons standards of care for cauda equina syndrome. Spine J. 2015;15:2–4.

35

Does Delaying Surgery Increase Mortality for Patients with Hip Fracture?

RUPERT WHARTON AND EDWARD IBRAHIM

> Delay in operation is associated with an increased risk of death but not readmission after a fractured neck of femur, even with adjustment for comorbidity.
>
> —Bottle et al.[1]

Citation: Bottle A, Aylin P. Mortality associated with delay in operation after hip fracture: observational study. BMJ. 2006;22;332(7547):947–51.

Research Question: Does delay in surgery of > 1 day increase mortality and/or readmission in patients aged > 65 years old with hip fracture?

Funding: Both authors received 50%–100% funding from Dr. Foster Ltd. Through a unit research grant. Dr. Foster Ltd. is a provider of healthcare information in the UK, monitoring the performance of the National Health Service and providing information to the public.

Year Study Began: 2001

Year Study Published: 2006

Study Location: All UK hospitals managing > 100 hip fractures (total 151)

Research base: Imperial College London

Who Was Studied: All patients aged > 65 years old admitted from their own home with a hip fracture in UK hospitals managing > 100 hip fractures over 3 years.

Who Was Excluded: Patients who were aged < 65 years old, living in an institution (nursing or care home) immediately prior, previously admitted for a hip fracture, or admitted to a trust managing < 100 cases over 3 years.

How Many Patients: 129 522

Study Overview: See Figure 35.1.

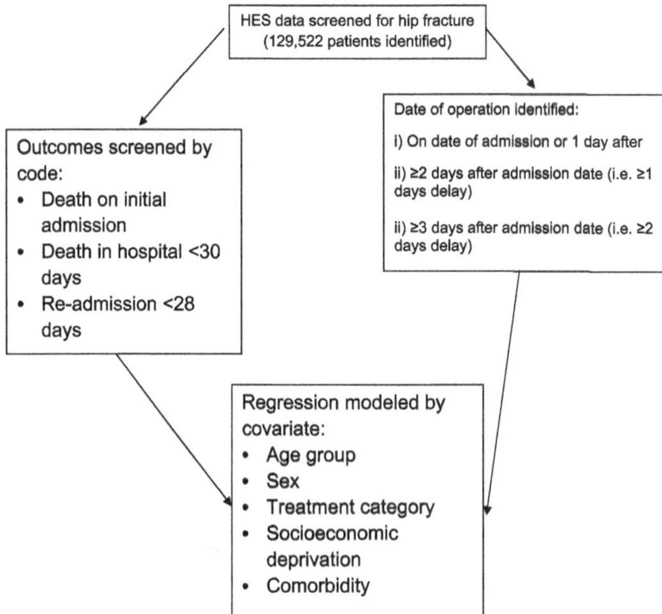

Figure 35.1. Summary of the study design.

Study Intervention: The authors used Hospital Episode Statistics (HES) data to identify patients with hip fracture allocated to categories based on treatment code entered (fixation, prosthetic replacement, other procedure, no procedure [i.e., medical management]).

Outcome measures consisted of the following:

- Any death in hospital during initial admission
- Death in hospital within < 30 days of initial admission
- Emergency readmission within < 28 days of discharge

Data were interrogated for operation date and categorized into either of the following:

- No delay (defined as surgery on the day of or 1 day after admission date)
- ≥ 1-day(s) delay
- ≥2-day delay

Logistic regression models were run for each outcome against the following:

- Patient age
- Sex
- Treatment category
- Socioeconomic deprivation
- Comorbidity

Chosen comorbidities included the following:

- Dementia
- Diabetes mellitus
- Chronic ischemic heart disease
- Chronic lower respiratory disease
- Heart failure
- Hypertension
- Renal failure
- Malignancy

These models were utilized to calculate the odds ration (OR) for mortality and readmission, as well as to predict the number of deaths that were attributable to delay.

Follow-Up: Inpatient stay after hip fracture, or 30 days if readmitted to hospital

Endpoints: Inpatient death during initial admission, death in hospital within < 30 days of initial admission, and emergency readmission within < 28 days of discharge.

RESULTS

- *Death rate*:
  - This was significantly increased with delay to operation of > 1 day after admission, even after adjustment for all measured factors (Tables 35.1 and 35.2, Figures 35.2 and 35.3).

- Delaying for > 1 day led to an estimated excess of 1742 deaths over the study duration of 3 years (9.4% of all deaths).
- *Risk factors*: Increasing age, renal failure, heart failure, and malignancy were also

identified as significant risk factors for mortality.

- *Hospitals*: There were no significant differences in delay rates between hospitals.
- *Re-admission*: There was no significant increase in risk for emergency readmission or readmission.
- < 30 days:
    - Because of delay to surgery
    - Because of the type of procedure performed (but this was not analyzed according to fracture type)

Table 35.1 OR FOR DEATH AND READMISSION FOR AGE, SEX, DEPRIVATION, AND COMORBIDITY

Factor	**Death in Hospital**	**Death in Hospital < 30 Days of Admission**	**Emergency Readmission < 28 Days**
Sex (male:female)	1.89 (1.82–1.97)	1.85 (1.78–1.92)	1.33 (1.26–1.39)
Age (within age groups)	1.5 (65 y)–9.52 (95 y)	1.38 (65 y)–8.49 (95 y)	1.12 (65 y)–1.63 (95 y)
Deprivation	1 (least)–1.19 (most)	1 (least)–1.18 (most)	1 (least)–1.32 (most)
Dementia	1.34 (1.28–1.41)	1.23 (1.16–1.30)	1.41 (1.33–1.50)
Heart failure	3.79 (3.59–4.00)	3.90 (3.68–4.13)	1.15 (1.04–1.27)
Renal failure	5.55 (5.12–6.03)	4.95 (4.56–5.39)	1.28 (1.09–1.51)
Lower respiratory tract infection	1.85 (1.75–1.96)	1.95 (1.83–2.07)	1.26 (1.17–1.36)
Chronic ischemic heart disease	1.89 (1.80–1.98)	2.12 (2.01–2.23)	1.26 (1.17–1.35)
Diabetes mellitus	1.14 (1.07–1.21)	1.06 (0.98–1.14)	1.24 (1.15–1.34)
Malignancy	3.02 (2.79–3.27)	2.81 (2.57–3.07)	1.14 (0.99–1.30)
Hypertension	0.88 (0.84–0.92)	0.87 (0.82–0.91)	0.93 (0.88–0.99)

95% CI has not been added to age and deprivation.

Table 35.2 ODDS RATIO (95% CI) FOR DELAY IN OPERATION (REPLACEMENT OR FIXATION ONLY; SIGNIFICANT) AND TYPE OF PROCEDURE (NOT SIGNIFICANT)

Factor	**Death in Hospital**	**Death in Hospital < 30 Days of Admission**	**Emergency Readmission < 28 Days**
> 1 day (vs. < 1 day)	1.27 (1.23–1.32)	1.25 (1.19–1.31)	1.04 (0.99–1.08)
> 2 days (vs. < 2 days)	1.43 (1.37–1.43)	1.36 (1.29–1.43)	1.04 (0.99–1.10)
Replacement	1.02 (0.98–1.06)	0.99 (0.95–1.04)	1.02 (0.97–1.06)
Fixation	1	1	1

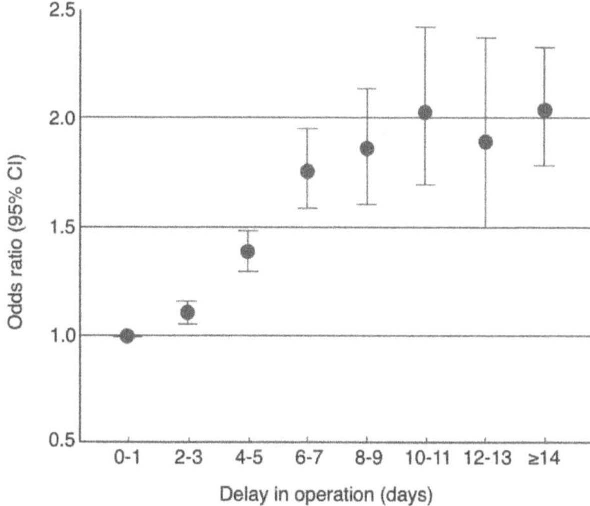

Figure 35.2. OR of death within hospital by operative delay relative to at most 1-day delay, after adjustment for age, sex, deprivation, type of procedure (fixation and replacement only), and selected comorbidities.

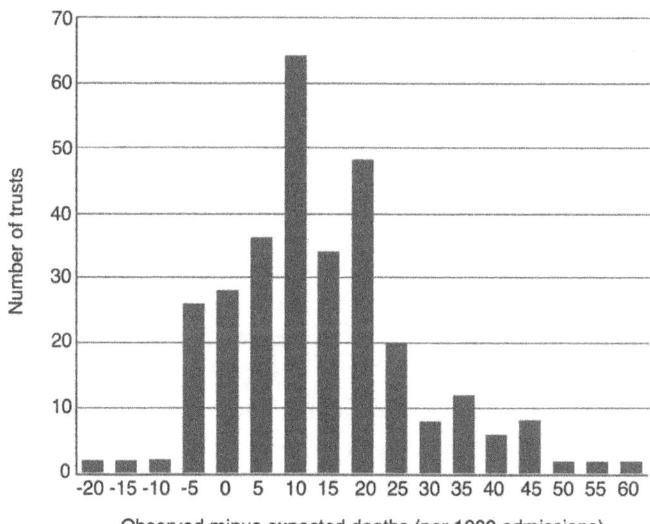

Figure 35.3. Mean annual difference between observed and expected deaths in the hospital per 1000 admissions by trust associated with an operative delay > 1 day.

Criticisms and Limitations: First, and most importantly, since this was not a randomized trial, it is only possible from this analysis to conclude that a delay in surgery for hip fracture is associated with higher mortality, not that it causes higher mortality. In addition, data quality from HES was reliant on the quality of data inputting, which is often imperfect in real-world clinical practice. Out-of-hospital deaths were not captured, which may affect true 30-day mortality.

Other Relevant Studies and Information:

- Single-center data (Peterborough, UK) including 6638 patients aged > 60 years found that worsening American Society of Anesthesiologists grade, increasing age, and extracapsular fracture increased the risk of 30-day mortality.[2] The same study found that increasing mobility, higher mini mental test score, and female gender improved survival. After adjusting for the above, surgery within < 12 hours conferred a survival benefit vs. surgery at 12–72 hours. Surgery at > 72 hours was not assessed.
- Scottish data suggested increased mortality with a delay of > 24 hours (8470 patients studied), but only if the delay was because of clinical concern, not for administrative reasons.[3] This finding may highlight the concern related to confounding.
- However, a similar study from northeastern Italy demonstrated no difference in mortality in 13 822 patient registry data, once medical confounders were controlled for.[4]
- Although there is conflict in the worldwide literature as to whether the outcome threshold is 12, 24, or 48 hours, the consensus is that when confounders are controlled for, delay in surgery increases mortality,[5–7] with 48 hours being the most critical cut-off.[8]
- The British Best Practice Tariff recommends surgery within < 36 hours after hip fracture, with 48 hours being a minimum standard.[9] American College of Surgeons guidelines support the 48-hour mark but present a call to arms to halve the time as a new target.[10]

Summary and Implications: This nonrandomized interrogation of the HES data set suggests that in patients aged > 65 years admitted from home with hip fractures, a delay to surgery of > 1 day after admission was associated with higher in-hospital mortality during the same admission or within < 30 days. Although a randomized trial would be required to prove that delays in surgery for hip fracture led to increased mortality, based on this and other compelling observational data, surgical guidelines recommend surgical treatment of hip fractures within < 48 hours of hospital admission. Though not definitive, this study adds weight to the argument that hip fracture surgery should be expedited in units managing acute trauma.

CLINICAL CASE: FAMILY REQUEST A DELAY IN SURGERY UNTIL THEY ARRIVE FROM ABROAD

Case History

A 70-year-old lady with chronic renal failure and stable ischemic heart disease is admitted with a fractured neck of femur sustained at home while cleaning her bathroom. No reversible medical conditions are identified. She is listed for surgery the next day. Her family lives abroad and wants to fly in to see her before the operation. They have requested that the operation be delayed until they have an opportunity to see her preoperatively. What is the risk of delaying her surgery based on this study?

Suggested Answer

National Institute of Clinical Excellence guidance, based on consensus evidence from studies such as this by Bottle and Aylin, suggests that early surgery reduces the risk of early mortality for patients with a hip fracture. The surgical team should be prioritizing her case over surgery that is not life or limb threatening. A delay beyond the next day of her admission would increase her risk of dying early in the hospital (odds ratio [OR] 1.27). A delay of a further day would increase this risk again (OR 1.43). This patient already has a high-risk stratification for mortality on this admission due to her medical comorbidities. A complete discussion with her family should therefore include an explanation that, although the surgery is high risk, an expeditious procedure will reduce the overall risk. All efforts should be made to converse with the family over the phone and documented within patient notes. It is also good medical practice to discuss the need for do not attempt resuscitation orders or any advanced directives/power of attorney for welfare and health with the patient, the patient's next of kin/family, and the orthogeriatric and anesthetic teams to ensure a multidisciplinary approach.

References

1. Bottle et al. Mortality associated with delay in operation after hip fracture: observational study. BMJ. 2006;332(7547):947–51.
2. Bretherton et al. Early surgery for patients with a fracture of the hip decreases 30-day mortality. Bone Joint J. 2015;97-B:104–8.
3. Mackenzie et al. Mortality associated with delay in operation after hip fracture: Scottish data provide additional information. BMJ. 2006;332(7549):1093.
4. Franzo et al. Mortality associated with delay in operation after hip fracture: . . . but Italian data seem to contradict study findings. BMJ. 2006;332(7549):1093.

5. Alvi et al. Time-to-surgery for definitive fixation of hip fractures: a look at outcomes based upon delay. Am J Orthop (Belle Mead NJ). 2018;9:47.
6. Leer-Salvese et al. Does time from fracture to surgery affect mortality and intraoperative medical complications for hip fracture patients? Bone Joint J. 2019;101-B:1129–37.
7. Nyholm et al. Time to surgery is associated with thirty-day and ninety-day mortality after proximal femoral fracture: a retrospective observational study on prospectively collected data from the Danish fracture database collaborators. J Bone Joint Surg Am. 2015;97(16):1333–9.
8. Rosso et al. Prognostic factors for mortality after hip fracture: operation within 48 hours is mandatory. Injury. 2016;47(Suppl 4):S91–7.
9. The Royal College of Physicians. National Hip Fracture Database (NHFD). Best Practice Tariff (BPT) for fragility hip fracture care user guide. 2010. https://www.nhfd.co.uk
10. American College of Surgeons and Orthopaedic Trauma Association. Committee on Trauma. ACS TQIP. Best practices in the management of orthopaedic trauma. 2015. https://www.facs.org/-/media/files/quality-programs/trauma/tqip/ortho_guidelines.ashx

36

Role of Surgery in Spinal Cord Compression Caused by Metastatic Cancer

ARASH AFRAMIAN, KAPIL SUGAND, HAMID HASSANY, AND REZA MOBASHERI

> Significantly more patients in the surgery group (42/50, 84%) than in the radiotherapy group (29/51, 57%) were able to walk after treatment (odds ratio 6·2 [95% CI 2·0–19·8] p=0·001). Patients treated with surgery also retained the ability to walk significantly longer than did those with radiotherapy alone.
>
> —PATCHELL ET AL.[1]

Citation: Patchell RA, Tibbs PA, Regine WF, Payne R, Saris S, Kryscio RJ, Mohiuddin M, Young B. Direct decompressive surgical resection in the treatment of spinal cord compression caused by metastatic cancer: a randomised trial. Lancet. 2005;366(9486):643–8.

Research Question: Should patients with metastatic epidural spinal cord compression be managed with radiotherapy and corticosteroids or with direct decompressive surgery prior to medical management?

Funding: Grants from the National Cancer Institute (RO1 CA55256) and the National Institute for Neurological Disorders and Stroke (K24 NS502180)

Year Study Began: 1992

Year Study Published: 2005

Study Location: USA; Bluegrass Neuro-Oncology Consortium with 7 participating institutions: University of Kentucky, MD Anderson, Brown University, University of Alabama-Birmingham, University of Michigan, University of Pittsburgh, University of South Florida

Who Was Studied: Adults aged at least 18 years with a tissue-proven diagnosis of cancer (not of central nervous system or spinal column origin) who also had magnetic resonance imaging (MRI) evidence of metastatic spinal cord compression (MSCC) and at least 1 neurological sign or symptom (including pain) but who were not totally paraplegic > 48 hours before study entry.

Who Was Excluded: Patients with a mass that compressed only the cauda equina or spinal roots and those with multiple discrete compressive lesions were excluded.

How Many Patients: 101

Study Overview: See Figure 36.1.

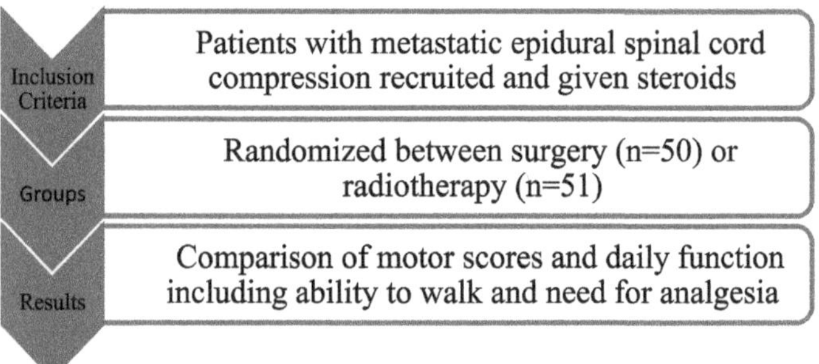

Figure 36.1. Overview of study design.

Study Intervention: All patients received steroids (dexamethasone) immediately and until commencement of randomized treatment. Those in the radiotherapy treatment group received 3 Gy × 10 fractions (total 30 Gy) through a port that encompassed 1 vertebral body above and below the visible lesion. Those in the surgery group had direct circumferential decompression of the spinal cord (with stabilization if spinal instability was present), followed by (adjuvant) radiotherapy for < 14 days, as in the radiation group.

Follow-Up: Median was 102 days in the surgery group and 93 days in the radiation group.

Endpoints: Primary outcome was ability to walk after treatment and how long walking persisted after treatment. Secondary outcomes were urinary continence, changes in functional scale and motor scores (i.e., Frankel[2] [assesses the severity and prognosis of spinal cord injury using 5 grades of sensory and motor scales] and American Spinal Injury Association[3] [ASIA; most widely accepted and employed clinical scoring system for spinal cord injury with motor and sensory components] scores), and use of corticosteroids and opioid analgesics.

Results: The patients treated with decompressive surgery performed better:

- *Primary outcome (Figure 36.2):*
  - Patients were significantly better able to regain (odds ratio 6.2, 95% CI: 2.0–19.8, $p = 0.001$) and to retain ($p = 0.0017$) the ability walk, and for a longer period of time.
  - The ability to retain walking ability was also true ($p = 0.024$) for those who could still walk at the time of surgery (94%, median 153 days) compared to the nonsurgical group (74%, median 54 days) after treatment.
  - Within the subgroup who were able to walk at entry to the study, 94% (32/34) continued to walk after treatment in the surgery group, compared to 74% (26/35) in the radiation group ($p = 0.024$).
- *Secondary outcomes:*
  - Continence, functional scale, and motor scores were all superior in the surgical group as shown in Table 36.1.
  - The surgical group needed less opioid analgesia (morphine daily equivalent dose in the surgery group was 0.4 mg [interquartile range (IQR): 0–0.6 mg] compared with 4.8 mg [IQR: 0–200 mg] in the radiation group, $p = 0.002$) and less ongoing corticosteroids (dexamethasone daily equivalent dose in the surgery group was 1.6 mg [IQR: 0.1–44 mg] compared with 4.2 mg [IQR: 0–50 mg] in the radiation group, $p = 0.0093$).
- The trial was terminated early by the supervising data safety and monitoring committee when it became clear that outcomes in the surgical group were superior.

Table 36.1 Summary of Key Findings

	Radiation Group	**Surgery Group**	**Relative Risk**[a]	**95% CI**[a]	***p* Value**[a]	**Significant Predictors**[b]**: Relative Risk (RR; 95% CI)**
Maintenance of continence	17 days	156 days	0.47	0.25–0.87	0.016	Surgery RR = 0.51 (0.29–0.90) Baseline Frankel score RR = 0.56 (0.30–0.73)
Maintenance of ASIA score	72 days	566 days	0.28	0.13–0.61	0.001	Surgery RR = 0.30 (0.14–0.62) Stable spine RR = 0.43 (0.22–0.83) Cervical spinal level RR = 0.49 (0.26–0.90) Baseline Frankel score RR = 0.65 (0.46–0.91)
Maintenance of Frankel score	72 days	566 days	0.24	0.11–0.54	0.0006	Surgery RR = 0.26 (0.12–0.54) Stable spine RR = 0.39 (0.20–0.75) Cervical spinal level RR = 0.53 (0.74–0.98) Baseline Frankel score RR = 0.62 (0.44–0.88)
Survival time	100 days	126 days	0.60	0.38–0.96	0.033	Surgery RR = 0.60 (0.40–0.92) Breast primary tumor RR = 0.29 (0.13–0.62) Lower thoracic spinal level RR = 0.65 (0.43–0.99)

[a] Based on a Cox model with all covariates included.

[b] Based on a Cox model with only significant predictors included (stepwise selection).

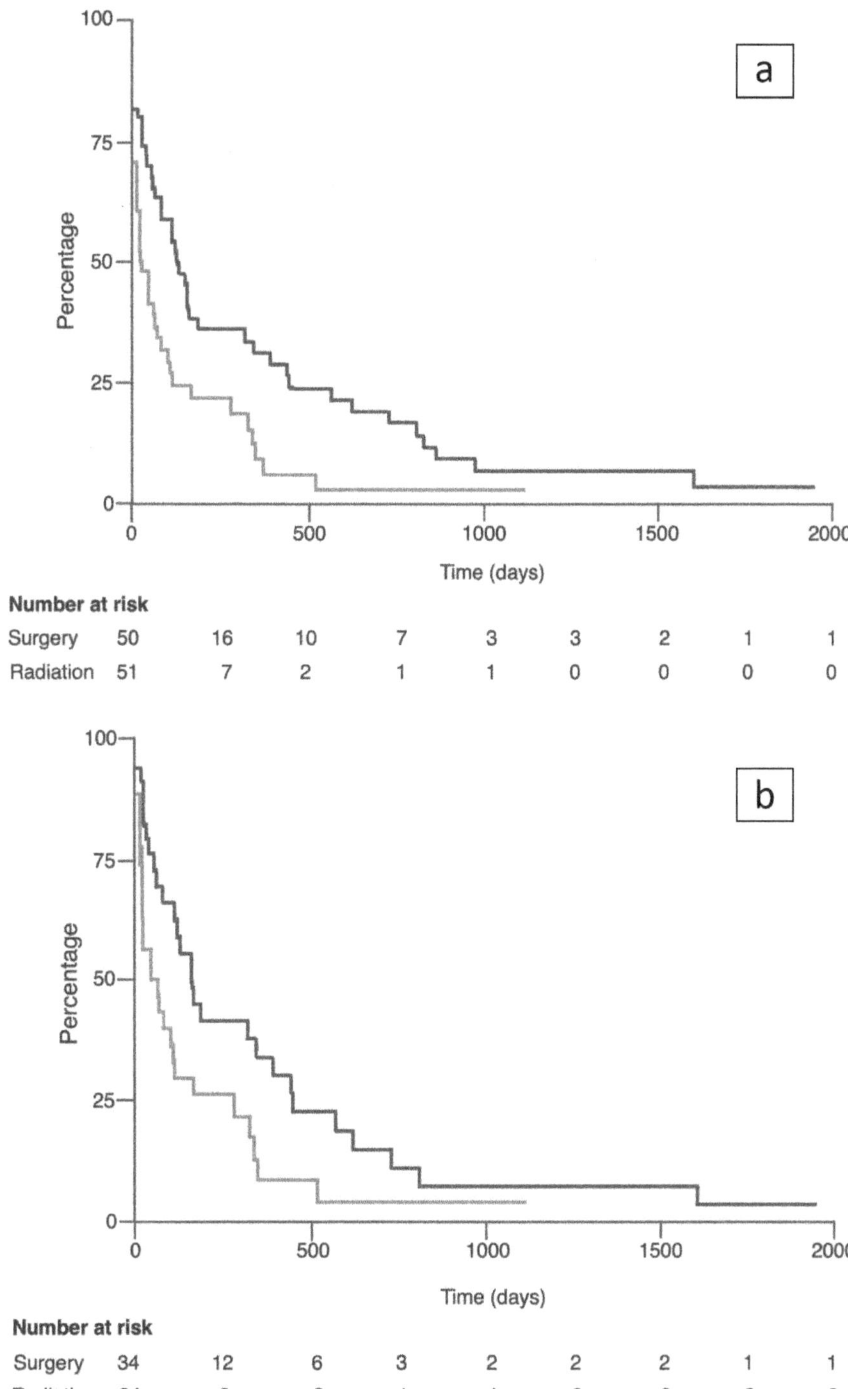

Figure 36.2. Kaplan-Meier estimates of length of time that (a) all study patients remained ambulatory after treatment and (b) patients who were ambulatory at study entry remained ambulatory after treatment.

Criticisms and Limitations: The patient population studied consisted of those for whom surgery would be regarded as a realistic treatment option. Patients with radiosensitive tumors, multiple areas of spinal cord compression, or total paraplegia for > 48 hours were excluded. Hence, results of this study cannot justify surgery in all patients with MSCC.

Other Relevant Studies and Information:

- Surgery has been shown in this study to be effective but is clearly more costly, and the incremental cost-effectiveness ratio was US$250,307 per quality-adjusted life year.[4]
- Primary tumor type and the ability to walk prior to treatment are both significant mediators to outcomes.[5,6]
- National Institute for Health and Care Excellence guidelines recommend surgery for patients with a life expectancy > 3 months using Tokuhashi (system for the preoperative evaluation of a patient's prognosis with a metastatic spinal tumor) scoring[7] (and if paraplegia/tetraplegia has been present for < 24 hours, unless spinal stabilization is required for pain relief).[8]

Summary and Implications: This landmark study provides evidence that surgical treatment of patients with spinal cord compression due to metastatic cancer leads to superior outcomes compared to radiation therapy alone. Patients in the surgical treatment arm experienced superior outcomes for all primary and secondary endpoints (i.e., ability to walk, continence and functional scores, and survival) vs. patients in the group receiving steroids and radiation therapy alone. Major guidelines now recommend surgical decompression for patients who are appropriate surgical candidates with spinal cord compression due to metastatic cancer.

CLINICAL CASE: MANAGEMENT OF MSCC

Case History

A 75-year-old man who is otherwise well presents with acute-onset and worsening atraumatic lumbago. He presents to the local Emergency Department with incomplete neurological compromise for the last few hours. An urgent MRI scan is performed and demonstrates a single-level thoracic vertebral metastasis impinging on the spinal cord. There are no other systemic metastases, but a primary tumor was found in the lung on a subsequent staging computed tomography (CT) scan. He presents with weakness and paresthesia of his lower limbs (without upper limb involvement) but is still ambulatory and has difficulty passing urine. Retained urine was confirmed on postmicturition bladder scan. His life expectancy is > 6 months. Based on the results of this study, how should this patient be treated?

Suggested Answer

The patient is in good general condition with a single-level vertebral metastasis but without major internal organs involved. CT of the chest, abdomen, and pelvis confirms a primary lung tumor. This has favorable outcomes for spinal surgery (few medical comorbidities, no known extraspinal metastases, and incomplete palsy) according to the data. This would give him a low Tokuhashi score[7] and a life expectancy > 6 months. His symptoms have been present for < 24 hours and therefore he should receive surgery, followed up with radiation and corticosteroids to improve his outcomes, and thus helping to preserve function. The data suggests that he is more likely to not only recover normal walking ability but also retain it for longer. Additionally, he is more likely to regain normal urinary continence with better functional and motor scores if he has surgery prior to adjuvant radiotherapy and steroid treatment. The evidence in his case would suggest urgent surgical decompression as well as stabilizing the spine as necessary.

References

1. Patchell et al. Direct decompressive surgical resection in the treatment of spinal cord compression caused by metastatic cancer: a randomised trial. Lancet. 2005;366(9486):643–8.
2. Frankel et al. The value of postural reduction in the initial management of closed injuries of the spine with paraplegia and tetraplegia. Paraplegia I. 1969;7:179–92.
3. Fehlings et al. Burns Essentials of Spinal Cord Injury: Basic Research to Clinical Practice. Denver, CO: Thieme Medical Publishers Inc.; 2013.
4. Furlan et al. The combined use of surgery and radiotherapy to treat patients with epidural cord compression due to metastatic disease: a cost-utility analysis. Neuro Oncol. 2012;14(5):631–40.
5. Helweg-Larsen et al. Prognostic factors in metastatic spinal cord compression: a prospective study using multivariate analysis of variables influencing survival and gait function in 153 patients. Int J Radiat Oncol Biol Phys. 2000;46(5):1163–9.
6. Sundaresan et al. Surgery for solitary metastases of the spine: rationale and results of treatment. Spine (Phila Pa 1976). 2002;27(16):1802–6.
7. Tokuhashi et al. A revised scoring system for preoperative evaluation of metastatic spine tumor prognosis. Spine (Phila Pa 1976). 2005;30(19):2186–91.
8. National Institute for Health and Care Excellence. Metastatic spinal cord compression overview. February 2019. https://www.pathways.nice.org.uk/pathways/metastatic-spinal-cord-compression

37

Comorbidities Predisposing to Failure of Intracapsular Hip Fracture Fixation

SOPHIA BURNS AND SIMON MELLOR

> We found that pre-existing renal failure, respiratory disease and alcohol abuse were the comorbidities most strongly predictive for failure following fixation of a hip fracture in young adults. These three risk factors predispose to poor bone quality and so these patients are often poor candidates for internal fixation.
>
> —DUCKWORTH ET AL.[1]

Citation: Duckworth AD, Bennet SJ, Aderinto J, Keating JF. Fixation of intracapsular fractures of the femoral neck in young patients: risk factors for failure. J Bone Joint Surg Br. 2011;93(6):811–6.

Research Question: How do comorbidities in patients under 60 years of age undergoing hip fracture fixation influence the risk for failure of fixation, non-union, and avascular necrosis (AVN) of the femoral head?

Funding: Nil

Year Study Began: 1995

Year Study Published: 2011

Study Location: Royal Infirmary of Edinburgh, Scotland

Who Was Studied: Patients were identified from trauma admissions between December 1995 and June 2008. Those ≤ 60 years with a Garden type III/IV intracapsular neck of femur (NOF) fracture who underwent cannulated screw fixation were included.

Who Was Excluded: Patients who presented ≥ 1 week postinjury.

How Many Patients: 122

Study Overview: See Figure 37.1.

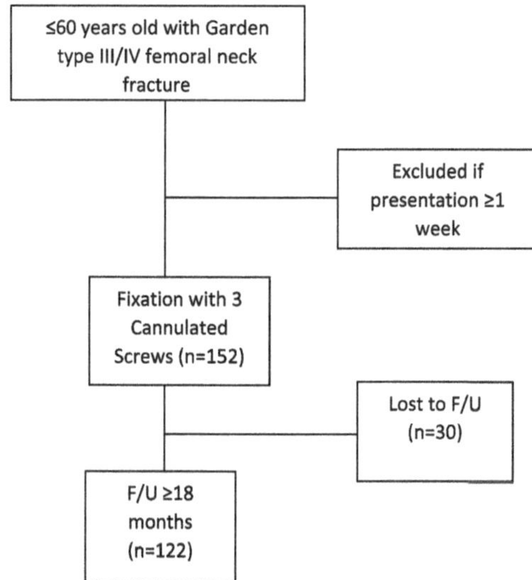

Figure 37.1. Summary of study design.

Study Intervention: All patients included in the study underwent fixation using 3 cannulated screws in an inverted triangle configuration. Capsulotomy or aspiration of intracapsular hematoma was not performed. Of those patients, only 2 underwent open reduction because a satisfactory reduction could not be achieved with closed technique. All patients were mobilized touch weight bearing for the first 6 weeks postoperatively followed by full weight bearing.

Follow-Up: At least 18 months

Endpoints: The primary outcomes assessed were union, failure of fixation, nonunion, and the development of AVN.

RESULTS (TABLE 37.1)

- *Complications:*
  - Complications occurred in 39 patients (32%) at a mean of 11 months.
  - The most common and earliest complication was loss of fixation (Figure 37.2 differentiates between acceptable and unacceptable parameters).
- *Nonunion*: 7.4% of cases ($n = 9$)
- *AVN:* 11.5% ($n = 14$)
- *Risk factors*:
  - Comorbid conditions predisposing to failure were identified in 30 (77%) patients who developed complications.
  - Alcohol excess ($p < 0.001$), renal failure ($p = 0.03$), liver failure ($p = 0.04$), and respiratory disease ($p = 0.03$) were the only significant medical comorbidities predictive of failure on multivariate binary logistic regression analysis.
- *Delay to fracture fixation*: The only significant surgical factor predictive of failure
- *Smoking*: Not found to be a risk factor for failure
- Figure 37.3 demonstrates the distribution of hip fractures in patients aged < 60 years by 10-year cohorts, and Figure 37.4 demonstrates the distribution of fractures by 10-year cohorts according to mechanism of injury.

Table 37.1 Summary of Key Findings

	No Failure (%)	**Failure (%)**	***p* Value**
Total (%)	83 (68)	39 (32) *Loss of fixation: 16 (13.1)* *Nonunion: 9 (7.4)* *AVN: 14 (11.5)*	N/A
Most Significant Predictors of Failure			
Alcohol excess	9 (11)	14 (36)	< 0.001
Delay in time to fixation (>24 h)	18 (22)	18 (46)	0.005
Chronic respiratory disease	3 (4)	5 (13)	0.03
Renal failure	0 (0)	3 (8)	0.03
Liver disease	1 (3)	4 (10)	0.04
Learning difficulties	9 (11)	9 (23)	0.07
Cerebral palsy	2 (2)	4 (10)	0.08
Pre-existing mobility problems	2 (1)	4 (10)	0.08
Not Predictive of Failure			
Smoking	19 (23)	12 (31)	0.35

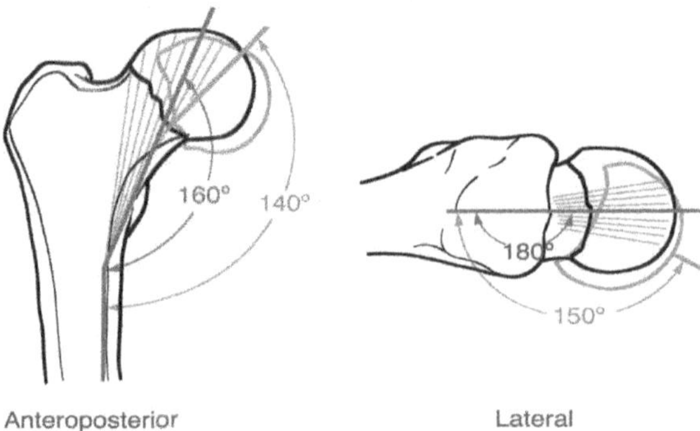

Figure 37.2. Garden alignment index, with an angle of 160–180 degrees on both anteroposterior and lateral radiographs considered satisfactory. The blue arrows indicate anatomical reduction, while the orange arrows represent unacceptable reduction positions.

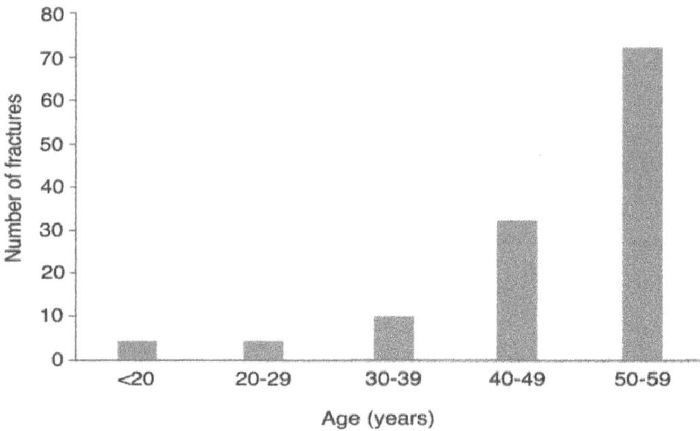

Figure 37.3. Bar chart showing the distribution of hip fractures in patients < 60 years of age by 10-year cohorts.

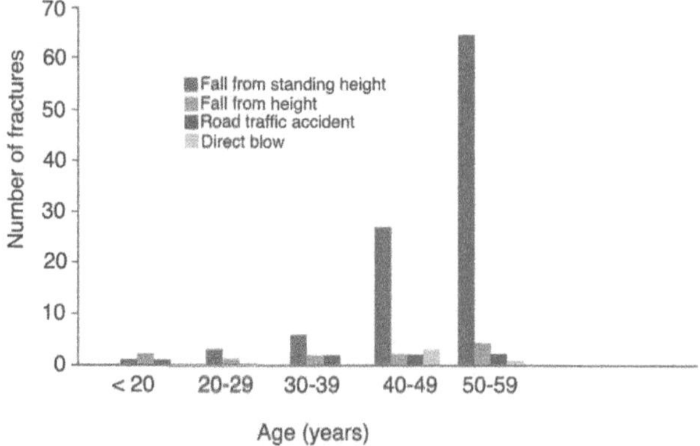

Figure 37.4. Bar chart showing the distribution of fractures by 10-year cohorts according to mechanism of injury.

Criticisms and Limitations: Follow-up was a minimum of 18 months per patient; however, union occurred at a mean of 58 months, raising questions about whether the study was of sufficient duration to adequately capture outcomes. In addition, only 39 patients (32%) had postreduction radiographs available to review.

Other Relevant Studies and Information:

- Consensus in the literature indicates that prompt anatomical reduction and internal fixation should be performed for patients aged < 60 years.[2]
- Most studies attribute failure of fixation, nonunion, and AVN to the fracture configuration and biomechanical stability of fixation. Huang et al. found that screw configurations other than an inverted triangle resulted in a significantly higher nonunion rate.[3]
- Alcohol excess and chronic kidney disease are recognized risk factors for reduced bone mineral density (BMD).[4,5] Schweitzer et al.[6] found that young patients who developed AVN were older and had suffered lower-energy trauma, suggesting reduced BMD. The correlation between reduced BMD and failure of fixation in younger patients is yet to be explored.

Summary and Implications: This study confirmed that delay to surgery was the surgical factor most significantly associated with failure of fixation ($p < 0.005$); however, medical comorbidities were more strongly predictive. The results of this study indicate that management of 40–60-year-old patients with displaced intracapsular NOF fractures following a low-energy fall should take into account their medical comorbidities. Arthroplasty should be considered as an alternative to cannulated screw fixation, especially if there is a history of alcohol excess, renal failure, liver failure, or respiratory disease due to increased risk of fixation failure.

CLINICAL CASE: YOUNG PATIENT WITH DISPLACED NOF FRACTURE

Case History

A 50-year-old woman is admitted with right hip pain and inability to mobilize following a low-energy fall in her garden yesterday evening. Pelvic anteroposterior radiograph shows the presence of a displaced, Garden III, intracapsular NOF fracture. The patient works as an administrator at the local school; she lives with her partner and is otherwise independently mobile. Though she denies any significant medical conditions, a detailed history reveals that she drinks a bottle of wine and 2 gin and tonics every evening; she also smokes 20 cigarettes a day and becomes breathless after a flight of stairs. She has had previous admissions for injuries while intoxicated. How should this patient be managed according to this study?

Suggested Answer

Duckworth et al.[1] found that medical comorbidities that reduce bone density, such as alcohol excess, renal disease, liver disease, and respiratory disease, are predictive of fracture fixation failure for displaced intracapsular NOF fractures. The patient is young, but her medical history suggests that she is at high risk for low BMD, and hence failure of fixation. The treating surgeon should counsel the patient on the risks of both fixation and arthroplasty, highlighting the potential for fixation failure, to come to an agreed-upon course of action. Services for smoking cessation, alcohol withdrawal, and substance misuse should be provided and a dual x-ray absorptiometry scan arranged following surgery. Secondary fracture prevention treatment should also be seriously considered.

References

1. Duckworth et al. Fixation of intracapsular fractures of the femoral neck in young patients: risk factors for failure. J Bone Joint Surg Br. 2011;93(6):811–6.
2. Robinson et al. Hip fractures in adults younger than 50 years of age. Epidemiology and results. Clin Orthop Relat Res. 1995 Mar;(312):238–46.
3. Huang et al. Displaced femoral neck fractures in young adults treated with closed reduction and internal fixation. Orthopedics. 2010;33:873.
4. Tucker et al. Effects of beer, wine, and liquor intakes on bone mineral density in older men and women. Am J Clin Nutr. 2009;89:1188–96.
5. Cunningham J et al. Osteoporosis Work Group. Osteoporosis in chronic kidney disease. Am J Kidney Dis. 2004;43:566–71.
6. Schweitzer et al. Factors associated with avascular necrosis of the femoral head and nonunion in patients younger than 65 years with displaced femoral neck fractures treated with reduction and internal fixation. Eur J Orthop Surg Traumatol. 2013;23:61–5.

38

Surgery versus Orthosis versus Watchful Waiting for Hallux Valgus

SHIRLEY ANNE LYLE AND SHELAIN PATEL

> Surgical osteotomy is an effective treatment for painful hallux valgus. Orthoses provide short-term symptomatic relief.
>
> —TORKKI ET AL.[1]

Citation: Torkki M, Malmivaara A, Seitsalo S, Hoikka V, Laippala P, Paavolainen P. Surgery vs orthosis vs watchful waiting for hallux valgus: a randomized controlled trial. JAMA. 2001;285(19):2474–80.

Research Question: Should patients with hallux valgus be treated with surgery, orthotics, or observation?

Funding: Finnish Office for Health Technology Assessment, Finnish Medical Foundation, Scientific Foundation of Jorvi Hospital, and Scientific Foundation of Mehiläinen Hospital

Year Study Began: 1997

Year Study Published: 2001

Study Location: 4 general community hospitals in Finland

Who Was Studied: Adults with a painful bunion with a hallux valgus angle (HVA) < 35 degrees and intermetatarsal angle (IMA) < 15 degrees.

Who Was Excluded: Patients with rheumatoid disease, pregnancy, age > 60 years, those using functional foot orthoses, and those with severe hallux valgus, hallux limitus, or previous hallux valgus surgery.

How Many Patients: 209

Study Overview: See Figure 38.1.

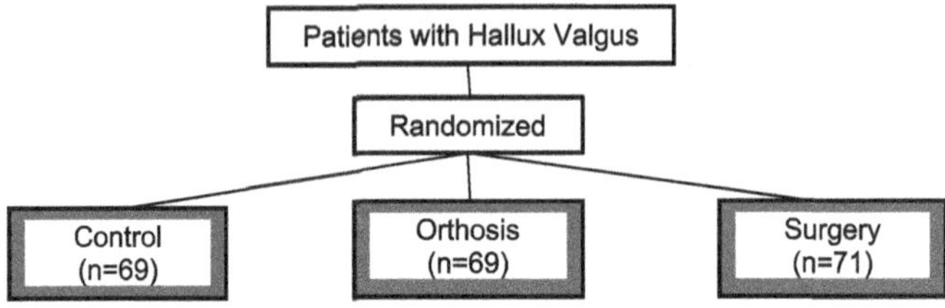

Figure 38.1. Summary of study design.

Study Intervention: Patients in the surgical group were treated with medial exostectomy, adductor release, and first metatarsal distal Chevron osteotomy without fixation (except 1 patient stabilized with a Kirschner wire). An abduction splint was used to hold the hallux for 6 weeks. Patients in the orthosis group were supplied with an individualized polypropylene orthosis made by negative cast technique. The control group was instructed to avoid surgery or use an orthosis during the follow-up (F/U) period.

Follow-Up: 12 months

Endpoints: Pain intensity during walking on a visual analog scale (VAS; 0–100), patient assessment of global improvement, number of painful days, cosmetic disturbance, footwear problems, functional status, and treatment satisfaction; all feet were scored by the hallux metatarsophalangeal scale of the American Orthopaedic Foot and Ankle Society[2] (AOFAS; clinical rating system combining objective and subjective metrics for pain, function, and alignment).

RESULTS

- At 6-month F/U:
  - *Pain:* The intensity of foot pain was less in the surgical and orthosis treatment groups than in the control group (Figure 38.2).
  - *Cosmesis:* The surgical group had the least cosmetic disturbance compared with the other 2 groups.

  - *Footwear problems:* The proportion of the those with footwear problems was significantly lowest in the surgical group.
  - *Satisfaction:* Satisfaction rates were lowest in the control group.
- At 1-year F/U:
  - *Treatment effect:* 83%, 46%, and 24% of patients in the surgery, orthosis, and control groups respectively felt that they were better than at the start of the evaluation.
  - *Pain:* Pain intensity improved in all groups, although the greatest improvement was observed in the surgical group (Figure 38.2).
  - *Functional outcome:* Surgery produced greater improvements in function and satisfaction with fewer painful days and footwear issues than orthosis or watchful waiting.
  - *Footwear problems and global assessment:* There was significant improvement in footwear problems ($p < 0.01$) and global assessment ($p < 0.001$) in the surgical group compared to both the control and orthosis groups.
- *Global assessment*: This was significantly better for the orthosis group vs. the control group ($p < 0.01$), but not better for footwear problems ($p = 0.5$).
- *Surgical correction:* Surgery significantly improved both HVA by a mean of 10.4 degrees and IMA by a mean of 3.7 degrees.
- *Complications:* Surgery was associated with 4 (4%) complications in 97 osteotomies:
  - 1 infection
  - 1 metatarsal fracture
  - 1 nerve injury
  - 1 recurrence
- *Cost:* The mean cost of treatment per patient within the control, orthosis, and surgery groups was $125, $221, and $930 respectively.

Table 38.1 Summary of Key Findings at 1 Year

Outcome	**Control**	**Orthosis**	**Surgery**
Intensity of foot paina	40	40	20
Global foot assessmentb	24%	46%	83%
No footwear problems	7.5%	4.5%	35.4%
AOFAS hallux metatarsophalangeal-interphalangeal scorec	66	64	75

[a] Mean score recorded on 100-mm VAS from 0 (no pain at all) to 100 (unbearable pain).
[b] Percentage of patients who self-report their foot was better than 1 year ago.
[c] Total scores ranges from 0 to 100. Higher scores indicate better functional ability.

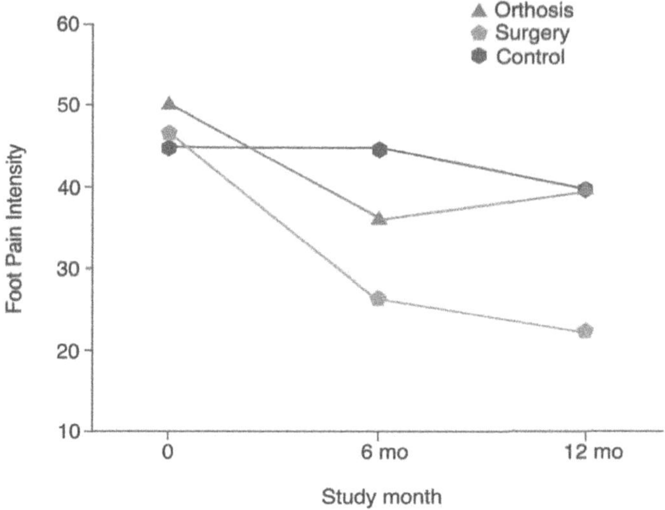

Figure 38.2. Mean intensity of foot pain. Visual analog scale scores from 0 to 100, where 100 depicts the most pain, at baseline and 6 and 12 months in the surgery, orthosis, and control groups.

Criticisms and Limitations: The study was not double blinded, so patient expectations might have influenced subjective outcome measures. The surgery employed in this study was a Chevron osteotomy, which is only one of many options available for hallux valgus correction, and surgical outcomes may vary depending on the surgical technique utilized. The F/U period was short at only 1 year, so long-term conclusions cannot be drawn. For the orthosis and control groups, neither the radiological findings nor the complications were reported. There were no reported statistical analyses for the outcomes of AOFAS or foot pain.

Other Relevant Studies and Information:

- Yamamoto et al.[3] showed that the quality of life (QOL) in untreated and symptomatic hallux valgus subjects is lower than that of the general population. However, QOL and clinical evaluation parameters do not correlate with the severity of deformity, so decision-making on treatment should be guided by clinical rather than radiographic assessment.

- Long-term results from a randomized study comparing 2 of the most widely used osteotomies for hallux valgus (Chevron and scarf) showed similar rates of clinical outcomes and recurrence at 14 years.[4]
- Minimally invasive hallux valgus surgery is becoming increasingly popular. Recent data supports its use as an alternative to traditional open surgery with less pain early on but comparable outcomes at between 1 and 2 years.[5,6]

Summary and Implications: This randomized controlled trial showed that surgery is more effective than orthosis or no intervention in treating patients with mild to moderate hallux valgus deformity. At 1 year the pain intensity decreased more in the surgical group (distal Chevron osteotomy) than in the control or the orthotic group. The surgical group also had fewer painful days, cosmetic disturbances, and footwear problems, as well as greater functional status and satisfaction. However, surgery is associated with complications and a higher cost of treatment. Since orthotics provide short-term relief (i.e., 6 months after which the effect fades), they may be an option in patients unsuitable or unwilling to undergo surgery and rehabilitation.

CLINICAL CASE: HALLUX VALGUS: WATCH, WAIT, OPERATE?

Case History

A 47-year-old woman with a history of mild hypertension is bothered by a painful bunion on her right foot, especially on walking. She finds it difficult to buy appropriate footwear. Weight-bearing dorsoplantar radiographs show an IMA of 12 degrees and an HVA of 26 degrees (Figure 38.3). The joint is congruent and correctable. She works as a shop assistant and wants treatment to reduce her pain. She is not keen on surgery due to fear of complications. She has done some research online and wonders whether any other conservative measures could be considered first. What treatment options should be offered to her according to this study?

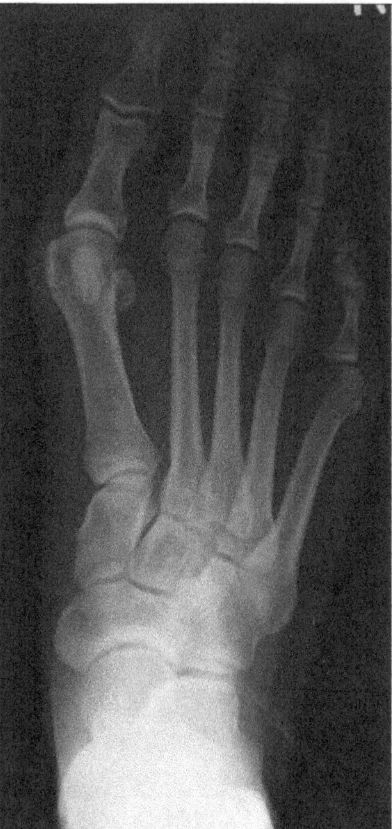

Figure 38.3. Plain radiograph of right foot.

Suggested Answer

This study has shown that although either watchful waiting or an orthosis provides subjective improvement in some patients at 1 year, surgical intervention is more likely to improve both her foot pain and function and reduce her footwear issues. She should be counseled about surgical intervention to correct the hallux valgus as well as being warned that she will have a period of protected weight bearing and be absent from work for 6 weeks on average. Surgical risks should not be ignored and may be important in her decision-making process.

References

1. Torkki et al. Surgery vs orthosis vs watchful waiting for hallux valgus: a randomized controlled trial. JAMA. 2001;285(19):2474–80.
2. Kitaoka et al. Clinical rating systems for the ankle-hindfoot, midfoot, hallux, and lesser toes. Foot Ankle Int. 1994;15:349–53.

3. Yamamoto et al. Quality of life in patients with untreated and symptomatic hallux valgus. Foot Ankle Int. 2016;37(11):1171–7.
4. Jeuken et al. Long-term follow-up of a randomized controlled trial comparing scarf to Chevron osteotomy in hallux valgus correction. Foot Ankle Int. 2016;37(7):687–95.
5. Lai et al. Clinical and radiological outcomes comparing percutaneous Chevron-akin osteotomies vs open scarf-akin osteotomies for hallux valgus. Foot Ankle Int. 2018;39(3):311–7.
6. Lee et al. Hallux valgus correction comparing percutaneous Chevron/akin (PECA) and open scarf/akin osteotomies. Foot Ankle Int. 2017;38(8):83846.

39

Isolated Medial Patellofemoral Repair Does Not Improve Patient Outcomes or Decrease the Rate of Patella Redislocation

SARA BOUTONG, KAPIL SUGAND, AND MUDASSAR AHMAD

> Delayed primary repair of the MPFL after primary patella dislocation does not reduce the risk of redislocation nor does it produce any significantly better subjective functional outcomes.
>
> —CHRISTIANSEN ET AL.[1]

Citation: Christiansen SE, Jakobsen BW, Lund B, Lind M. Isolated repair of the medial patellofemoral ligament in primary dislocation of the patella: a prospective randomized study. Arthroscopy. 2008;24(8):881–7.

Research Question: Does surgical intervention improve the clinical outcomes for patients presenting with a primary patella dislocation?

Year Study Began: 1998–2002

Year Study Published: 2008

Study Location: Aarhus University Hospital, Denmark

Who Was Studied: Patients aged 13–30 presenting with a first-time patella dislocation.

Who Was Excluded: All patients with a past history of patella dislocation, pain, or instability or any patients who were deemed unable to follow the instructions of any management plan.

How Many Patients: 77

Study Overview: See Figure 39.1.

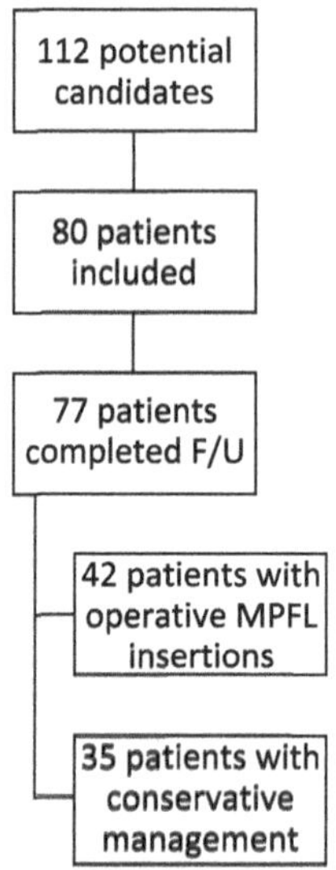

Figure 39.1. Study overview.

Study Intervention: Patella dislocation was diagnosed by either a locked dislocated patella or a history of acute knee trauma with hematoma, tenderness to palpation over the medial epicondyle, and a positive lateral patella apprehension test. Every patient had an evaluation of the joint by undergoing a diagnostic arthroscopy ± repair/excision of osteochondral defects. After the initial arthroscopy, patients were then randomized for repair of their medial patellofemoral ligament (MPFL; i.e., operative) or no further surgery (i.e., conservative) groups. The procedure used an incision over the adductor tubercle and the repair was made using a baseball stitch and 2 Mitek G2 anchors (DePuy Synthes, Warsaw, Indiana, USA) without repairing the vastus medialis oblique (VMO) or adductor magnus tendon. No other concurrent surgical interventions were done except for addressing osteochondral fragments with either fixation or debridement. All procedures were performed or supervised by the same surgeon. The postoperative rehabilitation protocol was the same for all patients, as follows:

- 0–2 weeks: 0–20-degree range of motion (ROM) and full weight bearing
- 2–6 weeks: free ROM + increased quadriceps exercises

Follow-Up: Clinic appointments at 2 and 6 weeks and 1 and 2 years (endpoint)

Endpoints: The primary endpoint was the incidence of patella redislocation within 2 years. Secondary endpoints were patient-reported outcome measures. The Kujala score[2] (or Anterior Knee Pain Scale, a 13-item self-report questionnaire that assesses subjective reactions to particular activities and symptoms known to correlate with anterior knee pain syndrome) and Knee injury and Osteoarthritis Outcome Score[3] (KOOS; knee-specific tool that was developed to assess the patients' opinions about their short- and long-term consequences of knee injury) were used to evaluate the clinical outcome.

RESULTS (TABLE 39.1)

- *Demographics:* There was no difference between the groups with respect to sex, body mass index, or age.
- *Baseline characteristics:* There was no difference between the groups with respect to hyperlaxity, femoropatellar dysplasia, or patella alta. At arthroscopy, no differences in the extent of intra-articular cartilage lesions were seen between groups.
- *Mean delay to surgery*: The mean delay to surgery was 50 days from presentation.
- *Chondral injury:* Chondral injury without osteochondral fracture defined as International Cartilage Regeneration and Joint Preservation Society (ICRS) injury grade 2–4 was seen on the patella in 24% (17/72) and on the trochlea in 7% (5/72). Of the 10 osteochondral lesions found, only 2 were suitable for refixation (i.e., 1 in each group), which was done by open technique using resorbable pins.
- *Redislocation rate:* There was no significant difference in the operative group (16.7%) vs. the nonoperative group (20%) at 2-year follow-up (F/U).
- *Time of redislocation (Figure 39.2):* Survival analysis elicited slightly but insignificantly earlier time of redislocation (at any time point) in the conservative group vs. the operative group.
- *KOOS:* There was an insignificant difference between both groups.

- *Kujala scores*
  - *Patellar instability subscore:* This was significantly higher in the operative group than in the conservative group (median [range] = 10 [6–10] vs. 6 [4–6]; $p = 0.007$).
  - *Overall score*: There was insignificant improvement for the operative group (85 vs. 78; $p = 0.07$).

Table 39.1 Key Results

	Operative Group	**Conservative Group**	***p* Value**
Redislocation rate (%)	7/42 (16.7%)	7/35 (20%)	NS
Kujala score (mean [SD])	84.6 (17.5)	78.1 (15.9)	0.07
Patellar instability score (median [range])	10 (6–10)	6 (4–6)	0.01
	KOOS score (mean [SD])		
Symptoms	80.9 (17.4)	80.2 (15.9)	NS
Pain	95.5 (6.9)	92.3 (7.9)	NS
Activities of daily living	94.7 (10.3)	91.1 (9.8)	NS
Sports and recreation	87.2 (11.1)	83.6 (11.4)	NS
Quality of life	90.4 (8.9)	87.7 (9.7)	NS

NS, not significant.

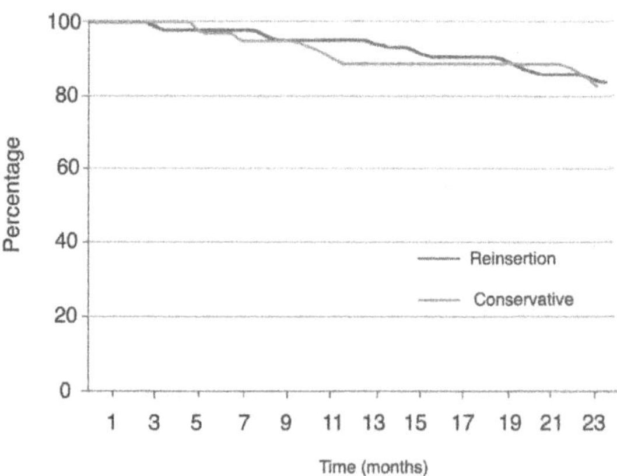

Figure 39.2. Kaplan-Maier survival curve of patients without redislocation during 2 years of F/U.

Criticisms and Limitations: This study excluded all patients with previous history or known trochlear dysplasia; thus, its inferences can only be speculatively applied to a high-risk subgroup.

Due to the infrastructure of the institution where the study was conducted, there was an inevitable delay to surgery (from days to months), and time to repair was not analyzed to observe for more favorable outcomes. The actual redislocation rate in the conservative treatment group was lower than the expected rate, making it more difficult to show a significant difference between both groups.

Other Relevant Studies and Information:

- Other comparable case studies containing a smaller number of patients may overestimate the success rates of MPFL repair, reporting excellent PROMs and redislocation rates.[4,5]
- 1 randomized controlled trial found results in accordance with the findings of this study; however, it cannot be compared directly as a different surgical procedure and technique were used.[6]
- Based on reviewing 70 publications by Krebs et al.[7] looking at study design, mean F/U, subjective and validated outcome measures, redislocation rates, and long-term symptoms, initial nonoperative management of a first-time traumatic patellar dislocation was recommended. However, there were exceptions in the presence of an osteochondral fracture, substantial disruption of the medial patellar stabilizers, a laterally subluxated patella with normal alignment of the contralateral knee, or a second dislocation and in patients not improving with appropriate rehabilitation.

Summary and Implications: For patients who present with a first-time patella dislocation, delayed isolated primary MPFL surgical repair using an anchor (to the adductor tubercle without repairing the VMO or adductor magnus tendon) does not reduce the risk of redislocation or provide significantly better subjective functional outcome scores. Only the specific subjective "patella stability score" was improved by MPFL repair compared with conservative treatment.

CLINICAL CASE: MPFL: SHOULD ISOLATED REPAIR BE UNDERTAKEN?

Case History

A 25-year-old female presents with a first-time dislocation of her patella following a fall during a netball match. She felt a pop at the front of her knee and has been unable to return to her physical activity due to episodes of instability. She is otherwise fit and well, without any previous history of patella instability, knee pain, or hypermobility. Her Beighton score is 2, she has a positive patellar apprehension test and is complaining of pinpoint tenderness over the medial facet. Magnetic resonance imaging scan confirms a complete rupture of the MPFL. Based on the results of this MPFL study, how should this patient be managed?

Suggested Answer

Christiansen et al.[1] conducted a prospective randomized study to demonstrate that delayed isolated repair of the MPFL makes no significant difference to patient outcomes (both KOOS and the overall Kujala scores) or redislocation rate. Only the patellar instability questionnaire of the Kujala score was significantly higher in the operative group. This patient fits the inclusion demographics of the MPFL study. Based on the findings of that study, this patient should not be offered delayed isolated MPFL reconstruction as management of her first-time patella dislocation but may be reserved for failed nonoperative intervention (i.e., rehabilitation with physical therapy and bracing) and recurrent redislocations.

References

1. Christiansen et al. Isolated repair of the medial patellofemoral ligament in primary dislocation of the patella: a prospective randomized study. Arthroscopy. 2008;24(8):881–7.
2. Kujala et al. Scoring of patellofemoral disorders. Arthroscopy. 1993;9(2):159–63.
3. Roos et al. The Knee injury and Osteoarthritis Outcome Score (KOOS): from joint injury to osteoarthritis. Health Qual Life Outcomes. 2003;1:64.
4. Ahmad et al. Immediate surgical repair of the medial patellar stabilisers for acute patellar dislocation. A review of eight cases. Am J Sports Med. 2000;28:804–10.
5. Sallay et al. Acute dislocation of the patella. A correlative pathoanatomic study. Am J Sports Med. 1998;24:52–60.
6. Nikku et al. Operative treatment of primary patellar dislocation does not improve medium-term outcome: a 7-year follow-up report and risk analysis of 127 randomized patients. Acta Orthop. 2005;76(5):699–704.
7. Krebs et al. The medial patellofemoral ligament: review of the literature. J Orthop. 2018;15(2):596–9.

40

A Meta-Analysis of Ankle Arthrodesis versus Replacement

LYDIA MILNES, KAPIL SUGAND, AND PALANISAMY RAMESH

> To our knowledge, this is the first systematic review of the intermediate and long-term outcomes of total ankle arthroplasty and ankle arthrodesis. Baseline differences in the patient populations and the small number of studies contributing to each analysis do not permit formal comparison between the two surgical procedures. However, the intermediate and long-term outcomes analyzed in this review do suggest that total ankle arthroplasty is comparable with ankle arthrodesis.
>
> —HADDAD ET AL.[1]

Citation: Haddad SL, Coetzee JC, Estok R, Fahrbach K, Banel D, Nalysnyk L. Intermediate and long-term outcomes of total ankle arthroplasty and ankle arthrodesis. J Bone Joint Surg Am. 2007;89:1899–905.

Research Question: How do the outcomes of total ankle arthroplasty (TAA) and arthrodesis compare?

Funding: DePuy funded this project

Year Study Began: 2005

Year Study Published: 2007

Study Location: USA (Glenview, Illinois, and Medford, Massachusetts)

Who Was Studied: The published literature was searched to include studies reporting on outcomes of TAA and ankle fusion; 49 studies were included.

Who Was Excluded: Any study with < 2-year follow-up (F/U) or with < 10 patients in the treatment arm were excluded.

How Many Patients: 2114

Study Overview: See Figure 40.1.

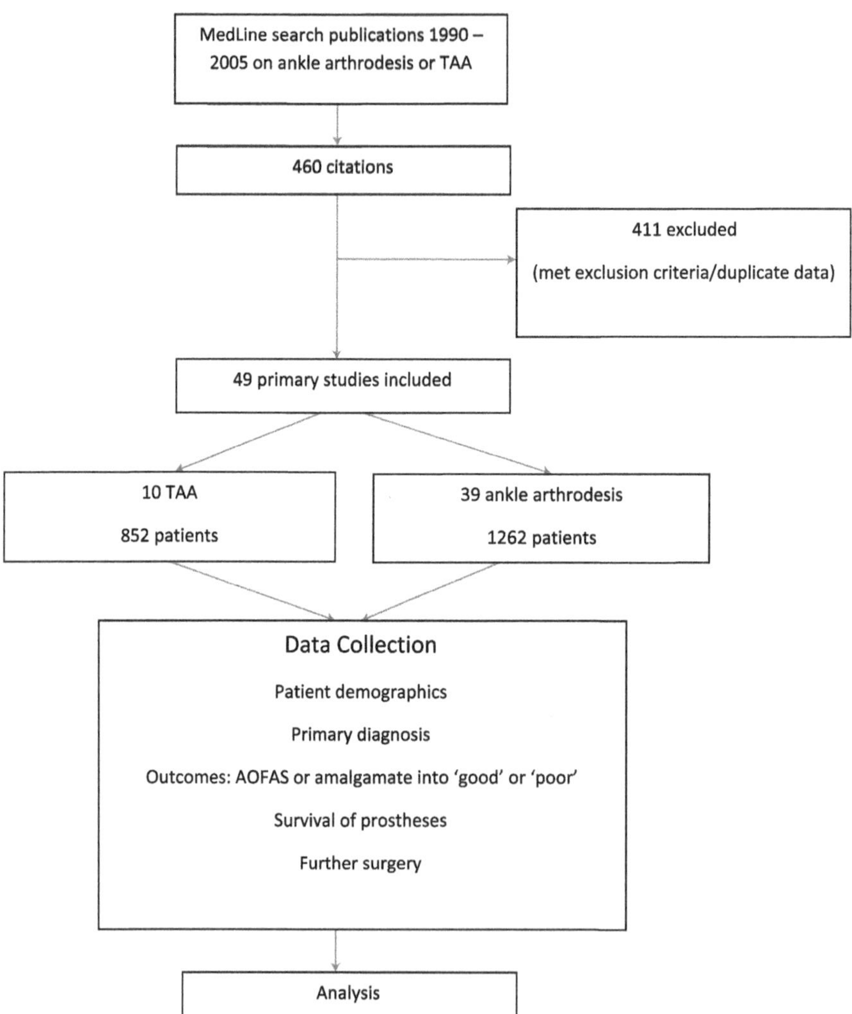

Figure 40.1. Overview of the study design.

Follow-Up: Approximately 5 years

Endpoints: American Orthopaedic Foot and Ankle Society (AOFAS) Ankle-Hindfoot Scale[2] (for function, alignment, pain, and range of motion [ROM]), which was mostly used for TAA evaluation; Mazur score[3] (most commonly used for arthrodesis); Kofoed scores[4] (for pain and function); ROM (overall and plantar/dorsiflexion); revision; conversion to arthrodesis; implant survival; and quality of life.

RESULTS (TABLES 40.1 AND 40.2)

- *TAA studies:* All 10 studies ($N = 852$) focused on second-generation implants.
- *F/U*: F/U ranged from 2 to 9 years in the studies of TAA and from 2 to 23 years in the studies of arthrodesis, but the average was circa 5 years.
- *Demographics:*
  - *Age (mean [range]):* Mean overall age was 53 (18–64) years. The patients treated with TAA were older at 58 (46–64) years compared to 50 (18–63) years in the arthrodesis group.
  - *Gender:* The TAA group consisted predominantly of females (59%), whereas the arthrodesis group consisted predominantly of males (52%).
- *Primary indication for surgery:* The primary indication was rheumatoid arthritis for TAA (39%) vs. posttraumatic arthritis for arthrodesis (57%).
- *Nonunion:* Arthrodesis had an overall 10% (95% CI: 7.4–12.1) nonunion rate.
- *Comparison studies:* No studies met the inclusion criteria directly comparing arthroplasty and arthrodesis.
- *Implant survival rates:* 5- and 10-year implant survival rates for TAA were 78% (95% CI: 69.0–87.6) and 77% (95% CI: 63.3–90.8) respectively.
- *Revision:*
  - *TAA*: The most common reason (28%) was loosening and/or subsidence.
  - *Arthrodesis:* 9% (95% CI: 5.5–11.6) underwent revision, primarily because of nonunion (the indication for 65% of all revisions of arthrodeses).

- *Conversion:* 5% (95% CI: 2.0–7.8) of TAA were converted to arthrodeses, with the main reason for conversion being loosening and/or subsidence (50% of all conversions).

Table 40.1 Meta-Analysis Mean Scores

		Meta-Analysis Mean (95% CI; %)	
		Arthroplasty	**Fusion**
AOFAS score (mean)		78.2 (71.9–84.5)[a]	75.6 (71.6–79.6)
Outcomes	*Excellent*	38 (0–96.8)[a]	30.7 (19.8–41.5)[a]
	Good	30.5 (21.0–39.9)	36.9 (26.4-47.3)[a]
	Fair	5.5 (0–16.9)[b]	13.3 (6.2–20.3)[a]
	Poor	24 (0–72.9)[a]	13.2 (7.6–18.7)[a]
Overall outcomes—binary	*Good (excellent and good)*	78.4 (61.9–95.0)[a]	72.6 (61.2–84.1)[a]
	Poor (fair and poor)	21.8 (4.9–38.6)[a]	27.4 (16.0–38.8)[a]
ROM	Plantarflexion	12.8° (5.1°–20.5°)[a]	16.8° (10.9°–22.7°)[b]
	Dorsiflexion	9.9° (5.6°–14.2°)[a]	0.1° (−7.9°–8.2°)[a]

[a] Significant heterogeneity ($p < 0.01$).
[b] Significant heterogeneity ($p < 0.10$).

Table 40.2 Mean Scores

		Mean (Points/°/%)		**Meta-Analysis Mean (95% CI)**	
		TAA	**Fusion**	**TAA**	**Fusion**
AOFAS Ankle-Hindfoot Scale score	*Total*	80.6	75.15	78.2 (71.9–84.5)[a]	75.6 (71.6–79.6)
	Pain	34.5			
	Function	37.4			
	Alignment	9.4			
Kofoed score	*Pain*	50.0	32.5		
	Function	21.0	15.7		
Mazur score			73.0		

Table 40.2 CONTINUED

		Mean (Points/°/%)		Meta-Analysis Mean (95% CI)	
		TAA	Fusion	TAA	Fusion
ROM	Overall	26.75°			
	Plantar flexion	15.23°	16.5°	12.8° (5.1°–20.5°)[a]	16.8° (10.9°–22.7°)[b]
	Dorsi flexion	11.25°	0.8°	9.9° (5.6°–14.2°)[a]	0.1° (−7.9°–8.2°)[a]
Revision surgery		7%	9%		
Required below-knee amputation		1%	5%		

[a] Significant heterogeneity ($p < 0.01$).
[b] Significant heterogeneity ($p < 0.1$).

Criticisms and Limitations: Direct comparative meta-analysis of arthroplasty vs. arthrodesis was not possible because there were no head-to-head trials. Three nonrandomized controlled trials of ankle arthrodesis compared different surgical techniques for arthrodesis. Only a pooled meta-analysis across all studies was conducted, with many studies being devoid of key data elements, including methodology reporting and baseline patient information, as well as variability of outcome reporting. Differences in patient populations, variability of surgical procedures, and differences in outcome valuation tools and F/U times may all be partially responsible for heterogeneity among these studies. Finally, sample sizes in many of the studies were small, patient characteristics were minimally described, and significant heterogeneity was detected in almost all of these meta-analyses.

Other Relevant Studies and Information:

- In 12 250 arthrodeses and 3002 TAA cases from the years 2002–2011, TAA was independently associated with a lower risk of blood transfusion, nonhome discharge, and overall complication. TAA was also independently associated with a higher hospitalization charge, but length of stay was similar between both groups. This study by Jiang et al.[5] showed no significant difference in risk for the majority of medical perioperative complications.
- Although a theoretical advantage of arthroplasty is improved ROM and subsequently gait, this has not been proved to be the case in postoperative gait analysis by Flavin et al.[6]

- A meta-analysis of 10 comparative studies reviewed by a South Korean team[7] indicated no significant differences between both procedures with respect to scores (AOFAS, SF-36, visual analog scale for pain, and patient satisfaction rate). The risk of reoperation and major surgical complications was significantly increased in the TAA group, but both operations could achieve similar clinical outcomes.
- Early results from a nonrandomized direct comparison by the Scandinavian Total Ankle Replacement (STAR) study[8] of the 2 interventions at 24 months have shown some improved function in the arthroplasty group.
- The British Orthopaedic Foot and Ankle Society (BOFAS)[9] and Finnish Registry[10] recommend that surgeons pool their resources or operate jointly where practical and that low volumes should be centralized to counteract the high number of technical errors in primary TAA.
- The BOFAS and Getting It Right First Time (GIRFT)[11] have commented that evidence is accumulating that patients with more severe polyarthropathy, often with deformity, gain more from TAA than from fusion (as long as bony and soft tissue deformities are managed to result in a functionally balanced foot). However, TAA requires F/U as per recommendations.

Summary and Implications: This meta-analysis involving studies of patients undergoing ankle arthrodesis and ankle replacement procedures found no significant differences in outcomes between both procedures. There is a paucity of methodologically rigorous data, however, and now that implant design has evolved, there is need for a powered randomized controlled trial to better assess which of these procedures leads to better surgical outcomes, and for which patients in particular.

CLINICAL CASE: ARTHROPLASTY VERSUS FUSION FOR ANKLE ARTHRITIS

Case History

A 55-year-old man who suffered an ankle fracture in his 30s has developed severe pain and stiffness gradually over the last few years. Standing radiographs reveal posttraumatic ankle joint osteoarthritis without significant deformity and with preservation of the subtalar joint. He is otherwise fit and well without a history of alcohol excess or smoking. He is relying on oral and topical analgesia on a daily basis, complains of nighttime pain, and has a reduced walking tolerance due to pain on full weight bearing. What management options should be offered to him according to the results of this meta-analysis?

Suggested Answer

This review did not show any clear advantage of one surgical option over the other; thus, both techniques would be reasonable choices. The patient needs to be counseled and consented for risks and outcomes of both procedures. Arthrodesis carries a 10% risk of nonunion, whereas TAA carries a risk of loosening/subsidence, which may require revision surgery. There are longer F/U studies on arthrodesis with subjects who are predominantly male and younger than the TAA subjects. Furthermore, TAA has been traditionally reserved for older and lower-demand patients with a good 5- and 10-year implant survival, which may improve with evolving generations of implant types.

References

1. Haddad et al. Intermediate and long-term outcomes of total ankle arthroplasty and ankle arthrodesis. J Bone Joint Surg Am. 2007;89:1899–905.
2. Ibrahim et al. Reliability and validity of the subjective component of the American Orthopaedic Foot and Ankle Society clinical rating scales. J Foot Ankle Surg. 2007;46(2):65–74.
3. Kaikkonen et al. A performance test protocol and scoring scale for the evaluation of ankle injuries. Am J Sports Med. 1994;22(4):462–9.
4. Kofoed. Cylindrical cemented ankle arthroplasty: a prospective series with long-term follow-up. Foot Ankle Int. 1995;16(8):474–9.
5. Jiang et al. Comparison of perioperative complications and hospitalization outcomes after ankle arthroplasty versus total ankle arthroplasty from 2002 to 2011. Foot Ankle Int. 2015;36(4):360–8.
6. Flavin et al. Comparison of gait after total ankle arthroplasty and ankle arthrodesis. Foot Ankle Int. 2013;34(10):1340–8.
7. Kim et al. Total ankle arthroplasty versus ankle arthrodesis for the treatment of end-stage arthritis: a meta-analysis of comparative studies. Int Orthop. 2017;41(1):101–9.
8. Saltzman et al. Prospective controlled trial of STAR total ankle replacement versus ankle fusion: initial results. Foot Ankle Int. 2009;30(70):579–96.
9. British Orthopaedic Foot and Ankle Society (BOFAS). BOFAS position statement on total ankle replacement. 2019. www.bofas.org.uk/Portals/0/Position%20Statements/BOFAS%20Statement%20on%20TAR%20.pdf?ver=8V10WJHt8JFkvV0bwSPaAw%3d%3d

10. British Orthopaedic Foot and Ankle Society (BOFAS). BOFAS GIRFT TAR document. 2020. www.bofas.org.uk/Portals/0/Position%20Statements/GIRFT%20Final%202020.pdf?ver=xjeqqoaXN24ekwGYXh8RkQ%3d%3d
11. Skyttä et al. Total ankle replacement: a population-based study of 515 cases from the Finnish Arthroplasty Register. Acta Orthop. 2010;81(1):114–8.

41

Long-Term Outcomes of Reverse Total Shoulder Arthroplasty

QUEN O. TANG, KAPIL SUGAND, AND DAOUD MAKKI

> We found that RTSA remained an effective therapeutic option with long-term implant survival rates (93% at 10 years) similar to those (previously) described. . . . Functional outcomes may be impacted by both the etiology of the shoulder dysfunction and time since implantation.
>
> —BACLE ET AL.[1]

Citation: Bacle G, Nové-Josserand L, Garaud P, Walch G. Long-term outcomes of reverse total shoulder arthroplasty: a follow-up of a previous study. J Bone Joint Surg Am. 2017;99(6):454–61.

Research Question: What is the prosthetic survivorship, clinical outcome, radiological assessment, and complication rate following reverse total shoulder arthroplasty (RTSA) at a minimum of 10 years after the original procedure?[2]

Funding: The authors did not receive any outside funding or grants in support of their research; 2 of the authors received, in any 1 year, payments or other benefits in excess of $10,000 from a commercial entity (Tornier).

Year Study Began: 1995

Year Study Published: 2017

Study Location: Lyon, France

Who Was Studied: All adults who underwent an RTSA between May 1995 and June 2003 (in the original study by Wall et al.[2]) for (1) rotator cuff tear arthropathy, (2) a failed previous arthroplasty, (3) a massive rotator cuff tear without osteoarthritis (OA), (4) posttraumatic glenohumeral OA with rotator cuff compromise, or (5) primary OA with rotator cuff compromise, with or without severe glenoid bone erosion.

Who Was Excluded: Patients who underwent RTSA following tumor resection, acute fracture, and rheumatoid arthritis were excluded from clinical and radiological evaluation but included in survivorship analysis.

How Many Patients: 240 prostheses in 232 patients

Study Overview: See Figure 41.1.

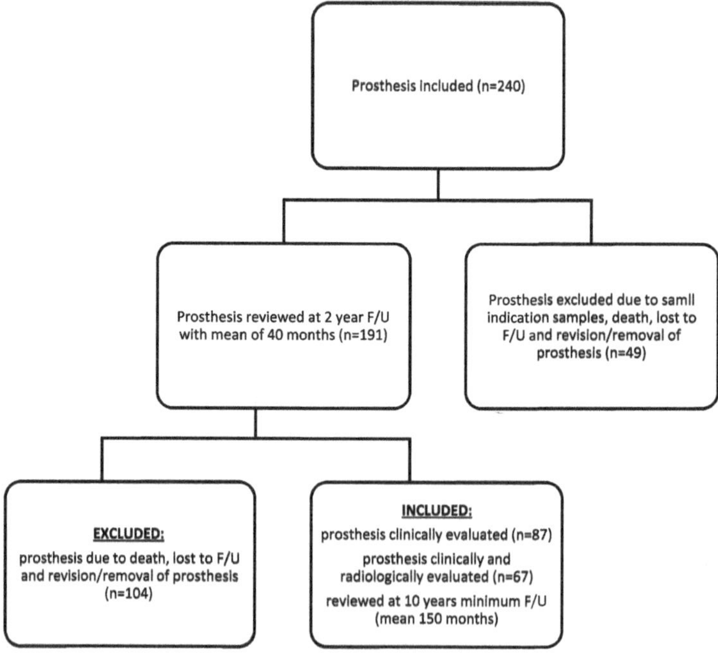

Figure 41.1. Summary of patient disposition and F/U.

Study Intervention: Data was collected retrospectively. The data consisted of clinical outcome, radiological assessment, complication rate, and implant survival. The original analysis[2] presented the data with at least 2-year follow-up (F/U; mean 39.9 months). The current study[1] presents data on the same cohort of patients with at least 10-year F/U (mean 150 months, range 121–241 months). Patients were grouped according to surgical indications, all of which involved a deficient rotator cuff: (1) rotator cuff tear arthropathy, (2) a failed previous arthroplasty (i.e., RTSA was a revision arthroplasty), (3) a massive rotator cuff tear without OA, (4) posttraumatic glenohumeral OA with rotator cuff compromise, or (5) primary OA with rotator cuff compromise and with or without severe glenoid bone erosion. Grammont-design prostheses were implanted through a deltopectoral approach, including 164 Delta-III (DePuy, Saint-Priest, France) and 27 Aequalis (Tornier) systems. Six shoulders required a custom glenoid implant due to bone loss. Only 1 humeral stem was uncemented. Postoperative complications were classified as early if they occurred within the first 2 years postoperatively and as delayed when they occurred after that.

Follow-Up: Minimum of 10 years with a mean of 150 months (range 121–241 months)

Endpoints: Clinical outcome was based on absolute and relative Constant scores[3] (scoring system defining the level of pain and the ability to carry out the normal activities of daily living [ADLs] to determine the functionality after the treatment of a shoulder injury; the test is divided into pain, ADLs, strength and range of motion [ROM], and active shoulder ROM). Radiographs were assessed for scapular notching (Sirveaux classification[4]), humeral radiolucent lines (Sperling[5] system modified by Lévigne et al.[6]), and loosening of implants (as described by Melis et al.[7]). Postoperative complications were classified as early (< 2 years) or delayed (> 2 years). A Kaplan-Meier survival analysis was performed with revision for any reason as the endpoint. Log-rank (Mantel-cox) was used to determine prosthetic survival among etiologies. Wilcoxon signed-rank tests were used to compare clinical outcomes (significance set at $p < 0.05$).

RESULTS

- *Constant score:*
  - The overall mean absolute (55 ± 16) and relative (86 ± 26) scores at final F/U improved significantly compared to preoperative scores. However, there was a significant decrease in the absolute scores

between medium- and long-term F/U both overall and in every subgroup (Table 41.1).
- The primary results from the earlier study conducted by Wall et al.[2] indicated an improvement in Constant scores (final vs. initial) according to pathologies ($p < 0.001$).
  - Rotator cuff tear arthropathy, revision arthroplasty, massive rotator cuff tear, posttraumatic OA, primary OA, other pathologies, and all-patient analysis with a F/U period between 34 and 43 months had improvement in all domains:
    - Total (64%–200%), pain (100%–323%), activity and mobility (44%–198%), and strength (180%–575%)
  - Only the revision arthroplasty and massive rotator cuff groups had significant changes for mobility, strength, and mean active anterior elevation in this F/U study by Bacle et al.[1]
- *ROM:* The overall mean active anterior elevation was significantly improved compared to preoperatively at medium- and long-term F/U; however, it decreased significantly between medium- and long-term F/U.
- *Pathology:* Rotator cuff tear arthropathy and primary OA as primary indications for RTSA were associated with the highest overall absolute Constant score at long-term F/U. Failed previous arthroplasty and posttraumatic OA were associated with the lowest Constant scores.
- *Radiology:* Of the 67 shoulders radiologically assessed at final F/U, 73% had scapular notching, with 61% of these classed as Sirveaux stage 1 or 2 and 39% as stage 3 or 4. There was no significant difference in long-term Constant scores between patients without notching or with a lower stage (0, 1, or 2) and those with a higher stage (3 or 4) of notching.
- *Complications:* Overall complications were recorded in 29% of patients, with 10% occurring after 2 years. Of the 10 delayed complications, 70% were due to unipolar prosthetic aseptic loosening (4 glenoid and 3 humeral side). No cases of glenoid loosening were secondary to progression of scapular notching.
- *Implant survival:* 12% of the original patients underwent revision surgery (half before and half after 2 years). Overall mean implant survival was 110.3 months (95% CI: 103.9–116.7), with 93% survival at 10 years. There was no difference in survival according to indication for RTSA (Figure 41.2).

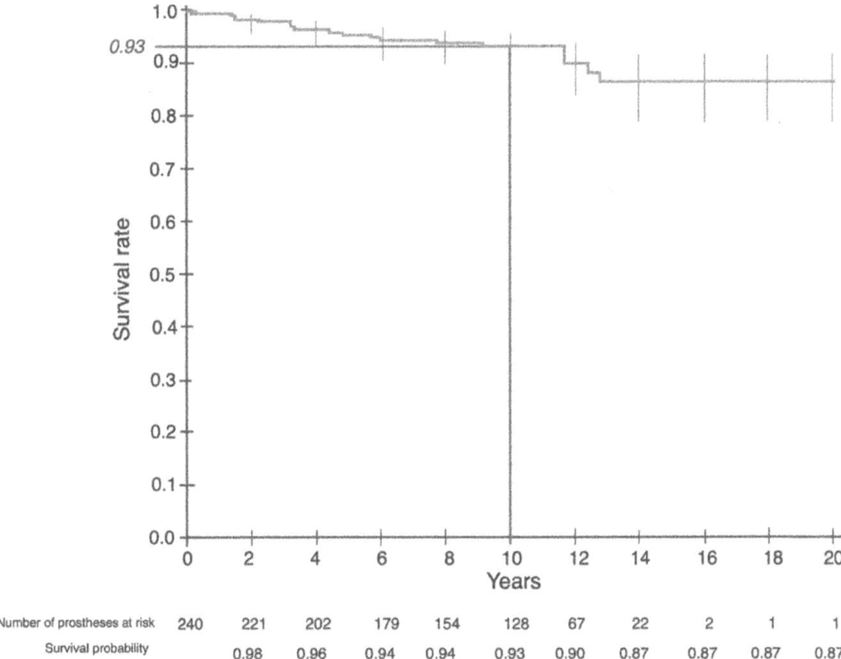

Figure 41.2. Kaplan-Meier survival curve, with 95% CI, with revision for any reason as the endpoint.

Table 41.1 SUMMARY OF KEY FINDINGS FROM THE STUDY BY BACLE ET AL.[1]

	Mean Constant Score and Standard Deviation		
	Absolute	**Relative**	**Mean Active Anterior Elevation and Standard Deviation (°)**
Preoperative	23 ± 12	33 ± 17	81 ± 43
Medium-term F/U	63 ± 14	90 ± 21	138 ± 26
Long-term F/U	55 ± 16	86 ± 26	131 ± 29
p value	< 0.001	0.025	< 0.001

Criticisms and Limitations: Although the current series presents the longest F/U for Grammont-style RTSAs, it is still a retrospective case series analysis (therapeutic level IV evidence) with 94 patients (50.5%) who died or were lost to F/U. The patient series also included a wide age range, making the results difficult to generalize to others. As these were retrospective studies, there was no possibility to directly compare between other treatments.

Other Relevant Studies and Information:

- A number of other studies assessing clinical outcome, radiological outcome, and implant survivorship of Grammont-style RTSAs have shown similar conclusions.[4,7–9]
- The finding of deterioration of functional outcome in patients who underwent a RTSA aged < 76 years is consistent with others[8,9] who recommended caution in the use of this prosthesis in younger patients.
- The British Elbow and Shoulder Society[10] recommend that RTSA should address OA on both the humeral and glenoid sides of the joint and be reserved for patients with cuff tear arthropathy or older patients with a torn or insufficient cuff.

Summary and Implications: This study found an overall 93% 10-year survivorship among patients undergoing a Grammont-style RTSA for indications relating to cuff deficiency. RTSA performed for rotator cuff tear arthropathy and primary OA appear to have better functional outcomes at 10 years compared to other indications.

CLINICAL CASE: A COMMON ASYMPTOMATIC RADIOLOGICAL SIGN IN RTSA

Case History

A 70-year-old female who is 4 years following a RTSA for posttraumatic OA was referred to your elective shoulder clinic as her family physician was concerned by the radiograph report. The patient complained of self-remitting pain following a fall but is no longer taking analgesia. Her radiograph shows scapular notching that has progressed slightly since her radiograph 2 years prior. Both the family physician and the patient are concerned regarding the degree of scapular notching. The patient asks whether this will affect her long-term clinical outcome. She would like to know how long her shoulder replacement should last for. Based on this current study, how should you advise this patient?

Suggested Answer

Scapular notching is a common radiographic finding following RTSA. The clinical importance of notching remains unclear, but certainly in the current study there appears to be no correlation between clinical functional outcome scores with notching of any severity at 10 years. Contrary to some earlier series that reported short-term complications of the glenoid component, the current study did not reveal such issues long term. In fact, it suggested that once the short-term complication period of 2 years had passed, the glenoid component is stable despite highly advanced scapular notching. The patient therefore should be reassured. She should also be informed that her prosthesis is expected to last at least 10 years (93% of the time), which has also been demonstrated in several other studies. The surgeon, however, should be cognizant that although the patient's long-term clinical outcome score is expected to improve, it will be comparatively less than those who had rotator cuff tear arthropathy and primary OA as indications for RTSA.

References

1. Bacle et al. Long-term outcomes of reverse total shoulder arthroplasty: a follow-up of a previous study. J Bone Joint Surg Am. 2017;99(6):454–61.
2. Wall et al. Reverse total shoulder arthroplasty: a review of results according to etiology. J Bone Joint Surg Am. 2007;89(7):1476–85.
3. Conboy et al. An evaluation of the Constant-Murley shoulder assessment. J Bone Joint Surg. 1996;78-B:229–32.
4. Sirveaux et al. Grammont inverted total shoulder arthroplasty in the treatment of glenohumeral osteoarthritis with massive rupture of the cuff. Results of a multicentre study of 80 shoulders. J Bone Joint Surg Br. 2004;86(3):388–95.
5. Sperling et al. Radiographic assessment of ingrowth total shoulder arthroplasty. J Shoulder Elbow Surg. 2000;9(6):507–13.
6. Lévigne et al. Scapular notching in reverse shoulder arthroplasty. J Shoulder Elbow Surg. 2008;17(6):925–35.
7. Melis et al. An evaluation of the radiological changes around the Grammont reverse geometry shoulder arthroplasty after eight to 12 years. J Bone Joint Surg Br. 2011;93(9):1240–6.
8. Guery et al. Reverse total shoulder arthroplasty. Survivorship analysis of eighty replacements followed for five to ten years. J Bone Joint Surg Am. 2006;88(8):1742–7.
9. Favard et al. Reverse prostheses in arthropathies with cuff tear: are survivorship and function maintained over time? Clin Orthop Relat Res. 2011;469(9):2469–75.
10. Thomas M et al. British Elbow and Shoulder Society (BESS). BESS/BOA Patient Care Pathways. Glenohumeral osteoarthritis. Shoulder Elbow. 2016;8(3):203–14.

42

Intramedullary Nailing or Percutaneous Plating in Fixing Distal Metaphyseal Fractures of the Tibia

REBECCA EMILY BEAMISH AND MATTHEW BARRY

> We conclude that both closed intramedullary nailing and percutaneous locked compression plate can be used to treat . . . type 43A distal metaphyseal fractures of the tibia. However, . . . nailing has the advantage of a shorter operating and radiation time and easier [implant] removal.
>
> —GUO ET AL.[1]

Citation: Guo JJ, Tang N, Yang HL, Tang TS. A prospective, randomized trial comparing percutaneous plating in the treatment of distal metaphyseal fractures of the tibia. J Bone Joint Surg Br. 2010;92-B:984–8.

Research Question: Do patients with distal metaphyseal tibial fractures recover better after closed intramedullary nailing (IMN) than after percutaneous locked compression plating (LCP), and what are the differences between both techniques with respect to operating time, imaging duration, wound complication rate, time to union, and mobility after 1-year follow-up (F/U)?

Funding: None stated

Year Study Began: 2005

Year Study Published: 2010

Study Location: First Affiliated Hospital of Soochow University, China

Who Was Studied: Patients with distal metaphyseal tibial fractures with the presence of a distal fragment at least 3 cm in length without incongruity of the articular surface corresponding to Orthopaedic Trauma Association type 43A fracture.

Who Was Excluded: Patients with open fractures (i.e., Gustilo and Anderson classification II or III), any cases where the fibula fracture was fixed, pathological fractures, nonosteoporotic osteopathies such as endocrine disorders and medical comorbidities (i.e., rheumatological disorders, diabetes mellitus, renal disease, and immunodeficiency states), and mental impairment or difficulty with communication.

How Many Patients: 111

Study Overview: See Figure 42.1.

Study Intervention: Distal metaphyseal (extra-articular) tibial fractures were managed either with closed IMN (S2 nailing system from Stryker, Duisburg, Germany) or with percutaneous locking compression plate (LCP, Synthes, Oberdorf, Switzerland) using a minimally invasive plate osteosynthesis (MIPO) technique. All operations were performed in a single center by the same group of senior surgeons. Postoperative care was the same with all patients immobilized in a below-knee cast for 3 weeks followed by range of motion exercises. Partial weightbearing was allowed once signs of radiographic union were seen.

Follow-Up: Clinical and radiographic F/U points were at 6-week intervals until bony union was achieved. Thereafter patients were reviewed at 3 and 6 months, and final F/U was at 12 months postoperatively.

Endpoints:

- *Intraoperatively*: Total radiation and operative times
- *Postoperatively*:
  - *Early*
    - Delayed wound healing
    - Infection
  - *Intermediate*
    - Time to union
    - Complications

- *Late*
  - Assessment of ankle function at 12 months utilizing the American Orthopaedic Foot and Ankle Society (AOFAS) scoring system[2] (standardized evaluation of the clinical status of the foot and ankle containing both subjective [patients' pain] and objective [alignment and functional] components)
  - A questionnaire concerning patient's wishes on implant removal

RESULTS (TABLES 42.1 AND 42.2)

- *Number of patients:* Out of the original 111 patients who were randomized for the study, 44 (39.6%) in the IMN group and 41 (36.9%) in the LCP group were reviewed at the 1-year F/U. Hence, 26 (30.5%) patients who had not reached the 1-year mark postoperatively were excluded from the final analysis as seen in Figure 42.1

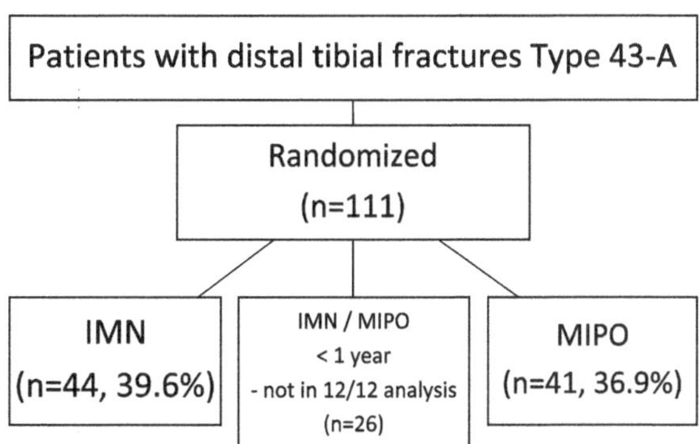

Figure 42.1. Summary of trial design.

- *Intraoperative outcomes*: The mean radiation and operating times were significantly lower in the IMN than in the LCP group.
- *Clinical and patient-reported outcome measures:* The IMN group had more pain but better function, alignment, and total AOFAS scores, although these differences were insignificant.
- *Implant removal:* 84.1% of the IMN group and 92.7% of the LCP group expressed a wish to have the implant removed, but only 47 (55.3%) had metalwork removed (23 in the IMN and 24 in the LCP group). There were no problems with removal of the nails but some difficulty with removing plates and screws in 9 (37.5%) patients.

Table 42.1 Summary of Main Study Outcomes with Final Scores at 1 Year Postoperatively

Outcome	IMN	MIPO	*p* Value
Mean radiation time (min)	2.12	3.0	< 0.001
Mean operating time (min)	81.2	97.9	< 0.001
Mean time to union (wk)	17.66	17.59	NS
Patients with wound problems (%)	6.8	14.6	
Mean total AOFAS score at 1 year	86.1	83.9	
Pain	325	31.5	
Function	44.3	43.2	
Alignment	9.3	9.3	

The 2 outcomes with significant differences were mean radiation and mean operating times (min), with lower times for IMN.

Table 42.2 Metalwork Removal Outcomes within the Study

Outcome	IMN	MIPO
Patient wishing to have metalwork removal (%)	84.9	92.7
Patients who had metalwork removed (%)	55.3	56.1
Difficulty of metalwork removal	None	9 patients with some difficulty—due to stripping of screw heads

The mean time for removal was 15.5 months (range 12–23 months).

Criticisms and Limitations: Six (75%) outcomes were insignificant, possibly due to type II error. There were wide exclusion criteria based on medical grounds such as pathological fractures, non-osteoporotic osteopathies from endocrine disorders, rheumatologic disorders, diabetes mellitus, renal disease, and immunodeficiency states, mental impairment, or difficulty in communication. In addition, 23.4% of patients were not included in the final analysis because they had not reached 1-year postoperative F/U by the time of the study. A consequence of the MIPO-LCP method was that the operation was delayed for up to 10 days if the leg was considerably swollen and bruised, although delayed operations appeared to have no influence on the final results. The majority of patients (84%–93%) wishing to have metalwork removed were reported; however, just over half of patients in both groups had metalwork removed. Along with pain and prominence, other reasons cited for metalwork removal were insurance and compensation related, which may be less applicable in other populations.

Other Relevant Studies and Information:

- Since this study was published in 2010, other studies[3–5] have been published with similar results and clinical outcomes. However, an earlier study[6] and subsequent meta-analysis[7] both reported plating to be associated with improved mechanical alignment, although not all of these studies used a locking plate, and F/U was too short in the majority to determine if this was clinically important.
- In 2017 the UK FixDT randomized clinical trial[8] was published, which also compared IMN and locking plate fixation. They had a larger population sample (i.e., 321 patients were randomized and 223 [69.5%] completed the study). There were no significant differences in outcome scores at early F/U time points, disability score at 3 months, and the Olerud-Molander Ankle Score at 3 and 6 months were all in favor of IMN.

Summary and Implications: The study suggested that IMN or MIPO can be used safely to manage distal tibial fractures, but IMN has the advantage of lower mean amount of radiation and operative times ($p < 0.001$). While there was no difference in alignment, this is at odds with other studies that found plating to be superior in that respect.[6,7] In terms of outcome scores, a trend was found in favor of IMN at 1 year, while the FixDT trial[8] found significant differences at 3 and 6 months, suggesting a possible type II error in the study by Guo et al.[1] (i.e., it may have been insufficiently powered with inadequate patient numbers to show this difference).

CLINICAL CASE: CLOSED INTRAMEDULLARY NAILING VERSUS PERCUTANEOUS PLATING IN DISTAL TIBIAL FRACTURE FIXATION

Case History

A 35-year-old male sustains an isolated, closed, neurovascularly intact, extra-articular (type 43A) distal tibial fracture after a hit and run. He is brought into the resus bay as a trauma call. There is minimal swelling and no sign of compartment syndrome. The patient is otherwise fit and well with no medical problems or regular medications. He is an ex-smoker with a 5-pack-year history. The patient is a self-employed manual laborer and is keen to return to work as soon as possible. He understands that he will need an operation to fix the fracture but is asking about operative options and risks of the procedure. How should this patient be managed based on the results of this study?

Suggested Answer

The study by Guo et al.[1] suggested that in a fit and well patient with a closed extra-articular distal tibial fracture, IMN fixation is recommended over plating. Their cited benefits included shorter mean amount of radiation and operative times alongside a trend toward better pain and functional outcomes at 1-year F/U. Although the differences were not significant, there were fewer patients with delayed wound healing, requesting for removal of metalwork, and problems with removal of metalwork in the IMN group, further supporting the choice of nailing over plating. Conversely, other studies[6,7] have suggested better mechanical alignment with plate fixation, which needs to be taken into account, but especially so for younger, fit, and active patients.

References

1. Guo et al. A prospective, randomised trial comparing percutaneous plating in the treatment of distal metaphyseal fractures of the tibia. J Bone Joint Surg Br. 2010;92-B:984–8.
2. Ibrahim et al. Reliability and validity of the subjective component of the American Orthopaedic Foot and Ankle Society clinical rating scales. J Foot Ankle Surg. 2007;46(2):65–74.
3. Li et al. Treatment of distal tibial shaft fractures by three different surgical methods: a randomized, prospective study. Int Orthop. 2014;38(6):1261–7.
4. Mauffrey et al. A randomised pilot trial of "locking plate" fixation versus intramedullary nailing for extra-articular fractures of the distal tibia. J Bone Joint Surg Br. 2012;94(5):704–8.
5. Li et al. Comparison of low, multidirectional locked nailing and plating in the treatment of distal tibial metadiaphyseal fractures. Int Orthop. 2012;36(7):1457–62.
6. Im et al. Distal metaphyseal fractures of tibia: a prospective randomized trial of closed reduction and intramedullary nail versus open reduction and plate and screw fixation. J Trauma. 2005;59:1219–23.
7. Kwok et al. Plate versus nail for distal tibial fractures: a systematic review and meta-analysis. J Orthop Trauma. 2014;28(9):542–8.
8. Costa et al. FixDT Trial Investigators. Effect of locking plate fixation vs intramedullary nail fixation on 6-month disability among adults with displaced fracture of the distal tibia. The UK FixDT Randomized Clinical Trial. JAMA. 2017;318(18):1767–76.

43

Metal-on-Metal Hip Failure

Do Metal Ion Blood Levels Predict Failure?

DONALD DAVIDSON, KAPIL SUGAND, AND HANI B. ABDUL-JABAR

> Blood metal ions (cobalt and chromium) have good discriminant ability to separate failed from well-functioning (MoM) hip replacements. The MHRA cut-off level of 7 ppb provides a specific test but has poor sensitivity.
>
> —HART ET AL.[1]

Citation: Hart AJ, Sabah SA, Bandi AS, Maggiore P, Tarassoli P, Sampson B, Skinner J. Sensitivity and specificity of blood cobalt and chromium metal ions for predicting failure of metal-on-metal hip replacement. J Bone Joint Surg Br. 2011;93(10):1308–13.

Research Question: Can cobalt and chromium blood ion levels discriminate between well-functioning and failing hip replacements in patients with metal-on-metal (MoM) bearing surfaces?

Funding: BOA through an industry consortium of 9 manufacturers: DePuy, Zimmer, Smith and Nephew, Biomet, JRI, Finsbury, Corin, Mathys, and Stryker

Year Study Began: 2007

Year Study Published: 2011

Study Location: Royal National Orthopaedic Hospital, UK

Who Was Studied: Adult patients with unilateral large-diameter MoM bearing total hip arthroplasty (THA). Participants were divided into "cases" (i.e., patients awaiting revision surgery for unexplained failed MoM hips) and "controls" (patients who were satisfied with their THA and experienced no pain symptoms).

Who Was Excluded: Bilateral MoM hip replacements, < 12 months postoperatively, abnormal renal function (no participants), overt prosthetic joint infection or another cause for explained hip replacement failure, and if the primary indication for surgery was anything other than osteoarthritis (OA).

How Many Patients: 176

Study Overview: See Figure 43.1.

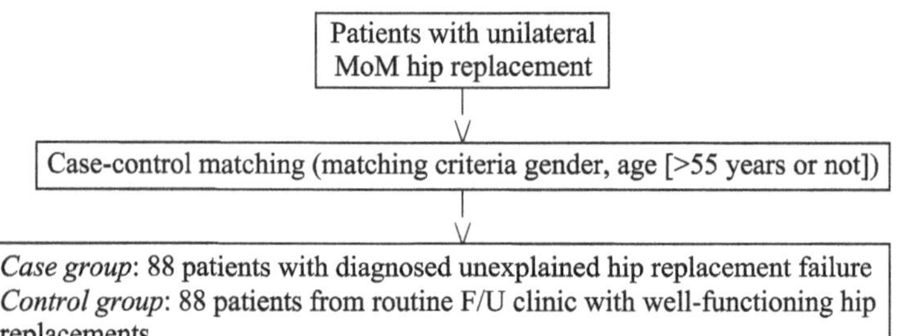

Figure 43.1. Study overview.

- *Case group*: 88 patients with diagnosed unexplained hip replacement failure
- *Control group*: 88 patients from routine follow-up clinic with well-functioning hip replacements

Study Intervention: All the patients in the pair-matched, case-control groups had their cobalt and chromium ion levels measured in a standardized manner; a blood sample was taken from an antecubital fossa vein using a 21-guage needle connected to a vacutainer system using trace element blood tubes containing sodium ethylenediaminetetraacetic acid (EDTA); the first 10 ml was used for inflammatory marker (C-reactive protein and erythrocyte sedimentation rate) measurement, and the second 10 ml was used for cobalt and chromium analysis. Cobalt and chromium measurements were made using dynamic reaction cell inductively coupled plasma mass spectrometry. The patients in the failed MoM hip group had their blood samples taken immediately prior to revision surgery.

Follow-Up: Patients were allocated based on the presence or absence of an unexplained failed MoM hip replacement. However, the final determination of "unexplained" failure was not made until after their revision surgery when the intraoperative findings and postoperative microbiological cultures were considered.

Endpoints: The main outcome was whether blood metal ion (cobalt and chromium) concentration could accurately predict failure of a unilateral MoM hip replacement and to determine the test characteristics (i.e., the ability to correctly identify failed and well-functioning hips). The authors also sought to determine the sensitivity and specificity of the 7 ppb whole blood concentration suggested by the Medicines and Healthcare products Regulatory Agency (MHRA; UK) as the upper limit of normal.

RESULTS (TABLE 43.1)

- *Blood metal ions:*
  - Patients with a failed MoM replacement had a median whole blood maximum cobalt or chromium concentration of 8.4 ppb compared to 2.4 ppb in the well-functioning group ($p < 0.001$).
  - *[Co]*: Patients with a failed MoM replacement had a median whole blood cobalt concentration of 6.9 ppb compared to 1.7 ppb in the well-functioning group ($p < 0.001$).
  - *[Cr]*: Patients with a failed MoM replacement had a median whole blood chromium concentration of 5 ppb compared to 2.3 ppb in the well-functioning group ($p < 0.001$).
- *Sensitivity:* At the MHRA cutoff of >7 ppb whole blood metal ion concentration, the sensitivity (the true-positive rate, i.e., the ability of a test to correctly identify patients with failed implants) was 49% for cobalt, 38% for chromium, and 52% for the maximum of cobalt or chromium.
- *Specificity:* At the MHRA cutoff of >7 ppb whole blood metal ion concentration, the specificity (the true-negative rate, i.e., the ability of a test to correctly identify patients who do not have a disease) was 90% for cobalt, 92% for chromium, and 89% for the maximum of cobalt or chromium.
- *Area under the curve (AUC)/receiver operating characteristic (ROC):* The AUC for the ROC curve (plotted sensitivity against [1-specificity]) describes the overall ability of the test to correctly predict diseased or healthy states: 1 is perfect prediction, 0.5 is as accurate as a coin toss,

and < 0.5 means the test is more likely to be incorrect than correct. The AUC for cobalt whole blood concentration was 0.74, for chromium was 0.69, and for the maximum of cobalt or chromium was 0.74.

- *Cutoff:* The optimum mathematical cutoff ion concentration (but potentially not the optimal clinical cutoff as this depends on the clinical purpose for the test) balancing maximal sensitivity and specificity based on the ROC was cobalt > 2.74 ppb (sensitivity 0.69 and specificity 0.87), chromium > 2.69 ppb (sensitivity 0.69 and specificity 0.68), and the maximum of cobalt or chromium > 4.97 ppb (sensitivity 0.63 and specificity 0.89).
- *Complications:* After surgery 54 patients (61%) were diagnosed with unexplained failure. Patient diagnosis was updated to explained failure due to aseptic loosening in 17 cases, prosthetic joint infection in 6, malalignment of components in 4, periprosthetic fracture in 4, and implant size mismatch in 3; when the explained failures were removed from the analysis, it made little difference to the results.

Table 43.1 Summary Diagnostic Test Characteristics (and CI) Using the MHRA 7 ppb Cutoff Value

Test	**Sensitivity (95% CI)**	**Specificity (95% CI)**
Cobalt > 7 ppb	0.49 (0.38–0.60)	0.90 (0.81–095)
Chromium > 7 ppb	0.38 (0.28–0.49)	0.92 (0.84–0.96)
Cobalt or chromium > 7 ppb	0.52 (0.41–0.63)	0.89 (0.80–0.94)

Criticisms and Limitations: This was a single-center study, and the findings may not be applicable to other settings or populations. The patients were matched on gender and poorly matched on age; other patient-specific or implant-specific factors were not considered. Several MoM hip bearing designs from different manufacturers were included and unevenly distributed between the cohorts.

Other Relevant Studies and Information:

- Prior to this study there was evidence that blood cobalt and chromium concentrations in patients with painful MoM hips were 2× than those with well-functioning MoM hips, although the ability to predict the implant failure rate based on the levels was unknown.[2]

- Other factors like implant positioning, female gender, and smaller head size have been demonstrated to increase metal ion concentration and MoM hip failure.[3,4]
- The identification of and ultimate decision to revise a failed MoM hip replacement is made after considering patient factors, radiological imaging, implant type and positioning, and blood metal ion levels. Blood metal ion levels do not solely predict outcome or oblige revision.[5–7]
- The MHRA surveillance protocol for the frequency of review appointments and the type of imaging assessment recommended for patients with MoM hip replacements differs depending on the device implanted (including implant design and size), patient sex, and whether the patient is symptomatic.[5] At each review, the MHRA recommends performing a functional assessment using the Oxford Hip Score (OHS), blood metal ion assessment, and an imaging assessment.[5] The MHRA recommends consideration of revision if imaging is abnormal and/or blood metal levels are rising and/or hip-related clinical function/OHS is deteriorating.[5]

Summary and Implications: Average blood metal (cobalt and chromium) ions are higher among patients with failed MoM hip replacements vs. those with well-functioning hips. The current metal ion concentration cutoff recommended by the MHRA for revision (≥ 7 ppb) demonstrates relatively low test sensitivity (~50%) but high specificity (~90%). In isolation, blood metal ion concentration is a poor screening test to determine if an MoM implant has failed; however, it may be an important adjunct with clinical and radiological assessment to guide management.

CLINICAL CASE: PAINFUL MOM HIP REPLACEMENT

Case History

A 55-year-old active man attends the clinic 5 years after his MoM bearing hip resurfacing. He was very happy with his hip; however, more recently he has started to develop groin pain, which negatively impacts on his activities. Plain radiographs of his hip at the appointment demonstrate the implants to be well positioned and no obvious worrying features. The whole blood metal ion concentration was determined to be 5 ppb for both chromium and cobalt, up from a level of 3 ppb and 2 ppb respectively the year before. Can the patient be reassured based on the whole blood metal ion concentrations?

Suggested Answer

This study demonstrated that blood metal ions are greater in patients with failing MoM hips than those with well-functioning MoM hips. However, blood metal ion levels alone are not sufficient to screen for the absence of a failing hip due to their relatively low sensitivity (i.e., the ability to detect true positives). Consequently, the patient cannot be reassured solely by blood concentrations being < 7 ppb. This patient has some concerning features, including worsening hip pain and function, as well as rising whole blood metal ion concentrations. As a result, and following the guidance from the MHRA, the patient requires cross-sectional imaging of his hip and ultimately consideration of the need for revision surgery if other causes of hip pain are excluded.

References

1. Hart et al. Sensitivity and specificity of blood cobalt and chromium metal ions for predicting failure of metal-on-metal hip replacement. J Bone Joint Surg Br. 2011;93(10):1308–13.
2. Hart et al. The painful metal-on-metal hip resurfacing. J Bone Joint Surg Br. 2009;91-B:738–44.
3. Langton et al. Early failure of metal-on-metal bearing in hip resurfacing and large-diameter total hip replacement: a consequence of excess wear. J Bone Joint Surg Br. 2010;92-B:38–46.
4. Langton et al. The effect of component size and orientation on the concentrations of metal ions after resurfacing arthroplasty of the hip. J Bone Joint Surg Br. 2008;90-B:1143–51.
5. MHRA Medical Device Alert, all metal-on-metal (MoM) hip replacements: updated advice for follow-up of patients, MDA/2017/018. June 29, 2017. www.assets.publishing.service.gov.uk/media/5954ca1ded915d0baa00009b/MDA-2017-018_Final.pdf
6. Kwon et al. Risk stratification algorithm for management of patients with metal-on-metal hip arthroplasty: consensus statement of the American Association of Hip and Knee Surgeons, the American Academy of Orthopaedic Surgeons, and the Hip Society. J Bone Joint Surg Am. 2014;96(1):e4.
7. Bolognesi et al. Metal-on-metal total hip arthroplasty: patient evaluation and treatment. J Am Acad Orthop Surg. 2015;23(12):724–31.

44

Dual Mobility and Large Femoral Head Diameter Are Implants for Safety in Total Hip Arthroplasty

AHMED MABROUK, BERNARD H. VAN DUREN, AND SAMEH A. SIDHOM

> The best implant of choice for short term that has lowest risk of revision and dislocation after total hip arthroplasty is dual mobility total hip arthroplasty (DMTHA) followed by big femoral head diameter total hip arthroplasty (BTHA). We recommend using dual mobility and big head as an implant for safety in total hip arthroplasty.
>
> —PITUCKANOTAI ET AL.[1]

Citation: Pituckanotai K, Arirachakaran A, Tuchinda H, Putananon C, Nualsalee N, Setrkraising K, Kongtharvonskul J. Risk of revision and dislocation in single, dual mobility and large femoral head total hip arthroplasty: systematic review and network meta-analysis. Eur J Orthop Surg Traumatol. 2018;28(3):445–55.

Research Question: Does the use of dual mobility and large femoral head diameter designs reduce the risk of postoperative dislocation and revision when compared to using conventional total hip arthroplasty (THA)?

Year Study Began: 2017

Year Study Published: 2017

Study Location: Thailand (but analysis included international studies)

Who Was Studied: Studies comparing postoperative dislocation and revision of dual mobility THA (DMTHA), big femoral head diameter THA (BTHA), constrained liner THA (CTHA), and standard THA (STHA) implants in THA (both primary and revision).

Who Was Excluded: Studies with insufficient data, case reports, abstracts, and review, and animal studies.

How Many Patients: 4084

Study Overview: See Figure 44.1.

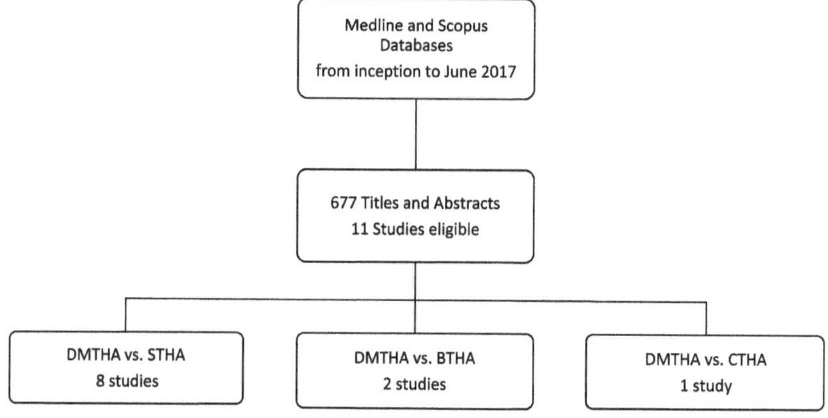

Figure 44.1. Flow chart showing an overview of the selection of the included study numbers and distribution.

Study Intervention: The PubMed/Medline and Scopus databases identified relevant studies based on titles and abstracts requiring the consensus of authors. In addition to the outcomes of interest (i.e., dislocation and revision rates), the number of subjects, continuous outcomes between groups and cross-tabulated frequencies between treatments, and all dichotomous outcomes were extracted. Two randomized controlled trials (RCTs) and 9 comparative studies met the inclusion criteria spanning over 6 nations, published between 2010 and 2017, and only 3 studies focused on revision surgery. A direct meta-analysis comparing the efficacy was made of all the treatment options (DMTHA [$n = 1068$; 26%],

BTHA [$n = 568$; 14%], CTHA [$n = 70$; 2%], STHA [$n = 2378$; 58%]). Relative risk (RR) of postoperative dislocation and revision of treatment comparisons was estimated and pooled for each study. A statistically significant Q-statistic or an $I^2 > 25\%$ was taken to indicate heterogeneity. A network meta-analysis assessed treatment effects between different implant options. The indirect comparisons between 2 implant options were performed by using information from common comparators; comparisons were weighted based on the number of subjects and number of studies included. A 2-stage meta-analysis was then applied to determine the relative effects of implant options.

Follow-Up: 0.5–11 years

Endpoints: Post-THA dislocation and revision as per original studies due to any reason (e.g., infection, fracture, dislocation, or aseptic loosening) or in any part (e.g., cup, stem, or insert).

RESULTS (TABLE 44.1)

- *Direct meta-analysis*: Compared to other treatment options, DMTHA may significantly lower the risk of dislocation by 75% (RR = 0.25; 95% CI: 0.12–0.51) and revision by 54% (RR = 0.46; 95% CI: 0.29–0.75) compared to STHA.
- *Network meta-analysis*: Treatment-ranking comparison between the different implants concluded that DMTHA had the lowest risk of revision and dislocation with a surface under the cumulative ranking curve of 80.8 and 80.2 respectively and a probability of being the best treatment of 46.5% and 46.7% respectively.
- *Dislocation analysis*: The number needed to treat (NNT) to prevent 1 STHA dislocation was 40 for DMTHA and 44 for BTHA. To prevent 1 STHA revision, the NNT was 34 for DMTHA and 27 for BTHA patients. For CTHA, there was an insignificantly higher risk with respect to revision and dislocation (when compared to DMTHA and BTHA).
- *Publication bias*: Based on a network funnel plot, no evidence of publication bias was reported.

Table 44.1 Table Overview of the Studies Included in the Meta-Analysis[1–11]

Study	Publication on Date	Study Location	Study Type		Implant Type & Numbers			F/U (y)	Primary/ Revision
				DMTHA	BTHA	CTHA	STHA		
Tarasevicius et al.	2010	Lithuania	Comparative	42	*	*	56	1	Primary
Bouchet et al.	2011	France	Comparative	105	*	*	108	—	Primary
Hernigou et al.	2016	France	Comparative	85	*	70	*	0.5	Primary
Haughom et al.	2016	USA	Comparative	24	365	*	*	—	Primary
Griffin et al.	2016	UK	RCT	9	10	*	*	2.5	Primary
Homma et al.	2016	Japan	Comparative	60	60	*	*	0.5	Primary
Jauregui et al.	2016	USA	Comparative	60	120	*	*	1	Revision
Chalmers et al.	2017	USA	Comparative	16	13	*	*	10	Revision
Catalli et al.	2017	Canada	RCT	12	*	*	12	11	Primary
Hernigou et al.	2017	France	Comparative	35	*	*	32	—	Revision
Tarasevicius et al.	2017	Lithuania	Comparative	620	*	*	2170	1	Primary
			Group Totals	**1068**	**568**	**70**	**2378**		
			Total Patients				**4084**		

Criticisms and Limitations: Overall, the quality of studies for the meta-analysis was not high. Only 2 of 11 included studies were level I studies (RCTs),[3,7] which only accounted for 43 of the total 4084 patients analyzed, and 2790 (68%) were drawn from a single study.[9] Among the implant types analyzed, there were low numbers for some of the groups; only a cohort of 70 CTHAs was included from a single study with at least 6-month follow-up (F/U).[6] The influence of a number of important factors such as approach, fixation, prosthesis design, and bearing couples was not taken into account. Many of the studies included reported short-term results (only 2 reported F/U ≥ 10 years[2,3]). The risks of loosening in mid- or long-term periods of DMTHA and CTHA in the high-risk population remain largely unquantified.

Other Relevant Studies and Information:

- Dual mobility articulations are a viable alternative to traditional bearing surfaces, with low rates of instability and good overall survivorship (96.6% at a mean of 5.4 years) in primary and revision THAs, and in those undertaken in patients with neck of femur fractures.[12]
- In all revision THA indications, DMTHA compared to standard implants has a significantly decreafed risk of postoperative dislocation without risk of early aseptic loosening at medium-term F/U.[13]
- In primary THA, a larger femoral head diameter was associated with a lower long-term cumulative risk of dislocation with all operative approaches, but the effect was greatest in association with the posterolateral approach.[14] A positive trend of decreasing femoral head diameter with increasing revision rate for dislocation was identified.[15]
- In contrast, the use of larger femoral heads did not notably reduce the prevalence of early dislocation after primary THA in high-risk patients compared to historical controls.[16]

Summary and Implications: In patients at a high risk of postoperative dislocation, the best implant of choice to reduce the risk in the short term appears to be DMTHA bearing surfaces followed by large femoral head diameter implants. However, because existing research has significant methodological flaws, the authors recommend further research with increased sample sizes, long-term F/U, and prospective RCTs.

CLINICAL CASE: IMPLANT DESIGN IN REVISION THA TO REDUCE DISLOCATION

Case Study

A 75-year-old male had a primary right THA for advanced osteoarthritis 7 years ago. Over the past 8 months he had 4 hospital admissions for dislocation requiring reduction under general anesthesia. On examination, there are no signs suggestive of infection, there is no leg length discrepancy, and he had no gross restriction to his range of motion and good power of the abductors. Serum inflammatory markers were within normal range. Radiographs show appropriate implant positioning and sizing with no evidence of loosening. Single-photon emission computed tomography scan confirmed abduction and anteversion of the cup within the safe zone, again without marked tracer uptake. What implant design features could be considered at revision to reduce the risk of further dislocation?

Suggested Answer

The use of a large femoral head diameter, a constrained liner, or DMTHA can all be considered to help reduce the risk of recurrent dislocation. Pituckanotai et al.[1] in their systematic review concluded that dual mobility and large femoral head designs were implants of safety. Their network analysis showed that only dual mobility implants significantly lowered the risk of dislocation by 75% and revision by 54% when compared to standard THA. Based on the study findings, a dual mobility implant would be the implant of choice to minimize risk of dislocation by large femoral head diameter implants. Constrained liners can be considered as a salvage option for patients with recurrent instability despite revision with either dual mobility or large femoral head diameter implants or in patients with significant comorbidities in whom all component revisions may present too great a risk.

References

1. Pituckanotai et al. Risk of revision and dislocation in single, dual mobility and large femoral head total hip arthroplasty: systematic review and network meta-analysis. Eur J Orthop Surg Traumatol Orthop Traumatol. 2018;28(3):445–55.
2. Chalmers et al. High failure rate of modular exchange with a specific design of a constrained liner in high-risk patients undergoing revision total hip arthroplasty. J Arthroplasty. 2016;31(9):1963–9.
3. Catelli et al. Does the dual-mobility hip prosthesis produce better joint kinematics during extreme hip flexion task? J Arthroplasty. 2017;32(10):3206–12.

4. Jauregui et al. Dual mobility cups: an effective prosthesis in revision total hip arthroplasties for preventing dislocations. Hip Int J Clin Exp Res Hip Pathol Ther. 2016;26(1):57–61.
5. Homma et al. Benefit and risk in short term after total hip arthroplasty by direct anterior approach combined with dual mobility cup. Eur J Orthop Surg Traumatol Orthop Traumatol. 2016;26(6):619–24.
6. Hernigou et al. Dual-mobility implants prevent hip dislocation following hip revision in obese patients. Int Orthop. 2017;41(3):469–73.
7. Griffin et al. A randomised feasibility study comparing total hip arthroplasty with and without dual mobility acetabular component in the treatment of displaced intracapsular fractures of the proximal femur: the Warwick Hip Trauma Evaluation Two: WHiTE Two. Bone Joint J. 2016;98-B(11):1431–5.
8. Haughom et al. Is there a benefit to head size greater than 36 mm in total hip arthroplasty? J Arthroplasty. 2016;31(1):152–5.
9. Tarasevicius et al. Short-term outcome after total hip arthroplasty using dual-mobility cup: report from Lithuanian Arthroplasty Register. Int Orthop. 2017;41(3):595–8.
10. Tarasevicius et al. Dual mobility cup reduces dislocation rate after arthroplasty for femoral neck fracture. BMC Musculoskelet Disord. 2010;11:175.
11. Bouchet et al. Posterior approach and dislocation rate: a 213 total hip replacements case-control study comparing the dual mobility cup with a conventional 28-mm metal head/polyethylene prosthesis. Orthop Traumatol Surg Res. 2011;97(1):2–7.
12. Darrith et al. Outcomes of dual mobility components in total hip arthroplasty: a systematic review of the literature. Bone Joint J. 2018;100-B(1):11–9.
13. Schmidt et al. Dual mobility cups in revision total hip arthroplasty: efficient strategy to decrease dislocation risk. J Arthroplasty. 2020;35(2):500–7.
14. Berry et al. Effect of femoral head diameter and operative approach on risk of dislocation after primary total hip arthroplasty. J Bone Joint Surg Am. 2005;87(11):2456–63.
15. Conroy et al. Risk factors for revision for early dislocation in total hip arthroplasty. J Arthroplasty. 2008;23(6):867–72.
16. Lachiewicz et al. Low early and late dislocation rates with 36- and 40-mm heads in patients at high risk for dislocation. Clin Orthop. 2013;471(2):439–43.

45

Arthroscopic Subacromial Decompression for Subacromial Shoulder Pain (CSAW)

A Multicenter, Pragmatic, Parallel Group, Placebo-Controlled, Three-Group, Randomized Surgical Trial

RAFIK NABIL FANOUS AND BEN GOODING

Study Nickname: CSAW—Can Shoulder Arthroscopy Work

> To our knowledge, this is the largest study to compare surgery with no treatment and is the first published trial of shoulder surgery to include a placebo comparison. Both types of surgery were better than no treatment, but the differences were not clinically significant, which questions the value of this type of surgery to patients.
>
> —Beard et al.[1]

Citation: Beard DJ, Rees JL, Cook JA, Rombach I, Cooper C, Merritt N, Shirkey BA, Donovan JL, Gwilym S, Savulescu J, Moser J, Gray A, Jepson M, Tracey I, Judge A, Wartolowska K, Carr AJ; CSAW Study Group. Arthroscopic subacromial decompression for subacromial shoulder pain (CSAW): a multicentre, pragmatic, parallel group, placebo-controlled, three-group, randomised surgical trial. Lancet. 2018;391(10118):329–38.

Research Question: Is arthroscopic subacromial decompression of the shoulder more effective than diagnostic arthroscopy or no treatment?

Funding: Arthritis Research UK, National Institute for Health Research Biomedical Research Centre, and Royal College of Surgeons (England)

Year Study Began: 2012

Year Study Published: 2018

Study Location: Multicenter across 31 hospitals

Who Was Studied: Patients with subacromial pain for > 3 months. All patients had an intact rotator cuff and had failed nonoperative treatment that had to include a period of physiotherapy and at least 1 steroid injection.

Who Was Excluded: Aged > 75 years, full-thickness rotator cuff tears, calcific tendonitis, other shoulder pathologies on imaging, previous surgery, previous septic arthritis or radiotherapy, inflammatory arthropathies, cervical spine pathology.

How Many Patients: 313

Study Overview: See Figure 45.1.

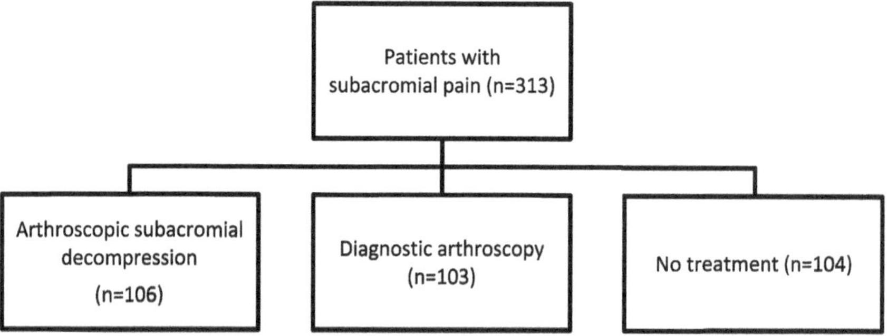

Figure 45.1. Overview of the study design.

Study Intervention: Patients were randomized to 1 of 3 arms: (1) arthroscopic subacromial decompression (i.e., active treatment), (2) diagnostic arthroscopy (i.e., placebo), or (3) no treatment (i.e., control group). All patients randomized to a surgical arm were masked as to the surgery they would receive. Patients randomized to a surgical arm had a standard postoperative physiotherapy regimen. Those in the no-treatment group had a shoulder specialist consultation at 3 months after randomization. Patients undergoing surgery who were found to have other pathology requiring intervention were treated as needed. The principal analysis was done according to the randomization (intention to treat).

Follow-Up: All patients were followed up at 6 and 12 months. Follow-up (F/U) periods were defined as time since randomization. It was expected that most patients would receive surgery within < 4 months of randomization; however, in all groups a percentage of patients had not received their intervention by the 6-month F/U.

Endpoints: Primary outcome measure was Oxford Shoulder Score[2] (OSS; patient-reported outcome measure on pain and function of shoulder related to surgical intervention) at 6 months. Secondary outcome measures were OSS at 12 months, modified Constant-Morley shoulder score, PainDETECT, Quantitative Sensory Testing, adverse events, EQ-5D-3L, EuroQol visual analog scale (VAS), patient expectations and satisfaction, and Hospital Anxiety and Depression Score.

RESULTS (TABLE 45.1)

- *Baseline:* The baseline characteristics of all 313 patients were well balanced.
- *Surgeon profile:* The median number of operations performed by each surgeon was 2 (range 1–6).
- *Allocations:* By 6 months, 23%, 42%, and 12% of the decompression, diagnostic arthroscopy, and no-treatment groups respectively had not received their allocated treatment.
- *Time to surgery:* Median time was 90, 82, and 217 days for the decompression, diagnostic arthroscopy, and no-treatment groups respectively.
- *OSS (Figure 45.2)*
  - All groups demonstrated an improvement at 6 and 12 months.
  - *At 6 months:*
    - There was no significant difference between the decompression and diagnostic arthroscopy groups.
    - Both surgical groups showed a small but insignificant improvement over the no-treatment group.
- *Other outcomes:*
  - Nearly all the secondary outcomes demonstrated a similar pattern to the primary outcome at 6 and 12 months.
  - Per-protocol analysis showed similar results, and the results were not sensitive to missing data.

Table 45.1 Summary of Key Results

	Mean Difference (95% CI); *p* Value		
	Decompression vs. Diagnostic Arthroscopy	**Decompression vs. No Treatment**	**Diagnostic Arthroscopy vs. No Treatment**
OSS (6 mo)	−1.3 (−3.9–1.3); 0.314	2.8 (0.5–5.2); 0.018	4.2 (1.8–6.6); 0.001
OSS (1 y)	0.3 (−2.9–3.5); 0.857	3.9 (0.7–7.1); 0.019	3.6 (0.6–6.6); 0.019
Constant-Morley (6 mo)	0.3 (−4.1–4.7); 0.897	9.3 (4.1–14.6); 0.001	9.1 (3.1–15.2); 0.004
Constant-Morley (1 y)	2.7 (−2.7–8.2); 0.308	8.3 (2.5–14.1); 0.006	4.9 (0.9–8.9); 0.017

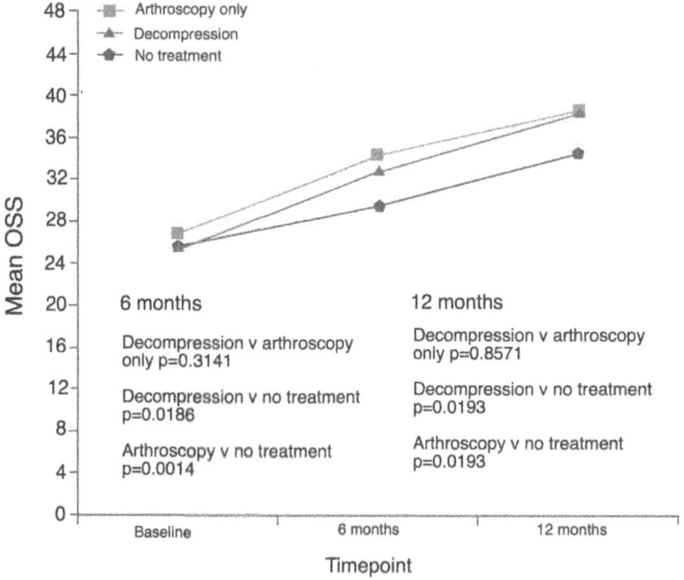

Figure 45.2. OSS in the intention-to-treat analyses. Data are mean (95% CI) shown at F/U timepoints.

Criticisms and Limitations: Of the 740 patients assessed for eligibility, only 313 (42.3%) were eligible. Of the 313 patients, only 274 (87.5%) provided 6-month F/U data for intention-to-treat analysis and only 207 for per-protocol analysis. Long waiting lists after randomization meant that some patients had not received surgery by the primary endpoint analysis and some had shorter F/U. At the primary endpoint, 23%, 42%, and 12% of the decompression, placebo, and no-treatment groups respectively had not received their assigned treatment.

Other Relevant Studies and Information:

- The FInnish subacromial IMPingement Arthroscopy Controlled Trial (FIMPACT)[3] study was similar to the CSAW trial. It was also multicenter and had the same treatment arms with 210 patients. Primary outcome was VAS pain score at 24 months. There was no significant difference or benefit seen between arthroscopic subacromial decompression and diagnostic arthroscopy at 2-year F/U.
- Haahr et al.[4] led a single-center study with 90 patients randomized to either the subacromial decompression or physiotherapy arm. Primary outcome was sick leave/ability to work at 1 year and then 4–8-year F/U. No difference was seen between both treatment options and hence exercises may be as efficient as subacromial decompression in patients with subacromial stage II impingement.
- A Cochrane systematic review[5] in 2019 analyzed 8 trials with a total of 1062 patients. Once again, the data does not support the use of subacromial decompression for rotator cuff disease.

Summary and Implications: This study is the largest randomized controlled trial to look at the efficacy of arthroscopic subacromial decompression. Evidence from the data suggests that there is no benefit to this intervention compared to diagnostic arthroscopy and an insignificantly small improvement compared to the nonoperative group. Nevertheless, these findings should be interpreted with caution, as some patients who do not improve with conservative management may ultimately benefit from surgery.

CLINICAL CASE: IMPINGEMENT PAIN

Case History

A 45-year-old right-hand-dominant manual laborer presents with a 4-month history of right shoulder impingement pain. He has tried exercises with a physiotherapist and had a steroid injection by his family physician, which provided 4 weeks of symptomatic relief. He is now dependent on oral analgesia on a daily basis. Ultrasound has not demonstrated any other shoulder pathology except for subacromial subdeltoid bursitis, and he is otherwise fit and well. He is an ex-smoker with a 2-pack-year history. He presents to you because he is unable to work and lift due to the pain leading to reduced range of motion. Based on the results from the CSAW trial, how should he be treated?

Suggested Answer

Based on the CSAW trial, this patient can be managed without surgical treatment at this point. This clinical vignette is the typical patient that CSAW aimed to address. A discussion should be had with the patient to explain the results of this trial and that the evidence shows no significant benefit to arthroscopic surgery over no treatment. CSAW and other similar trials do not clearly prove that there is no role for surgery, as the surgical cohorts improved significantly, and so a pragmatic approach should be taken for appropriate patient selection. Many surgeons would still advocate for surgery for patients with prolonged symptomatology affecting their quality of life and a confirmed diagnosis of mechanical impingement who have failed a conservative or no-treatment approach. Ultimately, the evidence ought to be presented to patients and they should be counseled for the potential benefits and risks of surgical intervention.

References

1. Beard et al. Arthroscopic subacromial decompression for subacromial shoulder pain (CSAW): a multicentre, pragmatic, parallel group, placebo-controlled, three-group, randomised surgical trial. Lancet. 2018;391(10118):329–38.
2. Younis et al. The range of the Oxford Shoulder Score in the asymptomatic population: a marker for post-operative improvement. Ann R Coll Surg Engl. 2011;93(8):629–33.
3. Paavola et al. Subacromial decompression versus diagnostic arthroscopy for shoulder impingement: randomised, placebo surgery controlled clinical trial. BMJ. 2018;362:k2860.
4. Haahr et al. Exercises may be as efficient as subacromial decompression in patients with subacromial stage II impingement: 4-8-years' follow-up in a prospective, randomized study. Scand J Rheumatol. 2006;35(3):224–8.
5. Karjalainen et al. Subacromial decompression surgery for rotator cuff disease. Cochrane Database Syst Rev. 2019;1(1):CD005619.

46

Patellar Resurfacing in Total Knee Arthroplasty

A Prospective, Randomized, Double-Blind Study with 5–7 Years of Follow-Up

ZAKIR HAIDER AND KESAVAN SRI-RAM

> There was no significant difference between groups treated with and without [patellar] resurfacing with regards to the overall Knee Society score or the pain and function subscores. Obesity, the degree of patella chondromalacia, and the presence of preoperative anterior knee pain did not predict postoperative clinical scores or . . . postoperative anterior knee pain.
>
> —BARRACK ET AL.[1]

Citation: Barrack RL, Bertot AJ, Wolfe MW, Waldman DA, Milicic M, Myers L. Patellar resurfacing in total knee arthroplasty. A prospective, randomized, double-blind study with five to seven years of follow-up. J Bone Joint Surg Am. 2001;83(9):1376–81.

Research Question: Do factors including obesity, degree of patellar chondromalacia, and the presence of preoperative anterior knee pain predict clinical outcome following total knee arthroplasty (TKA) with or without patellar resurfacing?

Funding: Zimmer Inc.

Year Study Began: 1992

Year Study Published: 2001

Study Location: 3 hospitals in the USA

Who Was Studied: Patients with severe knee osteoarthritis (OA) undergoing TKA after trial of nonoperative therapy.

Who Was Excluded: Patients who previously had undergone tibial osteotomy or extensor mechanism surgery or patients with a history of septic arthritis, osteomyelitis, medical disability limiting walking, disabling concomitant joint disease in another lower limb joint, inflammatory arthropathy, or significant clinical deformity.

How Many Patients: 67 patients (93 knees)

Study Overview: See Figure 46.1.

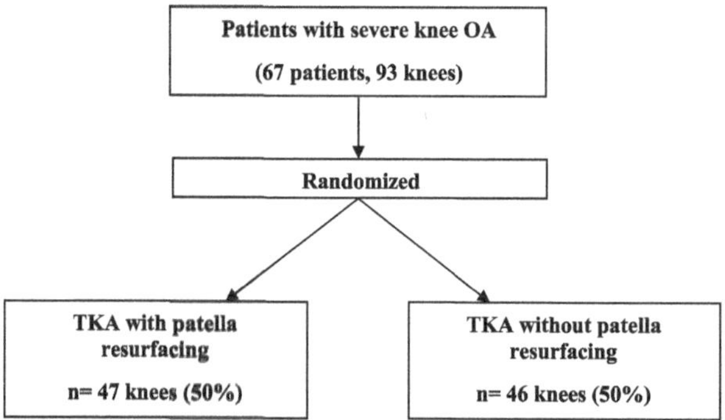

Figure 46.1. Summary of study design.

Study Intervention: Both groups received a cruciate retaining (CR) knee prosthesis—tibial/femoral components (Miller-Galante II; Zimmer, Warsaw, Indiana, USA) performed or supervised by 1 of the authors. In the patellar resurfacing group, a cemented, 3-peg, all-polyethylene component was used. In the nonpatellar resurfacing group, patellar arthroplasty was performed including removal of osteophytes, smoothing of fibrillated cartilage, and drilling of eburnated bone.

Follow-Up: Average 70.5 months

Endpoints: Knee Society Score[2] (KSS) with pain and function subscores and completion of patient questionnaire produced by authors evaluating overall satisfaction and patellofemoral symptoms.

RESULTS (TABLE 46.1)

- *Patient satisfaction:* 93% of patients in the patellar nonresurfacing group and 91% of patients in the patellar resurfacing group were satisfied with their operation.
- *KSS:*
  - No significant difference was found in postoperative KSS along with pain and function subscores between the patellar resurfacing and nonresurfacing groups.
  - Obesity and degree of patellar chondromalacia did not have a significant effect on postoperative KSS and subscores.
- *Functional outcome:* No significant difference was found between the patellar nonresurfacing and patella resurfacing groups on evaluation of postoperative patellofemoral function including exiting an automobile, rising from a chair, and climbing stairs.
- *Postoperative anterior knee pain:*
  - No significant difference was found in the incidence between the resurfaced patellar and nonresurfaced patellar group.
  - 7 (15.2%) TKAs without patella resurfacing were subsequently revised with patella resurfacing due to anterior knee pain. Follow-up of 5 knees found that although the average pain rating reduced at 2–4 years, in 4 out of 5 knees anterior knee pain had deteriorated again at 4–7 years.

Table 46.1 Summary of Key Findings

Outcome	**Non resurfaced Patellae**	**Resurfaced Patellae**	***p* Value**
	Postoperative Knee Society Scores		
Pain	88.5	88.3	0.77
Function	80.7	73.5	0.16
Overall	169.1	161.6	0.36
	Postoperative Patellofemoral Function Test		
Exiting automobile	8.1	7.5	0.36
Rising from chair	8.1	8.1	0.94
Stair climbing	7.9	7.9	0.99

Criticisms and Limitations: This study has low participant numbers, which may affect its validity. In addition, the study results are from 1 surgeon's operative technique and 1 type of prosthesis used. This in turn may have affected the applicability and reproducibility of results. No power calculation was mentioned even though this was a randomized controlled trial (RCT).

Other Relevant Studies and Information:

- A large body of evidence investigating patella resurfacing exists within the medical literature. However, this remains a controversial topic, with multiple meta-analyses of RCTs coming to conflicting conclusions as to which option is better.[3–7]
- In 2018 a systematic review[8] of 10 meta-analyses found outcomes between patellar resurfacing and nonresurfacing to be comparable with no clear superiority of either group. A higher risk of reoperation was noted in the nonresurfacing group. However, the authors explained that this should be interpreted with caution due to methodological limitations of the meta-analyses and the surgeon's tendencies to perform secondary patellar resurfacing in patients with painful TKA.
- Meta-analyses[9,10] of RCTs evaluating the effect on the patella denervation in TKA without patella resurfacing have provided conflicting evidence with regard to anterior knee pain and postoperative function.
- Minimal research has been performed with low patient numbers assessing patella denervation in patella resurfacing and therefore no clear conclusions can be determined.
- National Institute for Health and Care Excellence guidelines[11] recommend that by conducting patellar resurfacing during a primary total knee replacement (TKR), the need for further surgeries may be reduced, as well as the financial burden. This also reflects on the National Joint Registry (NJR), as a secondary patellar resurfacing for anterior knee pain is defined as "revision surgery." Hence, the NJR and Hospital Episode Statistics approximate that only a fifth to a third of primary TKRs have concomitant patella resurfacing.

Summary and Implications: No significant differences were found between patients who underwent TKA with or without patellar resurfacing in postoperative KSS or evaluation of patellofemoral function. Moreover, obesity, degree of patella chondromalacia, and preoperative anterior knee pain did not have a significant effect on postoperative knee scores, patellofemoral-related function, or postoperative anterior knee pain. Thus, surgeons should carefully consider offering patellar resurfacing to patients and be mindful that factors such as obesity or preoperative anterior knee pain may not predict postoperative patient outcomes or satisfaction as accurately as previously thought.

CLINICAL CASE: PATELLAR RESURFACING IN TKA

Case History

A 75-year-old lady presents to the clinic with a 2-year history of worsening pain in her right knee. Her pain wakes her up at night, gives her difficulty when climbing stairs, and limits her daily activities. She has plain radiographs that reveal significant arthritic changes in all compartments of her knee. The patient is counseled for a knee replacement without patella resurfacing. The patient recalls that her friends have had knee replacements and their surgeons also changed their "knee cap." She challenges her surgeon on why she will not have the same done. She feels short-changed and is concerned about suboptimal care. Based upon current evidence, how should her question be addressed?

Suggested Answer

One could first explain to the patient that different surgeons employ different techniques when performing a TKR. It would be prudent to explain that a large amount of research has been performed looking into TKR with and without patellar resurfacing. However, there is no clear answer as to which is better, and outcomes are comparable. One could also explain that patellar resurfacing is not risk free and complications can occur such as patellar fracture and possible need for patellectomy if unable to fix, thus requiring a posterior-stabilized (PS) implant. If a knee replacement is performed without patellar resurfacing and the patient experiences anterior knee pain that the surgeon thinks is related to the patellofemoral compartment, there is the option to have a secondary patellar resurfacing procedure, although this also does not guarantee complete resolution of anterior knee pain. Conversely, it is difficult to revise if the patient develops anterior knee pain after having their patella already resurfaced during the primary operation.

References

1. Barrack et al. Patellar resurfacing in total knee arthroplasty. A prospective, randomized, double-blind study with five to seven years of follow-up. J Bone Joint Surg Am. 2001;83(9):1376–81.
2. Insall et al. Rationale of the Knee Society clinical rating system. Clin Orthop Relat Res. 1989;248:13–14.

3. Pavlouet et al. Patellar resurfacing in total knee arthroplasty: does design matter? A meta-analysis of 7075 cases. J Bone Joint Surg Am. 2011;93(14):1301–9.
4. Pilling et al. Patellar resurfacing in primary total knee replacement: a meta-analysis. J Bone Joint Surg Am. 2012;94(24):2270–8.
5. Tang et al. A meta-analysis of patellar replacement in total knee arthroplasty for patients with knee osteoarthritis. J Arthroplasty. 2018;33(3): 960–7.
6. Chen et al. Patellar resurfacing versus non-resurfacing in total knee arthroplasty: a meta-analysis of randomized controlled trials. Int Orthop. 2013;37(6):1075–83.
7. Pakoset et al. Patellar resurfacing in total knee arthroplasty: a meta-analysis. J Bone Joint Surg Am. 2005;87(7):1438–45.
8. Grassi et al. Patellar resurfacing versus patellar retention in primary total knee arthroplasty: a systematic review of overlapping meta-analyses. Knee Surg Sports Traumatol Arthrosc. 2018;26(11):3206–18.
9. Li et al. Patellar denervation in total knee arthroplasty without patellar resurfacing and post operative anterior knee pain: a meta-analysis of randomized controlled trials. J Arthroplasty. 2014; 29(12): 2309–13.
10. Cheng et al. Patellar denervation with electrocautery in total knee arthroplasty without patellar resurfacing: a meta-analysis. Knee Surg Sports Traumatol Arthrosc. 2014;22(11):2648–54.
11. National Institute for Health and Care Excellence. Resource impact report: joint replacement (primary): hip, knee and shoulder (NG157). June 2020. https://www.nice.org.uk/guidance/ng157/resources/resource-impact-report-pdf-8708810221

47

Operative versus Nonoperative Treatment for Calcaneal Fractures

CHANG PARK, KAPIL SUGAND, CENK OGUZ, AND GARTH ALLARDICE

Study Nickname: The UK Heel Fracture trial (UK HeFT)

> Surgery by open reduction and internal fixation in patients with typical displaced calcaneal fractures does not improve outcomes compared with non-operative care.
>
> —Griffin et al.[1]

Citation: Griffin D, Parsons N, Shaw E, Kulikov Y, Hutchinson C, Thorogood M, Lamb SE; UK Heel Fracture Trial Investigators. Operative versus non-operative treatment for closed, displaced, intra-articular fractures of the calcaneus: randomised controlled trial. BMJ. 2014;349:g4483.

Research Question: Does the surgical treatment of displaced intra-articular calcaneal fractures improve the outcomes of pain and function as compared to non-operative treatment?

Funding: Arthritis Research Grant

Year Study Began: 2007

Year Study Published: 2014

Study Location: Multicentered with 22 sites in the UK

Who Was Studied: Adults with a closed displaced intra-articular calcaneal fracture < 3 weeks old. Fractures with displacement measured to be at least 2 mm in the posterior facet of the subtalar joint.

Who Was Excluded: Those with a gross deformity, other significant leg injury, not fit for surgery, or unable to consent were excluded.

How Many Patients: 151

Study Overview: See Figure 47.1.

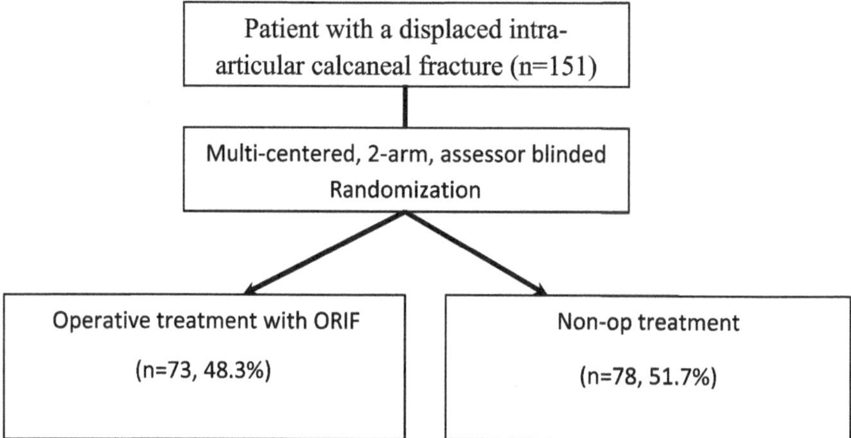

Figure 47.1. Summary of UK HeFT study design.

Study Intervention: Those treated nonoperatively wore a temporary splint and were non–weight bearing for 6 weeks and partial weight bearing for an additional 6 weeks. Patients in the operative treatment group underwent open reduction and internal fixation (ORIF) with interfragmentary screws and application of a neutralization plate to the lateral wall. This was performed within < 3 weeks of injury through an extensile lateral approach. Postoperative they had the same removable splint and same weight-bearing regimen as the nonoperative arm. Both treatment arms had a standardized physiotherapy regimen.

Follow-Up: Total of 2 years

Endpoints: Primary endpoint was patient-reported pain and function with the Kerr-Atkins Calcaneal Fracture Score[2] (KACFS; for pain and function after calcaneal fracture). Secondary endpoints consisted of complications, functionality with the AOFAS score[3] (standardized evaluation of the clinical status of the foot and ankle containing both subjective [patients' pain] and objective [alignment and functional] components), health and quality of life (QOL) outcomes, and gait analysis.

RESULTS (TABLE 47.1)

- *Primary endpoint (Figure 47.2):* There was no significant difference in the KACFS of pain and function at 2 years between the operative (69.8) and nonoperative groups (65.7).
- *Effect size:* Unadjusted effect size was 4.1 (95% CI: −3.4–11.5, $p = 0.28$).
- *Fracture severity:* Fracture severity (according to Sanders classification) had no effect on postoperative outcomes of pain and the KACFS ($p = 0.697$).
- *Secondary outcomes:* There was no significant difference in any secondary outcomes between the 2 interventions, including general health, QOL, hindfoot pain, and function or gait analysis (Figure 47.3).
- *Complications:* Those undergoing surgery had more complications and reoperations (17/73; 23%) than those managed nonoperatively (3/78; 4%) with an estimated odds ratio of 7.5 (95% CI: 2.0–41.8, Fischer's exact test $p < 0.001$). The most common operative complication was surgical site infection ($n = 19$, 26%).
- *Reoperation:* 11 (15%) patients required reoperation (commonly to treat infection and also for removal of painful metalwork) in the operative group.

Table 47.1 Summary of UK HeFT Key Findings

Outcome	Number	Operative Treatment	Number	Nonoperative Treatment	Difference (Adjusted 95% CI)	*p* Value
			Primary Outcome			
KACFS	69	69.8	74	65.7	0.0 (−7.1–7.0)	0.993
			Secondary Outcomes			
AOFAS	54	79.2	60	76.8	0.1 (−6.5–6.7)	0.976
Walking speed (m/s)	54	1.19	58	1..05	0.05 (−0.02–0.17)	0.137

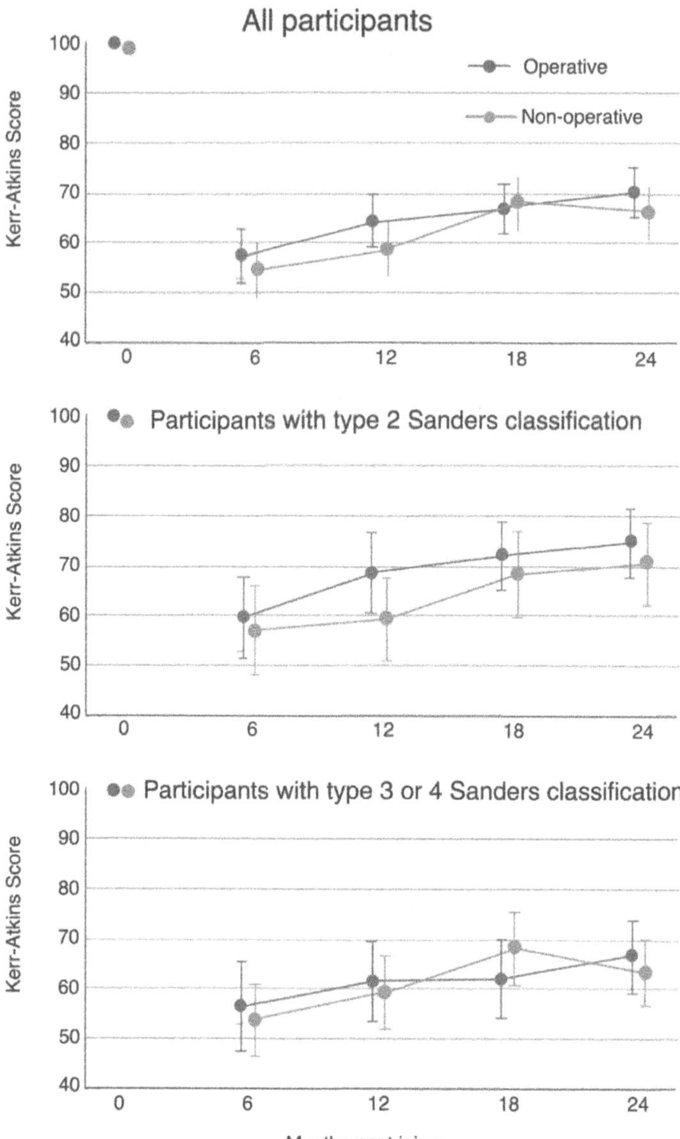

Figure 47.2. KACFS for calcaneal fracture and 95% CI at baseline (before injury) and 6, 12, 18, and 24 months after injury for all participants with fractures under the Sanders classification.

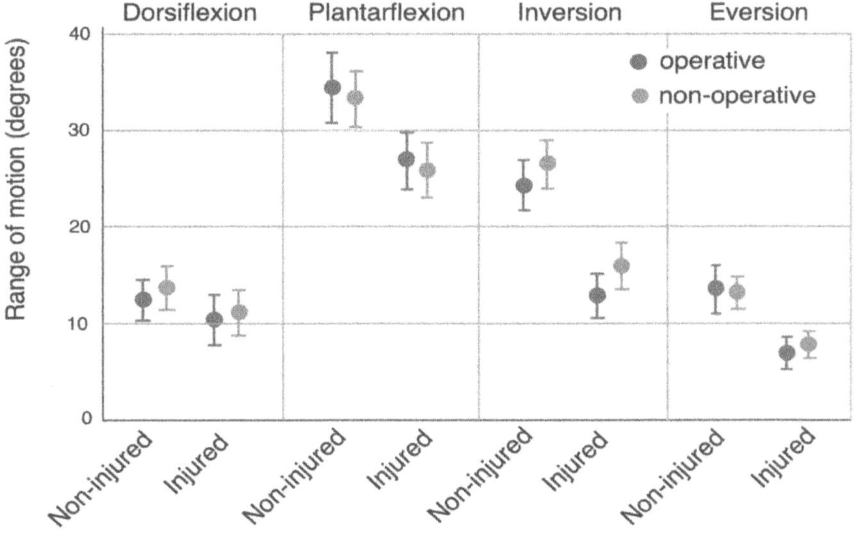

Figure 47.3. ROM in degrees (group means and 95% CI) and gait symmetry data at 24 months postinjury for injured and noninjured feet.

Criticisms and Limitations: The trial had a low recruitment rate (30%) and therefore the results may not be generalizable to the overall population. The sample size was low and the follow-up (F/U) period was only 2 years, which may not identify future sequelae (e.g., subtalar arthrosis necessitating arthrodesis). Newer percutaneous and arthroscopic methods of fixation were also excluded, which may have affected the severity and rates of postoperative complications.

Other Relevant Studies and Information:

- A recent Cochrane review has called for further research as there was insufficient quality of evidence to support operative vs. nonoperative treatment of displaced intra-articular calcaneal fractures.[4]
- There have been 3 randomized controlled trials (RCTs) with 1 reporting benefits from operative treatment by a functional questionnaire (87/100 vs. 55/100, $p < 0.001$); however, it had only 30 patients with 13% lost to F/U at a mean of only 15 months.[5]
- 2 further trials support the UK HeFT study with no difference in outcomes when comparing operative vs. nonoperative treatment.[6,7]

- Recent evidence suggests that minimally invasive and percutaneous approaches to the calcaneus may reduce the risk of operative complications when compared to ORIF.[8–10]

Summary and Implications: In patients with intra-articular displaced closed calcaneal fractures, there was no difference in the primary outcomes of pain and the KACFS between operative and nonoperative intervention at 2 years. Complications and reoperations were more common in the operatively treated group. Thus, nonoperative management of these fractures may result in similar outcomes while avoiding the risks of surgery. Ongoing research is exploring newer minimally invasive and percutaneous techniques on rates of long-term complications.

CASE STUDY: MANAGING ACUTE CALCANEAL FRACTURE

Case History

A 38-year-old builder falls from a height and sustains a left closed intra-articular calcaneal fracture. In the clinic 4 days postinjury, on plain film radiographs there is 3 mm of displacement of the posterior articular surface, and this is better defined on a computed tomography scan. The anterior and middle facet remains congruent and minimally displaced. He is otherwise well and is a nonsmoker, and this is an isolated injury. He wishes to return to work as soon as possible, as he is self-employed. He asks about the benefits of operative intervention and the implication of the injury in the longer term. Based on the UK HeFT results, should this be operatively managed, and how should this patient be counseled?

Suggested Answer

The UK HeFT results have shown that in its multicentered RCT there was no difference in function, pain, and QOL between operative and nonoperative treatments. In those undergoing operative management there is a significantly increased risk of surgical site infection and reoperation than those managed nonoperatively. Therefore, the UK HeFT trial recommends that this patient should be consented for the safer and equally effective nonoperative management. However, more recent minimally invasive surgical (MIS) techniques may reduce the risk of operative complications when compared to the traditional open approach studied in the UK HeFT study, and these should be considered in the management of this patient. There should be a frank discussion about the needs of the patient and the experiential skill of the surgeon with MIS technique.

References

1. Griffin et al. UK Heel Fracture Trial Investigators. Operative versus non-operative treatment for closed, displaced, intra-articular fractures of the calcaneus: randomised controlled trial. BMJ. 2014;349:g4483.
2. Kerr et al. Assessing outcome following calcaneal fracture: a rational scoring system. Injury. 1996;27(1):35–8.
3. Ibrahim et al. Reliability and validity of the subjective component of the American Orthopaedic Foot and Ankle Society clinical rating scales. J Foot Ankle Surg. 2007;46(2):65–74.
4. Bruce et al. Surgical versus conservative interventions for displaced intra-articular calcaneal fractures. Cochrane Database Syst Rev. 2013;(1):CD008628.
5. Thordarson et al. Operative vs. nonoperative treatment of intra-articular fractures of the calcaneus: a prospective randomized trial. Foot Ankle Int. 1996;17(1):2–9.
6. Buckley et al. Operative compared with nonoperative treatment of displaced intra-articular calcaneal fractures: a prospective, randomized, controlled multicenter trial. J Bone Joint Surg Am. 2002;84(10):1733–44.
7. Ågren et al. Operative versus nonoperative treatment of displaced intra-articular calcaneal fractures: a prospective, randomized, controlled multicenter trial. J Bone Joint Surg Am. 2013;95(15):1351–7.
8. van Hoeve et al. Outcome of minimally invasive open and percutaneous techniques for repair of calcaneal fractures: a systematic review. J Foot Ankle Surg. 2016;55(6):1256–63.
9. Marouby et al. Percutaneous arthroscopic calcaneal osteosynthesis for displaced intra-articular calcaneal fractures: systematic review and surgical technique. Foot Ankle Surg. 2020;26(5):503–8.
10. Basile et al. Comparison between sinus tarsi approach and extensile lateral approach for treatment of closed displaced intra-articular calcaneal fractures: a multicenter prospective study. J Foot Ankle Surg. 2016;55(3):513–21.

48

Bisphosphonates and Fractures of the Subtrochanteric or Diaphyseal Femur

BORNA GUEVEL AND ARJUNA IMBULDENIYA

> The occurrence of fracture of the subtrochanteric or diaphyseal femur was very rare, even among women who had been treated with bisphosphonates for as long as 10 years. There was no significant increase in risk associated with bisphosphonate use.
>
> —BLACK ET AL.[1]

Citation: Black DM, Kelly MP, Genant HK, Palermo L, Eastell R, Bucci-Rechtweg C, Cauley J, Leung PC, Boonen S, Santora A, De Papp A, Bauer DC. Bisphosphonates and fractures of the subtrochanteric or diaphyseal femur. N Engl J Med. 2002;347(23):1825–33.

Research Question: Is there a relationship between bisphosphonates and atypical fractures of the femoral shaft?

Funding: University of California, San Francisco (UCSF), Merck, Novartis

Year Study Began: 2008

Year Study Published: 2010

Study Location: University of California, San Francisco, USA

Who Was Studied: Hip or femur fractures from 3 bisphosphonate randomized controlled trials were reviewed. All patients were women aged > 55 years with osteoporosis.

Who Was Excluded: Subcapital fractures, neck of femur (NOF) fractures, periprosthetic fractures, and pathologic and high-energy fractures were excluded.

How Many Patients: 284 (2%) hip or femur fractures reviewed among 14 195 women across the 3 trials. A total of 12 (4.2%) fractures in 10 patients were classified as occurring in the subtrochanteric or diaphyseal femur.

Study Overview: See Figure 48.1.

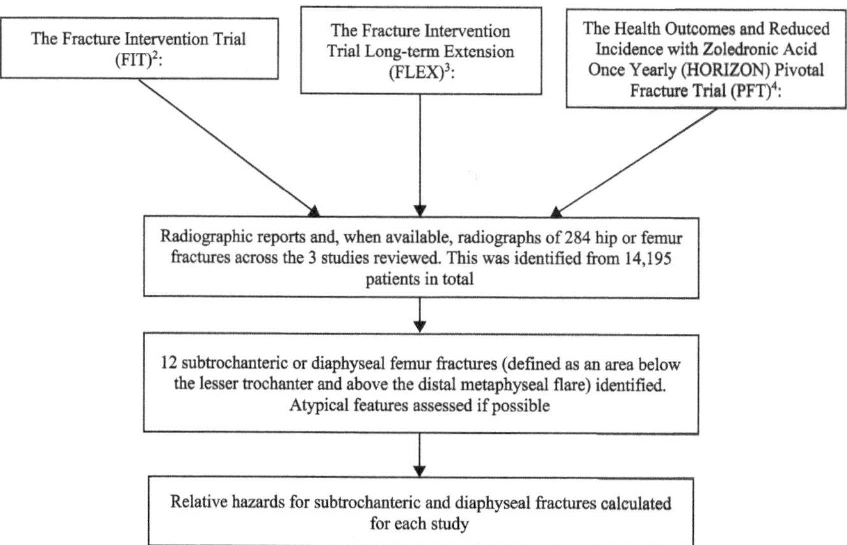

Figure 48.1. Summary of study design.

Study Intervention: In the Fracture Intervention Trial (FIT)[2] study, women aged 55–81 years with low femoral neck bone mineral density (BMD) were randomly assigned to receive 5 mg of daily alendronate or placebo for the first 2 years and then 10 mg thereafter. The FLEX[3] trial was a continuation of FIT where women originally assigned to receive alendronate treatment were randomized to receive either 5 further years of 5 mg or 10 mg alendronate or 5 years of placebo. In the HORIZON PFT study,[4] women aged 65–89 years with low femoral neck BMD were randomly assigned to either a 5-mg zoledronic acid infusion at 0, 12, and 24 months or placebo.

Follow-Up: In FIT, follow-up (F/U) was 3–4.5 years; in the FLEX trial, F/U was 10 years; and in HORIZON PFT, F/U was 3 years.

Endpoints: Primary outcome was a fracture confined to the area below the lesser trochanter and above the distal metaphyseal flare. Secondary outcomes were any atypical features associated with the fracture, the level of bone metabolism markers before the fracture, and any prodromal history of bone pain. The bone turnover markers measured were serum C-terminal telopeptide of type 1 collagen (CTX), serum procollagen type 1 N-propeptide (P1NP), serum bone-specific alkaline phosphatase (BSAP), and serum N-terminal telopeptide of type 1 collagen (NTX).

RESULTS (TABLE 48.1)

- *Inclusion*:
  - Among the 14 195 women analyzed across the 3 trials, 284 hip and femur fractures were identified (2%).
  - 12 of the fractures in 10 patients were identified as subtrochanteric or diaphyseal (4.2%).
- *Turnover markers:* CTX was below the premenopausal range in 2 patients, and P1NP in 1 (although both patients had a normal BSAP). NTX was within normal range in the 3 patients in whom it was measured.
- *Prodromal symptoms:* 3 patients described hip pain prior to fracture; 1 patient had a spiral fracture on radiography, but this was not deemed "atypical."
- *Age*: Mean age was 73.7 years.
- *Timing*: Mean time from randomization to fracture was 918.2 days.
- *Rate:* Overall rate for subtrochanteric or diaphyseal fractures over the 3 studies was 2.3 per 10 000 patient years.
- *Fracture risk with bisphosphonates:*
  - There was no significant increase in subtrochanteric fracture risk for patients on bisphosphonates compared to control across all 3 trials.
  - FIT and HORIZON had a significant decrease in NOF fracture risk in the bisphosphonate group compared to control.

Table 48.1 Summary of Key Findings

Study	Study Medication	Number of Subtrochanteric or Diaphyseal Fractures	Per 10,000 Patient-Years	Relative Hazard (95% CI)	*p* Value
FIT	*Placebo*	1	0.8	1.03	0.98
	Alendronate	1	0.8	(0.06–16.46)	
FLEX	*Alendronate/ placebo*	1	4.7	1.33 (0.12–14.67)	0.82
	Alendronate/ alendronate	2	6.3		
HORIZON	*Placebo*	2	1.9	1.50	0.65
PFT	*Zoledronic acid*	3	2.8	(0.25–9.00)	

Criticisms and Limitations: Only 1 radiograph for the 12 fractures of interest was available, which meant that the study could not independently verify the atypical features associated with prolonged use of bisphosphonates. As only 12 fractures were evaluated, the statistical power of the study was low and so drawing definitive conclusions about treatment is difficult, reflected in wide confidence intervals for the relative hazards.

Other Relevant Studies and Information:

- Subsequent nationwide case-control and cohort studies showed an association between long-term bisphosphonate use and atypical subtrochanteric fractures but once again confirmed a low absolute risk.[5,6]
- A review of 13 different controlled trials confirmed the efficacy of bisphosphates in reducing osteoporotic fractures and their long-term protective effects.[7]
- Future use of bisphosphonates was highlighted in a 2011 population-based retrospective cohort study, which noted a lower rate of revision for patients undergoing primary total hip arthroplasty or total knee replacement in bisphosphonate users compared to nonusers.[8]

Summary and Implications: Subtrochanteric or diaphyseal femur fractures following bisphosphonate use are rare. Although subsequent larger studies[5,6] have highlighted an association between bisphosphonate use and these atypical fractures, the overall consensus is that many more common osteoporotic fractures are prevented by bisphosphonates than caused by the drugs.[1,5,6] These results suggest that bisphosphonates should continue to be prescribed, but patients on long-term therapy should be re-evaluated and monitored.

CASE HISTORY: BISPHOSPHONATES AFTER OSTEOPOROTIC NOF FRACTURE

Case History

A 67-year-old lady sustained an NOF fragility fracture and is deemed high risk for further fractures based on her BMD measurements and Fracture Risk Assessment tool (FRAX)[9] scores. After undergoing a hip hemiarthroplasty to treat her fracture, she is recommended to start on a secondary bone protection regimen consisting of weekly oral alendronate for prophylaxis. However, the patient has raised concerns and is considering not taking the medication. Her grandchild, who is a medical student, has read that these medications can increase the chance of sustaining certain types of other fractures. Based on the results of this study, how should this patient be counseled?

Suggested Answer

The study states that the absolute risk of a subtrochanteric or diaphyseal femur fracture secondary to bisphosphonate use is extremely low, a finding that has been replicated in subsequent studies. Using data from 3 trials, this study states that treating 1000 patients with bisphosphonates for 3 years would prevent 100 fractures compared to the risk of sustaining 1.4 subtrochanteric or diaphyseal fractures per 1000 patients treated. The patient ought to be reassured with the results from this study but should also be cautioned to ensure that she is reviewed for the need for continued treatment every 3–5 years depending on BMD as per National Institute for Health and Care Excellence (NICE) guidelines.[10] NICE advised that this is to reduce the potential long-term skeletal adverse effects associated with bisphosphonates, such as atypical subtrochanteric fractures. It is based in part on the FLEX trial, which highlighted that apart from clinical vertebral fractures, discontinuing alendronate after 5 years did not incur a higher risk of fragility fractures.

References

1. Black et al. Bisphosphonates and fractures of the subtrochanteric or diaphyseal femur. N Engl J Med. 2002;347(23):1825–33.
2. Black et al. Randomised trial of effect of alendronate on risk of fracture in women with existing vertebral fractures. Fracture Intervention Trial Research Group. Lancet. 1996;348(9041):1535–41.
3. Black et al. FLEX Research Group. Effects of continuing or stopping alendronate after 5 years of treatment: the Fracture Intervention Trial Long-term Extension (FLEX): a randomized trial. JAMA. 2006;296(24):2927–38.
4. Grbic et al. Health Outcomes and Reduced Incidence with Zoledronic Acid Once Yearly Pivotal Fracture Trial Research Group. Incidence of osteonecrosis of the jaw in women with postmenopausal osteoporosis in the health outcomes and reduced incidence with zoledronic acid once yearly pivotal fracture trial. J Am Dent Assoc. 2008;139(1):32–40.
5. Park-Wyllie et al. Bisphosphonate use and the risk of subtrochanteric or femoral shaft fractures in older women. JAMA. 2011;305(8):783–9.
6. Schilcher et al. Bisphosphonate use and atypical fractures of the femoral shaft. N Engl J Med. 2011;364:1728–37.
7. Bilezikian et al. Efficacy of bisphosphonates in reducing fracture risk in postmenopausal osteoporosis. Am J Med. 2009;122(2 Suppl):S14–21.
8. Prietro-Alhambra et al. Association between bisphosphonate use and implant survival after primary total arthroplasty of the knee or hip: population based retrospective cohort study. BMJ. 2011;343:d7222.
9. Kanis et al. FRAX® and its applications to clinical practice. Bone. 2009;44:734–43.
10. National Institute for Health and Care Excellence. Osteoporosis—prevention of fragility fractures. Scenario: management. April 2023. https://cks.nice.org.uk/topics/osteoporosis-prevention-of-fragility-fractures/management/management/

49

Compartment Monitoring in Tibial Fractures

IRFAN MERCHANT, KAPIL SUGAND, AND JOHN PAUL MURPHY

> In our series, the use of a differential pressure of 30 mmHg as a threshold for fasciotomy led to no missed cases of acute compartment syndrome. We recommended that decompression should be performed if the differential pressure level drops to under 30 mmHg.
>
> —McQueen et al.[1]

Citation: McQueen MM, Court-Brown CM. Compartment monitoring in tibial fractures. The pressure threshold for decompression. J Bone Joint Surg Br. 1996;78(1):99–104.

Research Question: Should decompression be performed when compartmental tissue pressure rises to within 30 mmHg of the diastolic blood pressure?

Funding: Royal Infirmary of Edinburgh, Scotland

Year Study Began: 1991–1994

Year Study Published: 1996

Study Location: Edinburgh, Scotland

Who Was Studied: Patients with tibial diaphyseal fractures

Who Was Excluded: None

How Many Patients: 116

Study Overview: See Figure 49.1.

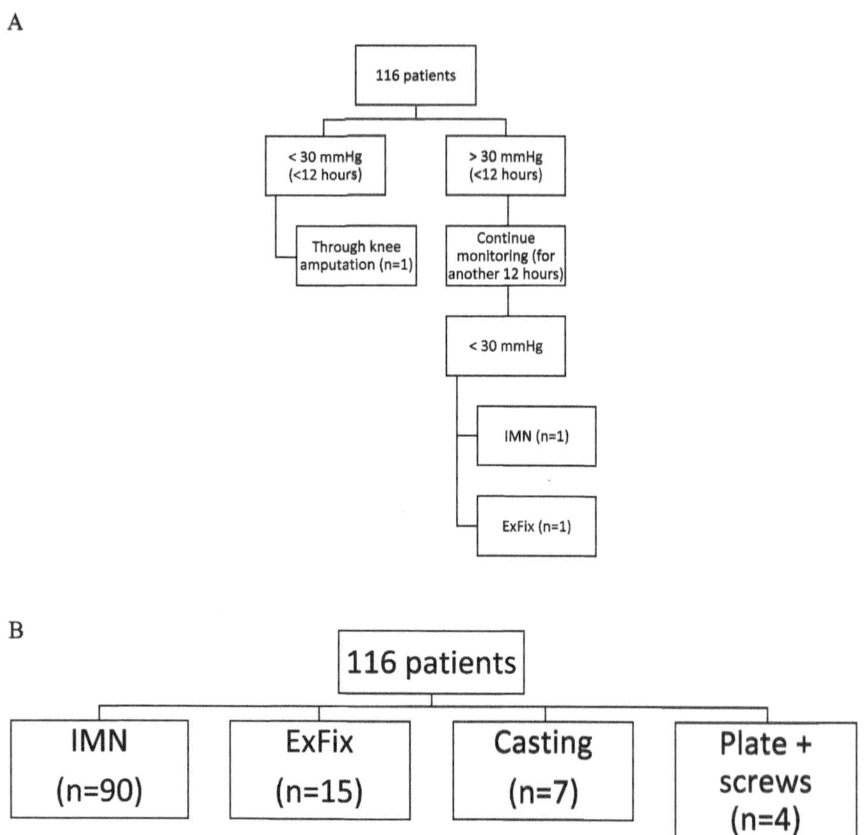

Figure 49.1. Summary of study design: (a) number requiring fasciotomies and (b) treatment plans.

Study Intervention: This study examined 116 patients with tibial diaphyseal fractures who had anterior compartment monitoring for 24 hours. On continuous monitoring the patients were identified with having a differential pressure either > 30 mmHg or < 30 mmHg. The patients with a differential pressure (i.e., ΔP) < 30 mmHg difference between compartmental pressure and diastolic blood pressure were taken to the theater for a 4-compartment leg fasciotomy. Compartmental monitoring of the patients was split into 2 × 12-hour periods.

In the first 12-hour period 1 patient was found to have differential pressure < 30 mmHg who progressed to requiring a fasciotomy. In the second 12-hour period 2 patients were found to have differential pressures < 30 mmHg, who both also progressed to having fasciotomies.

Follow-Up: Mean of 15 months (6–59)

Endpoints: Primary outcome was patients with a ΔP < 30 mmHg between compartmental pressure and diastolic blood pressure requiring a 4-compartment leg fasciotomy. Secondary outcome was that an absolute compartmental pressure measurement of 30 mmHg as a threshold for decompression is unreliable despite it being recommended by many authors.

RESULTS (TABLES 49.1 AND 49.2)

- *Demographics:* During 19 months of follow-up (F/U), there were 92 males and 24 females with an average age of 33 years (14–85).
- *Impact of surgical delay on pressures:* ΔP was lower (including in the first 12 hours postoperatively) as delay to surgery increased.
- *Impact of fracture grade on pressures:* As mode of injury did not significantly predict ΔP when adjusted for grade, only fracture grade was demonstrated to have the strongest influence on ΔP.
- *Effect of treatment on pressures:* There were no significant differences between the mean pressure levels of the different treatment groups (Figure 49.1b).
- *F/U:* At 6 months, no patient had any late sequelae of acute compartment syndrome and therefore it is unlikely for any patient to have been missed.

Table 49.1 Summary of Results

Timing	Fasciotomy Due to ΔP < 30 mmHg	Absolute Pressures (mmHg) > 30	> 40	> 50	Other Surgery (i.e., Fixation/ Casting)
0–12 hours	1 (0.9%)	53 (46%)	30 (26%)	4 (3.4%)	
12–24 hours	2 (1.7%)	28 (24%)	7 (6%)	2 (1.7%)	
< 24 hours					72 (62.1%)
> 24 hours					44 (37.9%)

Table 49.2 Correlations Observed from the Study

Correlations		
Negative	**Nil**	**Positive**
ΔP and fracture grade in the first 12 hours ($p < 0.02$), which became even stronger in the second 12 hours ($p < 0.001$)	Absolute pressures and either fracture grade or high- or low-energy injury Delay to surgery and ΔP in the second 12 hours	High-energy injury and lower ΔP ($p < 0.002$)
ΔP in the first 12 hours and the delay before operation ($p < 0.05$)	Delay to surgery and absolute or differential pressures in the second 12 hours postoperatively Either absolute or differential pressures and open or closed fractures	Fracture grade and mode of injury highly correlated ($p < 0.001$)

Criticisms and Limitations: A larger number of patients would provide a more comprehensive data set and therefore result, since only 3 (2.6%) patients ended up undergoing a leg fasciotomy. A larger data set may also include patients who have had their operation delayed for > 48 hours, therefore giving a different interpretation of the results. The trial does not include other causes of compartment syndrome, such as burns or crush injuries.

Other Relevant Studies and Information:

- Multiple authors have recommended an absolute compartment pressure of 30 mmHg as a threshold for decompression.[2]
- Others have suggested that open fractures may allow the compartments to decompress, therefore preventing compartment syndrome,[3] but clinically open fractures can still lead to compartment syndrome, so vigilant monitoring is mandatory.
- 36 patients in another study with crush injuries were included in a randomized double-blind trial < 24 hours postoperative and treated with hyperbaric oxygen or placebo. Hyperbaric oxygen was effective in improving wound healing and preventing further surgeries.[4]
- The British Orthopaedic Association and British Association of Plastic, Reconstructive, and Aesthetic Surgeons have published the British Orthopaedic Association Standards for Trauma guidelines[5,6] on the diagnosis and management of compartment syndromes in limbs.

They support the $\Delta P < 30$ mmHg threshold, absolute compartment pressure > 40 mmHg, 2-incision/4-compartment decompression of the leg, and operating within < 1 hour of the decision to proceed to surgery. However, in the absence of reliable evidence, it is the opinion of the American Academy of Orthopaedic Surgeons[7] that fasciotomy technique (e.g., 1 vs. 2 incision or its placement) is less important than achieving complete decompression of the affected compartments.

Summary and Implications: This study showed that absolute compartment pressures are not reliable when diagnosing compartment syndrome among patients with tibial fractures. However, when using differential pressures of ≤ 30 mmHg as a threshold for 4-part compartment fasciotomy, all cases of compartment syndrome were identified in the 116 patients included in the study. A 6-month F/U showed no sequelae of compartment syndrome, indicating that no patients were missed in being diagnosed. These findings suggest that 30 mmHg is an appropriate threshold to use when assessing the need for fasciotomy among patients with tibial fractures.

CLINICAL CASE: COMPARTMENT SYNDROME IN AN INTUBATED AND SEDATED PATIENT

Case History

A 29-year-old fit male attended the Emergency Department with polytrauma after being involved in a road traffic collision. He was hit by direct impact while crossing the road and sustained a closed midshaft tibial fracture. Within 24 hours of resuscitation and stabilization he was treated with intramedullary tibial nailing as part of damage control orthopaedics. He was then admitted to Intensive Treatment Unit (ITU), still sedated, intubated, and ventilated for his brain injury. He was found to have increased leg swelling with blistering and tense compartments 12 hours postoperatively. As he was not able to communicate, his monitor indicated distress and pain on passive stretch of the compartments with worsening tachycardia, tachypnea, and hypotension. The nurses are now drawing up morphine almost every hour to help the patient settle. How should this patient be managed, and what is the differential diagnosis?

Suggested Answer

The patient was assessed by ITU physicians and the attending/consultant orthopaedic surgeon. He was found to have intact pulses. In an ideal scenario, the surgeon would examine for neurological deficit with pain on passive stretch and when palpating the anterior, lateral, and posterior leg compartments. This patient is requiring more morphine, which needs to be assessed and monitored. Since this patient is sedated, the clinical findings will determine the need for surgery since compartment syndrome is ultimately a clinical diagnosis that may be confirmed with the assistance of intracompartmental pressure monitoring. There was no obvious signs of infection and the wounds were intact. The anterior compartment was measured using a handheld manometer, which showed a pressure of 55 mmHg with the diastolic blood pressure being 80 mmHg (i.e., $\Delta P < 30$ mmHg). Although the differentials were deep venous thrombosis or vascular injury, a diagnosis of compartment syndrome was made and a fasciotomy was performed. All 4 compartments were decompressed with significant muscle bulging but no signs of necrosis. The wounds were left open. Forty-eight hours later the wounds were primarily closed by plastic surgeons.

References

1. McQueen et al. Compartment monitoring in tibial fractures. The pressure threshold for decompression. J Bone Joint Surg Br. 1996;78(1):99–104.
2. Mubarak et al. Acute compartment syndromes: diagnosis and treatment with the aid of the wick catheter. J Bone Joint Surg Am. 1978;60-A:1091–5.
3. Rorabeck et al. Anterior tibial-compartment syndrome complicating fractures of the shaft of the tibia. J Bone Joint Surg Am. 1976;58-A:549–50.
4. Bouachour et al. Hyperbaric oxygen therapy in the management of crush injuries: a randomized double-blind placebo-controlled clinical trial. J Trauma. 1996;41(2):333–9.
5. British Orthopaedic Association (BOA). British Orthopaedic Association Standards for Trauma (BOAST). Diagnosis and management of compartment syndrome of the limbs. December 2016. https://www.boa.ac.uk/static/0d37694f-1cad-40d5-b4c10 32eef7486ff/de4cfbe1-6ef3-443d-a7f2a0ee491d2229/diagnosis%20and%20management%20of%20compartment%20syndrome%20of%20the%20limbs.pdf
6. British Orthopaedic Association (BOA) and British Association of Plastic, Reconstructive, and Aesthetic Surgeons (BAPRAS). Audit Standards for Trauma. British Orthopaedic Association Standards for Trauma (BOAST). Open fractures. December 2017. https://www.boa.ac.uk/static/3b91ad0a-9081-4253-92f7d90e8 df0fb2c/29bf80f1-1cb6-46b7-afc761119341447f/open%20fractures.pdf
7. American Academy of Orthopaedic Surgeons (AAOS). Management of acute compartment syndrome: evidence-based clinical practice guideline. December 2018. https://www.aaos.org/globalassets/quality-and-practice- resources/dod/acs-cpg-final_approval-version-10-11-19

50

A Multicenter, Prospective, Randomized, Controlled Trial of Open Reduction—Internal Fixation versus Total Elbow Arthroplasty for Displaced Intra-Articular Distal Humeral Fractures in Elderly Patients

YASMEEN KHAN, KAPIL SUGAND, AND DAVID AHEARNE

> Total elbow arthroplasty (TEA) may result in decreased reoperation rates, considering that 25% of fractures randomized to open reduction and internal fixation (ORIF) were not amenable to internal fixation. TEA is a preferred alternative for ORIF in elderly patients with complex distal humeral fractures that are not amenable to stable fixation.
>
> —McKee et al.[1]

Citation: McKee MD, Veillette CJ, Hall JA, Schemitsch EH, Wild LM, McCormack R, Perey B, Goetz T, Zomar M, Moon K, Mandel S, Petit S, Guy P, Leung I. A multicenter, prospective, randomized, controlled trial of open reduction—internal fixation versus total elbow arthroplasty for displaced intra-articular distal humeral fractures in elderly patients. J Shoulder Elbow Surg. 2009;18(1):3–12.

Research question: Should patients with complex intra-articular distal humeral fractures be treated with open reduction and internal fixation (ORIF) or total elbow arthroplasty (TEA)?

Funding: Orthopedic Trauma Association and Zimmer (Warsaw, IN, USA)

Year Study Began: 2001

Year Study Published: 2009

Study location: 4 university-affiliated Canadian academic medical centers

Who was studied: Adults aged > 65 years old with displaced, comminuted, intra-articular humeral fractures; closed fractures; or Gustilo type I open fractures treated locally and regionally < 12 hours postinjury; definitive surgery that was performed < 21 days of the injury.

Who was excluded: Extra-articular fractures; nonoperative management; Gustilo grade I open fractures > 12 hours postinjury; Gustilo grade II/IIIa/IIIb/IIIc fractures; previous ipsilateral distal humeral fractures; pathologic fractures; definitive surgery > 21 days after injury; severe joint disease; significant comorbidity; and noncooperative patients.

How many people: 40

Study Overview: See Figure 50.1.

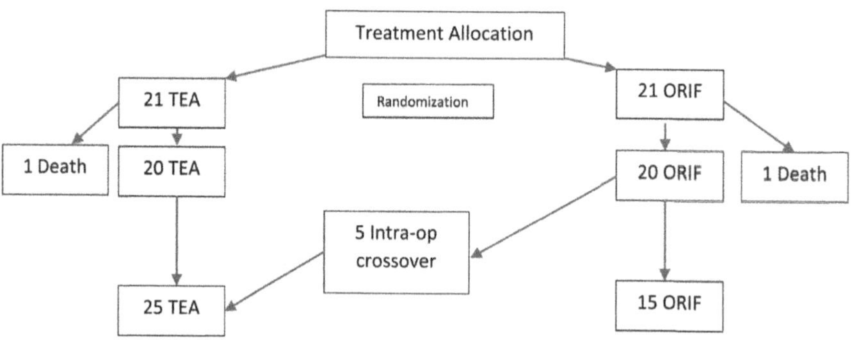

Figure 50.1. Summary of study design.

Study Intervention: Preoperative prophylactic antibiotics were given to all patients, and all procedures were performed with the patient under general anesthesia. All surgeries followed standardized protocols. ORIF was performed via a posterior approach with anatomic reduction of the fracture. A midline triceps split or triceps-sparing approach was used for TEA, and a midline triceps split or olecranon osteotomy was used for ORIF. With the triceps-sparing approach, the surgeon uses the working space created by the condylar resection to perform TEA without detaching the triceps from the olecranon.

Follow up: 2 years

Endpoint: Mayo Elbow Performance Score[2] (MEPS; an instrument used to assess the pathological limitations of the elbow during activities of daily living using 4 subscales: pain, range of motion [ROM], stability, and daily function) and Disabilities of the Arm, Shoulder, and Hand[3] (DASH; self-administered outcome tool to measure self-rated upper-extremity disability and symptoms consisting of mainly 30-item disability/symptom scale) score were determined at 6 weeks, 3 months, 6 months, 12 months, and 2 years. Complication type, duration, management, and treatment requiring reoperation were recorded.

RESULTS

- *Demographics*: Data was collected on 40 patients who had AO/Orthopaedic Trauma Association (OTA) type 13C fractures of the distal humerus confirmed intraoperatively. Two patients died before follow-up (F/U), and 5 patients originally randomized to the ORIF group were converted to TEA. There was no significant difference between the demographics and baseline preinjury scores.
- *Clinical outcomes:* There was a significantly decreased operating time (mean 32 minutes; $p = 0.001$) in the TEA group. Length of stay was less in the TEA group (9.3 vs. 7.7 days; $p = 0.5$).
- *Complications:* Complications were similar in both groups as seen in Table 50.1; 26% of patients had symptoms of ulnar neuropathy, which was the most common overall complication in both groups.
- *Questionnaire results:* Mean MEPS was significantly improved in patients who had a TEA vs. ORIF at 3, 6, and 12 months as well as at 2 years (Table 50.2, Figure 50.2). DASH score showed a significant improvement for TEA between 6 weeks and 6 months ($p < 0.04$), but not at 12 months or 2 years ($p < 0.18$).
- *Function:* There was improved motion in the TEA group for mean extension and flexion. Arc of motion of flexion-extension was not significantly different between both groups at 2 years.

- *Reoperation rate:* Revision surgery was required after the original procedure in 7 (17%) patients, 4 (27%) who had ORIF and 2 (12%) who had TEA, but these remained insignificant ($p = 0.2$).

Table 50.1 Complications in Patients Undergoing ORIF and TEA

Complication	**ORIF ($n = 15$)**	**TEA ($n = 5$)**
	Ulnar nerve	
Sensory deficit	5 (23.8%)	3 (16.7%)
Motor deficit	1 (4.8%)	2 (11.1%)
Radial nerve palsy (temporary)	1 (4.8%)	0
Wound complication	2 (9.5%)	4 (22.2%)
Posttraumatic stiffness	2 (4.8%)	3 (16.7%)
Malalignment > 5°	3 (14.3%)	1 (5.6%)
Incongruent reduction > 2 mm	4 (19%)	0
Nonunion	1 (4.8%)	0
	Infection	
Deep	0	1 (5.6%)
Superficial	1 (4.8%)	1 (5.6%)
Type III heterotopic ossification	1 (4.8%)	3 (16.7%)
Total	**21**	**18**

Table 50.2 Summary of Key Findings

Outcome	**ORIF**	**TEA**	
Numbers in groups	15	25	
	MEPS		
3 months	83	65	$p = 0.01$
6 months	86	68	$p = 0.003$
12 months	88	72	$p = 0.007$
2 years	86	73	$p = 0.015$
	DASH		
6 weeks	43	77	$p = 0.02$
6 months	31	47	$p = 0.04$
12 months	31	47	$p = 0.07$
2 years	32	43	$p = 0.18$
Reoperation rate	4	3	
Complication rate	21	18	

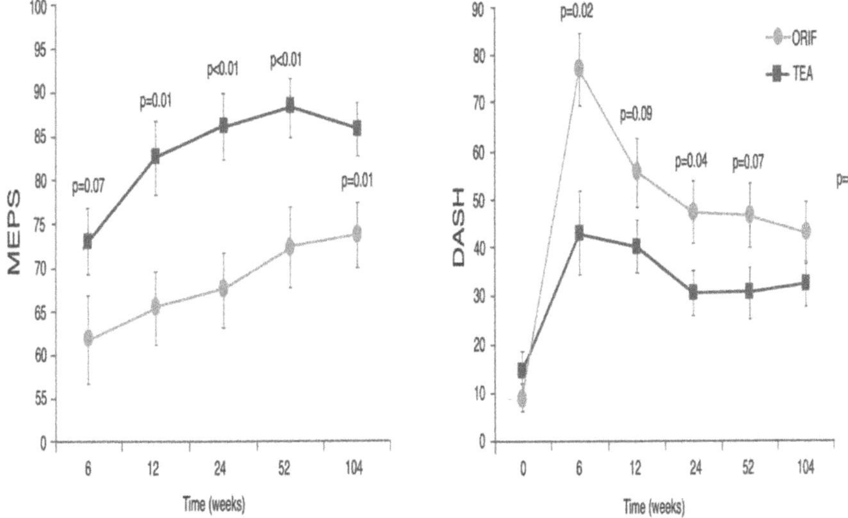

Figure 50.2. MEPS was significantly improved at 3 months (83 vs. 65, $p = 0.01$), 6 months (86 vs. 68, $p = 0.003$), 12 months (88 vs. 72, $p = 0.007$), and 2 years (86 vs. 73, $p = 0.015$) in patients with TEA (purple line) compared with ORIF (orange line). DASH scores showed a significant improvement for TEA (purple line) compared with ORIF (orange line) between 6 weeks (43 vs. 77, $p = 0.02$) and 6 months (31 vs. 47, $p = 0.04$) but not at 12 months (31 vs. 47, $p = 0.07$) and 2 years (32 vs. 43, $p = 0.18$). Error bars represent standard error.

Criticisms and Limitations: The sample size was relatively small, with a F/U of only 2 years. For the TEA group, this study also identified a reduced reoperation rate (12% vs. 27%; $p = 0.20$) and a 12-degree improvement in flexion-extension arc compared with the ORIF group, though this difference did not reach significance ($p = 0.19$), possibly due to the small sample size.

Other Relevant Studies and Information:

- TEA has been found to be a viable treatment option for carefully selected distal intra-articular humerus fractures in elderly patients with associated comorbidities such as rheumatoid arthritis, osteoporosis, and conditions requiring the use of systemic steroids. This procedure is not an alternative to osteosynthesis in younger patients.[4–7]

- A prospective, multicenter clinical study[8] ($n = 46$) with a 4-year F/U using the Discovery Elbow System (Biomet Inc., Warsaw, Indiana, USA) demonstrated a significant improvement in both pain and functional scores, but this was not compared to another treatment.
- Cemented linked semiconstrained elbow arthroplasty (Coonrad-Morrey prosthesis; $n = 461$) provides satisfactory clinical results in the treatment of rheumatoid arthritis with a reasonable rate of survivorship free of mechanical failure at 20 years,[9] which was supported by another comparative study.[10]
- The British Elbow and Shoulder Society (BESS) has published consensus best practice guidelines reviewing its literature, suitability, and implementation.[11]

Summary and Implications: This randomized prospective trial compared the efficacy of ORIF vs. TEA for comminuted distal humeral fractures in patients aged > 65 years. Primary semiconstrained TEA was superior to ORIF as measured by both surgeon-based (MEPS) and patient-based (DASH) outcome scores, especially in the early postoperative period. Operative time was shorter by a mean of 32 minutes in the TEA group. There were trends toward a reduced reoperation rate and improved ROM in the TEA group, albeit insignificant. Based on this and other research, clinical practice guidelines favor TEA in patients > 65 years of age with intra-articular distal humeral fractures, particularly in those with fractures not amenable to fixation.

CLINICAL CASE: ORIF VERSUS TEA IN THE TREATMENT OF AO/OTA TYPE 13C FRACTURE IN THE ELDERLY PATIENT

Case History

A 70-year-old woman with a history of rheumatoid arthritis, osteoporosis, and diabetes mellitus sustained a closed intra-articular distal humeral fracture. She sustained a low-energy mechanical fall onto her nondominant hand. Following the fall, she was taken by ambulance to her local Emergency Department where a primary and secondary survey were performed. Here radiograph can be seen in Figure 50.3. This was an isolated injury without neurovascular compromise. Based on the results of the multicenter, prospective, randomized, controlled trial of ORIF vs. TEA for displaced intra-articular distal humeral fractures in elderly patients, how should this patient be treated?

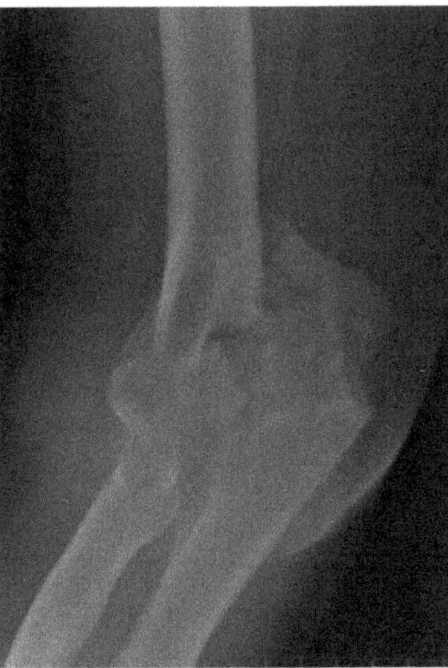

Figure 50.3. Anteroposterior radiograph of elbow.

Suggested Answer

This study showed that TEA has a role in the treatment of comminuted distal humerus fractures in the population > 65 years of age. TEA results in a shorter operating time and duration in the hospital. Whereas the DASH score only favored TEA in the short-term postoperative period, TEA demonstrated a more predictable and improved short- to long-term outcome. However, 2 years is not a long-term functional outcome compared with ORIF based on MEPS. TEA is both justifiable and a preferred alternative option to ORIF, especially for those fractures not amenable to stable fixation. This has been supported by related studies and BESS best practice recommendations.

References

1. McKee et al. A multicenter, prospective, randomized, controlled trial of open reduction internal fixation versus total elbow arthroplasty for displaced intra-articular distal humeral fractures in elderly patients. J Shoulder Elbow Surg. 2009;18(1):3–12.
2. Longo et al. Rating systems for evaluation of the elbow. Brit Med Bull. 2008;87(1):131–61.
3. Beaton et al. Measuring the whole or the parts?: validity, reliability, and responsiveness of the Disabilities of the Arm, Shoulder and Hand outcome measure in different regions of the upper extremity. J Hand Ther. 2001;14(2):128–42.
4. Armstrong et al. Total elbow arthroplasty and distal humerus elbow fracture. Hand Clin. 2004;20:475–83.

5. Cobb et al. Total elbow arthroplasty as primary treatment for distal humeral fractures in elderly patients. J Bone Joint Surg Am. 1997;79:826–32.
6. Frankle et al. A comparison of open reduction and internal fixation and primary total elbow arthroplasty in the treatment of intraarticular distal humerus fractures in women older than age 65. J Orthop Trauma. 2003;17:473–80.
7. Ray et al. Total elbow arthroplasty as primary treatment for distal humeral fractures in elderly patients. Injury. 2000;31(9):687–92.
8. Hastings 2nd et al. A prospective multicenter clinical study of the Discovery elbow. J Shoulder Elbow Surg. 2014;23(5):e95–107.
9. Sanchez-Sotelo et al. Primary linked semiconstrained total elbow arthroplasty for rheumatoid arthritis: a single-institution experience with 461 elbows over three decades. J Bone Joint Surg Am. 2016;98(20):1741–8.
10. Little et al. Outcomes of total elbow arthroplasty for rheumatoid arthritis: comparative study of three implants. J Bone Joint Surg Am. 2005;87(11):2439–48.
11. British Elbow and Shoulder Society. BESS Surgical Procedure Guidelines: the provision of primary and revision elbow replacement surgery in the NHS. 2018. https://bess.ac.uk/download/1420/surgical-procedure-guidelines/6230/total-elbow-replacement-spg-2018.pdf

INDEX

For the benefit of digital users, indexed terms that span two pages (e.g., 52–53) may, on occasion, appear on only one of those pages.

Tables and figures are indicated by *t* and *f* following the page number